Optical Coherence Tomography Angiography for Choroidal and Vitreoretinal Disorders
Part 2

Edited By

Miguel A. Quiroz-Reyes
Oftalmologia Integral ABC, Retina Department
Medical and Surgical Assistance Institution (Nonprofit Organization)
Affiliated with the Postgraduate Studies Division
National Autonomous University of Mexico
Mexico City, Mexico

&

Virgilio Lima-Gomez
Ophthalmology Service, Hospital Juarez de Mexico
Public Assistance Institution (Nonprofit Organization)
Mexico City, Mexico

Optical Coherence Tomography Angiography for Choroidal and Vitreoretinal Disorders – Part 2

Editors: Miguel A. Quiroz-Reyes & Virgilio Lima-Gomez

ISBN (Online): 978-981-5196-65-8

ISBN (Print): 978-981-5196-66-5

ISBN (Paperback): 978-981-5196-67-2

First published in 2023.

need for a court order if at any point you breach any terms of this License Agreement. In no event will any delay or failure by Bentham Science Publishers in enforcing your compliance with this License Agreement constitute a waiver of any of its rights.

3. You acknowledge that you have read this License Agreement, and agree to be bound by its terms and conditions. To the extent that any other terms and conditions presented on any website of Bentham Science Publishers conflict with, or are inconsistent with, the terms and conditions set out in this License Agreement, you acknowledge that the terms and conditions set out in this License Agreement shall prevail.

Bentham Science Publishers Pte. Ltd.
80 Robinson Road #02-00
Singapore 068898
Singapore
Email: subscriptions@benthamscience.net

BENTHAM SCIENCE

CONTENTS

FOREWORD

There is no doubt that serendipity plays an important role in many scientific developments. One very clear example is the evolution of Ophthalmic Coherence Tomography (OCT) in Ophthalmology.

In the early 1970s, Michel Duguay at the AT & T Bell Laboratories published "Light photographed in flight", where he proposed that echoes of light could be used to examine biological tissue. In the mid-1970s, Erich Ippen, of Massachusetts Institute of Technology (MIT), further developed femtosecond optics. Both discoveries built the foundation of the concept called optical reflectivity, with the idea that light interference could be used to obtain a non-invasive "biopsy" of translucid tissues. In the late 1980s, corneal refractive surgery was at its summit. It required an accurate measurement of corneal thickness. James Fujimoto of MIT collaborated with Ophthalmologists Joel Schuman, David Huang and Carmen Puliafito to refine this measurement, using low-coherence interferometry with only partial success. Nevertheless, in a poorly focused image of the cornea, Huang noticed what appeared to be an optical section of the retina in the background. Instead of dismissing this poorly defined image as useless, Huang continued experimenting until he was able to obtain an optical transverse image of the retina. Thus, retinal and choroidal OCT was born. Today OCT constitutes the most important ancillary test and standard of care in Ophthalmic practice, not only in vitreoretinal pathology, but also in glaucoma and problems of the anterior segment.

More recently, swept-source OCT, which can produce 500,000 scans per second and OCT angiography, employing motion contrast imaging, allow us to image retinal capillaries and the smallest neo-vessels in the retinal tissues. Also, enhanced penetration has allowed to provide detailed visualization of the choroid. New technologies are in constant development, such as visible light OCT (visOCT) and adaptive optics (AO-OCT) will allow further details and deeper penetration.

In this particular section of the book, after a review of general principles and advances of OCT and OCTa use in vitreoretinal disorders, all the contributors and coauthors engage in describing to us the normal and pathological parameters of macular and choroidal perfusion patterns, followed by a description and findings in several vitreoretinal and choroidal pathological disorders.

There is no doubt that all the new and described findings in this book will widen our knowledge and be of benefit to our ailing patients.

Alexander Dalma M.D.
Dr. Dalma y Asociados, UNAM
Ciudad de Mexico, Mexico

PREFACE

Optical coherence tomography angiography is one of the most important recent innovations in ophthalmology. The book you have in your hands represents the collaborative efforts of a select team of subject matter experts. This book aims to be a practical, patient-centered guide complemented with a clinical approach and demonstrative clinical cases to assist ophthalmologists and ophthalmology trainees in the evaluation of newly developed perfusion concepts and the diagnosis and management of patients presenting with a wide spectrum of diseases of the retina and choroid, as well as the role of perfusion parameters in the pathogenesis of diverse diseases. As mentioned briefly before, this book describes the journey from basic ophthalmology principles to the most sophisticated current aspects and advances that have resulted in the development of superb technological innovations. We have gone from fundus fluorescein angiography imaging to the evaluation of the perfusional indices of retinochoroidal structures using noninvasive and noncontact imaging techniques that allow a high histopathological correlation of structural tissue characterization with microvascular evaluation on tissue perfusion.

Written by leading international experts in the field, *Optical Coherence Tomography Angiography for Choroidal and Vitreoretinal Disorders* serves as a practical tool for daily work in a retina clinic, helping you through the first steps of perfusion investigation and clinical evaluation, correlation management and treatment decisions for these complex patients. Each chapter details distinct diseases of the retina or choroid, with a focus on signs and perfusion; optical coherent tomography is emphasized, and the chapters are illustrated with many multipaneled images, such that the book may be used as a reference for deciding on diagnostic and treatment options.

This book dissects the basics of angiography by optical coherence tomography and explains the differences in the clinical utility of optical coherence tomography as well as its complementarity. This gives us a broad explanation of the nomenclature and normal perfusional findings in healthy populations.

Several chapters explain macular perfusional findings in different vitreoretinal and choroidal pathologies, including vascular entities commonly seen in daily practice, such as diabetic retinopathy, hemorrhagic and ischemic infarctions of the retina due to vascular disorders, and choroidal pathological neovascularization; most importantly, perfusion parameters are evaluated by quantification and binarization of the different vascular plexuses at the retinal and choroidal level. Additionally, certain tractional entities are evaluated from the point of view of their microstructural findings and perfusional postoperative outcomes, associating them with the final vision.

Some chapters deal with new antivascular endothelial growth factor molecules and new extended-release delivery devices and provide a comparative evaluation of the therapeutic effect on perfusion. In this way, multiple complex pathological disorders of the retina and choroid are more efficiently diagnosed, followed by natural and treated medical or surgical evolution according to the specific cause and consequently, as mentioned before, monitored in response to specific treatments.

We hope that this book, from a multitude of experts, contributes pertinently to academia and achieves the objective of serving as a guide both in the diagnosis and clinical decision-making that those of us who are dedicated to the difficult but beautiful and challenging practice of clinical and surgical retina care perform on a daily basis.

Miguel A. Quiroz-Reyes, MD
Oftalmologia Integral ABC, Retina Department
Medical and Surgical Assistance Institution (Nonprofit Organization)
Affiliated with the Postgraduate Studies Division
National Autonomous University of Mexico
Mexico City, Mexico

&

Virgilio Lima-Gomez, MD
Ophthalmology Service, Hospital Juarez de Mexico
Public Assistance Institution (Nonprofit Organization)
Mexico City, Mexico

List of Contributors

Alejandra Nieto-Jordan	Institute of Ophthalmology, Fundacion Conde de Valenciana, Private Assistance Institution (Nonprofit Organization), Mexico City, Mexico
Aftab Taiyab	Department of Pathology and Molecular Medicine, McMaster University, Hamilton, Canada
Caleb Llacctarimay, MD	Hospital Nacional Sergio E. Bernales, Lima, Peru
Erick A. Quiroz-Gonzalez	Oftalmologia Integral ABC, Retina Department, Medical and Surgical Assistance Institution (Nonprofit Organization), Affiliated with the Postgraduate Studies Division, National Autonomous University of Mexico, Mexico City, Mexico Institute of Ophthalmology, Fundacion Conde de Valenciana, Private Assistance Institution (Nonprofit Organization), Mexico City, Mexico
Felipe Esparza-Correa	Institute of Ophthalmology, Fundacion Conde de Valenciana, Private Assistance Institution (Nonprofit Organization), Mexico City, Mexico
Geraint J. Parfitt	School of Optometry & Vision Sciences, Cardiff University, Cardiff, United Kingdom
Jose A. Roca-Fernandez, MD	Cayetano Heredia University, Lima, Peru Retina Division, Ricardo Palma Clinic, Lima, Peru
Jorge Morales-Navarro	Institute of Ophthalmology, Fundacion Conde de Valenciana, Private Assistance Institution (Nonprofit Organization), Mexico City, Mexico
Jorge E. Aceves-Velazquez	Institute of Ophthalmology, Fundacion Conde de Valenciana, Private Assistance Institution (Nonprofit Organization), Mexico City, Mexico
Juan Pablo Dávila-Gonzalez	Dalma y Asociados SC. Mexico City, Mexico
José Dalma-Weiszhausz	Asociacion para prevenir la Ceguera en Mexico, Mexico City, Mexico
Jennifer H. Kim-Lee	Institute of Ophthalmology, Fundacion Conde de Valenciana, Private Assistance Institution (Nonprofit Organization), Mexico City, Mexico
Miguel A. Quiroz-Reyes, MD	Oftalmologia Integral ABC, Retina Department, Medical and Surgical Assistance Institution (Nonprofit Organization), Affiliated with the Postgraduate Studies Division, National Autonomous University of Mexico, Mexico City, Mexico
Margarita Montano	Oftalmologia Integral ABC, Retina Department, Medical and Surgical Assistance Institution (Nonprofit Organization), Affiliated with the Postgraduate Studies Division, National Autonomous University of Mexico, Mexico City, Mexico
Miguel A. Quiroz-Gonzalez	Oftalmologia Integral ABC, Retina Department, Medical and Surgical Assistance Institution (Nonprofit Organization), Affiliated with the Postgraduate Studies Division, National Autonomous University of Mexico, Mexico City, Mexico
M. Naveed Yasin	Department of Ophthalmology, The University of Auckland, Auckland, New Zealand Department of Pathology and Molecular Medicine, McMaster University, Hamilton, Canada

Nathaly V. Huaman-Mendez, MD	Retina Division, Ricardo Palma Clinic, Lima, Peru
Sanjay Marasini	Department of Ophthalmology, The University of Auckland, Auckland, New Zealand
Virgilio Lima-Gomez, MD	Ophthalmology Service, Hospital Juarez de Mexico, Public Assistance Institution (Nonprofit Organization), Mexico City, Mexico
Zixuan Shao	Division of Chemistry and Chemical Engineering, California Institute of Technology, Pasadena, CA, USA

CHAPTER 1

Sequelae and Macular Perfusion Repercussions in Obstructive Venous Vascular Phenomena of the Retina

Geraint J. Parfitt[1] and **Miguel A. Quiroz-Reyes, MD**[2,*]

[1] *School of Optometry & Vision Sciences, Cardiff University, Cardiff, United Kingdom*

[2] *Oftalmologia Integral ABC, Retina Department, Medical and Surgical Assistance Institution (Nonprofit Organization), Affiliated with the Postgraduate Studies Division, National Autonomous University of Mexico, Mexico City, Mexico*

Abstract: Venous drainage from the retina merges into the central retinal vein and can be obstructed in the branch veins that drain the retinal quadrants, or the central retinal vein itself, which are termed Branch Retinal Vein Occlusion (BRVO) and Central Retinal Vein Occlusion (CRVO), respectively. Obstruction of retinal venous drainage often leads to a sudden or progressive increase in distal venous and capillary pressure with loss of vision and visual field defects. The extent of visual impairment correlates with the location and severity of the venous occlusion and how it impacts perfusion in the retina. Macular edema or retinal ischemia secondary to retinal vein occlusion is responsible for vision loss in retinal vein occlusions, and the advent of anti-VEGF therapeutics has revolutionized the management of vascular disease in the retina.

In this chapter, we review our current understanding of retinal vein occlusions and how OCT-Angiography (OCT-A) is being used clinically in the diagnosis and management of obstructive venous vascular phenomena. The benefits of using OCT-A in the diagnosis and management of CRVO and BRVO over conventional approaches, such as Fundus Fluorescein Angiography (FFA), are discussed. The current limitations of OCT-A and recent advances in the technology are also covered here. Finally, we assess how OCT-A can play a role in the development of new therapeutics to tackle one of the major causes of vision loss worldwide.

* **Corresponding author Miguel A. Quiroz-Reyes, MD:** Oftalmologia Integral ABC, Retina Department, Medical and Surgical Assistance Institution (Nonprofit Organization), Affiliated with the Postgraduate Studies Division, National Autonomous University of Mexico, Mexico City, Mexico; Tel: +525 5217 2732; Fax: +525 55 1664 7180; E-mails: drquiroz@prodigy.net.mx and drquirozreyes7@gmail.com

Keywords: Binarized, Branch retinal vein occlusion, Central retinal vein occlusion, Deep capillary plexus, Hemiretinal vein occlusion, Optical coherence tomography angiography, Macular edema, Neovascularization, Relative afferent pupillary defect, Retinal ischemia, Retinal vein occlusion, Skeletonization, Superficial capillary plexus.

INTRODUCTION

The retina is a highly metabolic tissue that requires a large volume of arterial blood inflow, and venous drainage, to prevent retinal hypoxia and the subsequent cell viability and vision loss. Arterial blood vessels of the retina supply oxygen to the inner neurons through the superficial capillary plexus (SCP), whereas the avascular region comprised of photoreceptors and retinal pigment epithelium relies on the choriocapillaris and deep capillary plexus (DCP) for providing oxygen by diffusion. Venous drainage of retinal blood vessels converges at the central retinal vein, which passes through the lamina cribrosa of the optic nerve head, and then drains into the superior ophthalmic vein or cavernous sinus. Central retinal vein occlusion (CRVO) and branch retinal vein occlusion (BRVO) are defined as a blockage of the veinous drainage from the eye in either the central vein, or one of the four branch veins that drain each quadrant of the retina, respectively.

Obstructive Venous Vascular Phenomena of the Retina and Optical Coherence Tomography Angiography (OCT-A)

Retinal vein occlusion (RVO) is the second most prevalent vascular pathology in the retina after diabetic retinopathy [1] and is a major contributor to vision loss. Currently, there is an estimated 16 million adults affected by RVO [1], and the prevalence of venous retinal occlusion is approximately 0.7% to 1.6%, according to a previous study conducted in Australia [2]. RVO can be subdivided into central retinal vein occlusion (CRVO); hemi-retinal vein occlusion (HRVO); or branch retinal vein occlusion (BRVO), according to the site of venous obstruction. It is predicted that 2.5 million people are affected by CRVO, while 13.9 million are affected by BRVO [3]. The prevalence and five-year incidence of BRVO are both 0.6%, while CRVO prevalence is found to be lower at 0.1%, with a five-year incidence of 0.2% [4]. The incidence of CRVO in the non-affected eye is 7% within four years [5]. The prognosis of RVO is mainly dependent on the region, extent, duration, and intensity of retinal ischemia as retinal neurons become starved of oxygen [1].

RVO can be diagnosed by a combination of fundus features, including retinal vascular dilation and tortuosity, cotton-wool exudates, flame-shaped retinal hemorrhages, optic disc swelling, and macular edema. Retinal hemorrhages will be present in all four quadrants of the fundus in CRVO, while they are confined to either the superior or inferior hemisphere of the fundus in HRVO. On the other hand, BRVO is characterized by hemorrhages localized to the area drained by the occluded branch retinal vein [6]. Vision loss is a consequence of macular edema or retinal ischemia secondary to RVO and retinal hypoxia. This chapter outlines how OCT-A is being used to evaluate obstructive venous vascular phenomena of the retina and their sequelae.

Optical Coherence Tomography (OCT) is a non-invasive imaging technique that uses low-coherence interferometry to obtain high-resolution, cross-sectional images of biological tissues *in vivo*, such as the retina. It is particularly valuable for imaging transparent or semi-transparent tissues and plays a crucial role in ophthalmology for diagnosing and monitoring retinal disease. OCT is based on the principles of interferometry and utilizes light waves to measure the time delay and intensity of backscattered or reflected light from tissue structures.

The basic setup of an OCT system consists of a light source, interferometer, sample arm, reference arm, and detector. Typically, a near-infrared light source with a broad bandwidth, such as a superluminescent diode or femtosecond laser, is used. The light is split into two paths: the sample arm, directed towards the tissue being imaged, and the reference arm, directed towards a mirror. The light beams recombine, and interference between the light waves from the sample and reference arms occurs. The interference signal is captured by a high-speed detector, such as a charge-coupled device (CCD) camera. By measuring the intensity of the interference pattern as a function of the reference arm mirror position, information about the depth or distance from the reference mirror to different tissue structures can be obtained. This depth-resolved information is used to construct cross-sectional images of the retina.

Low-coherence interferometry, a fundamental principle underlying OCT, was invented by physicist Endre M. György in 1965. In the early 1990s, David Huang, Carmen Puliafilto, James Fujimoto, and their colleagues developed the first Time-Domain OCT (TD-OCT) system for ophthalmic imaging [7], and commercial TD-OCT systems first became available in 1996. Maciej Wojtkowski's research team introduced Spectral-Domain OCT (SD-OCT), also known as Fourier-Domain OCT, which uses a spectrometer to measure the spectrum of backscattered light and enables faster imaging with higher resolution [8]. One of the key advantages of OCT is its high resolution, which allows for detailed visualization of tissue microstructures. The axial resolution of OCT is determined by the coherence length of the light source, while the lateral resolution is determined by the focusing optics and the beam diameter. With modern OCT systems, axial resolutions on the order of a few microns and lateral resolutions in the range of 10-20 μm can be achieved.

The latest innovations in OCT imaging include Swept-Source OCT (SS-OCT) and full-field OCT [9], which can increase the imaging depth and field of view. SS-OCT is an alternative to SD-OCT that employs a tuneable laser as its light source. Instead of using a spectrometer, SS-OCT measures the interference signal by sweeping the wavelength of the laser rapidly. It provides deeper penetration into the tissue and is particularly useful for imaging structures like the choroid. The extended imaging range SS-OCT systems utilize longer-wavelength light sources, typically around 1,050 nm, compared to the standard wavelength of around 800 nm used in conventional OCT systems. The longer wavelength allows for increased tissue penetration, enabling better visualization of structures beyond the retina, such as the choroid and sclera.

The resolution of OCT imaging is continually being improved by modifications such as changing the central wavelength and increasing the light source bandwidth. For example, the use of an 853nm central wavelength with 3 μm axial-resolution has been achieved in comparison to conventional OCT, which uses an 880nm central wavelength and has 7 μm axial-resolution [10]. The next major improvement in OCT image analysis will be ushered in with artificial intelligence (A.I.), which promises to objectively identify and quantify changes in retinal structure with increased speed. A.I. based segmentation of sub- and intra-retinal fluid or pigment epithelial detachment has shown huge potential to define these biomarkers of exudative macular degeneration accurately and much faster than human experts [11].

OCT-A enables visualization of the retinal vasculature in greater detail than previously possible and has already been used to great effect in the diagnosis and management of retinal vascular disease in ophthalmology, including retinal vein occlusions, diabetic retinopathy, and age-related macular degeneration. In comparison to fundus fluorescein angiography (FFA), which has been used in the clinic for over 50 years, OCT-A can resolve the fine microvasculature of the superficial and deep retinal plexus without dyes and is, therefore, an emerging approach for retinal diagnostics with significant advantages (Fig. **1**). When FFA is used to image the retinal vasculature, the superficial vascular plexus can only be observed and not the underlying vasculature in deeper retinal layers. OCT-A is an effective imaging technique that produces depth-resolved images of retinal and choroidal vasculature to show the different retinal vascular layers and has a superior demarcation of the foveal avascular zone (FAZ) when compared to FFA. OCT-A's limitations are the lack of normalized patient data, issues that arise from projection artifacts, and its difficulty to detect low-flow lesions or pathologies

[12]. Angiography is important in the precise diagnostics of RVO for the delineation of ischemic areas and is typically confirmed using FFA, which is the current standard of care. However, FFA is limited in its ability to image the FAZ, which can impact a clear prognosis [13].

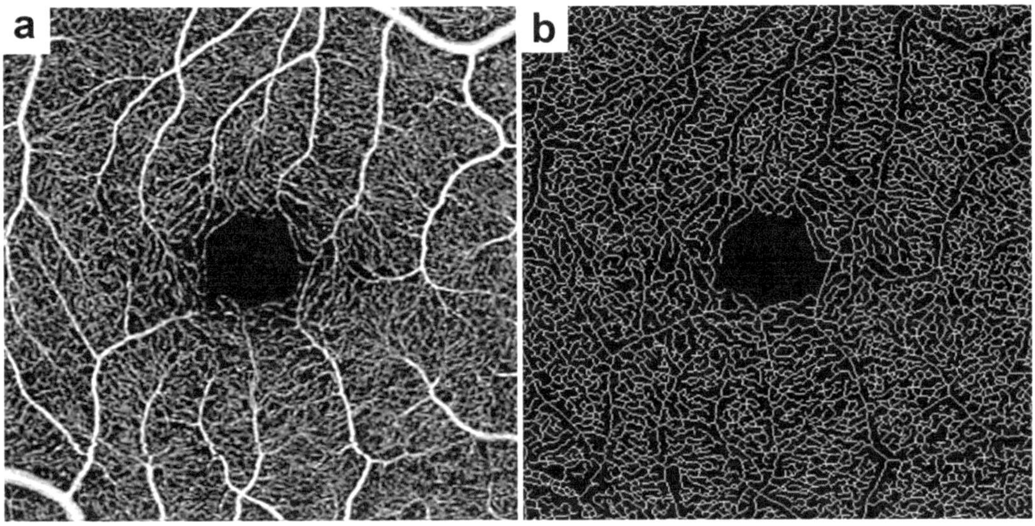

Fig. (1). OCT-A image of healthy retinal vasculature (**a**) and a binarized image showing the blood vessel skeleton (**b**). The foveal avascular zone is positioned centrally. Image kindly provided with permission by Kyle Green, M.D.

Central Retinal Vein Occlusion (CRVO)

CRVO involves an obstruction of the central retinal vein at, or proximal to, the collagenous lamina cribrosa of the optic nerve head. It is most likely to be caused by the occurrence of a thrombus, and it is thought that CRVO pathogenesis adheres to the principles of Virchow's triad for thrombogenesis, which are hypercoagulability; hemodynamic changes (stasis, turbulence); and endothelial injury or dysfunction. The central artery and vein share an outer fibrous connective tissue (adventitia), so any atherosclerotic changes in the central retinal artery may compress the vein at arteriovenous crossings posterior to the lamina cribrosa, which can lead to CRVO. Therefore, CRVO is often directly related to atherosclerosis and changes in the central retinal artery [14].

Thrombosis within retinal veins leads to obstruction of the blood flow that is drained from the eye and an increase in intraluminal pressure. The high intraluminal pressure induces the transudation of blood and an increase in interstitial fluid and proteins within the retina, causing an increase in the interstitial oncotic pressure. In turn, tissue edema results because of the elevated interstitial oncotic pressure, which prevents capillary perfusion and causes retinal ischemia [6]. Retinal ischemia can lead to retinal ganglion cell (RGC) death, and the extent of RGC loss is related to the severity and duration of ischemia. RGCs are neurons that transmit visual information through the optic nerve to the visual cortex and cannot regenerate after injury and cell death.

CRVO can be further subdivided into ischemic (non-perfused) and non-ischemic (perfused) subtypes, with each type having distinct clinical features and ischemic CRVO more likely to cause vision loss. Even patients defined as non-ischemic will have some degree of retinal ischemia to varying levels [15]. The level and severity of retinal ischemia can be determined by the extent of vision loss, the reduction of retinal capillary perfusion in fluorescein angiography, and electroretinograms (ERGs) showing reduced b-wave amplitudes and a reduced b:a-wave ratio. As mentioned above, macular edema is a critical factor in the changes to visual acuity caused by RVO.

Etiology

Age is the most important factor for CRVO, as 90% of cases occur in patients over 55 years of age. Systemic hypertension is also considered to be one of the biggest risk factors for the development of CRVO [16, 17], and retinal arterial changes associated with hypertension, such as arteriovenous nicking, have shown a consistent correlation with an increased chance of RVO [2, 4, 18]. Hyperlipidemia is also considered a risk factor as it was found to be twice as prevalent in RVO (both CRVO and BRVO) when compared with controls [19]. For example, at least 35% of patients with CRVO had a total cholesterol level of >6.5 mmol/l, regardless of their age. Other cardiovascular factors contributing to CRVO pathogenesis include diabetes mellitus, smoking, and obesity, although the evidence supporting these contributors has been inconsistent. Myeloproliferative disorders that increase blood viscosity have also been shown to be associated with CRVO, however, they are uncommon [6].

Glaucoma and increased intraocular pressure (IOP) have been established as potential risk factors for CRVO [1], with a reported adjusted odds ratio (OR) of 5.4 in CRVO for a history of glaucoma, according to one study [17]. Another study confirmed that 22% of patients with CRVO had an elevated IOP of >22mm Hg [20]. One report found that the risk of CRVO in glaucoma patients is increased by up to 10-fold [21]. It is speculated that deformity of the lamina cribrosa caused by the elevated IOP contributes to compression of the central retinal vein and the increased chances of venous occlusion in glaucoma.

Inflammation of the retina has been found to contribute to the pathophysiology of retinal vein occlusions. It has previously been shown that increased expression of the cytokines interleukin (IL) 6 and 8, monocyte chemoattractant protein-1, and vascular endothelial growth factor (VEGF) was associated with CRVO [22, 23]. It is not well understood how these inflammatory factors contribute to RVO pathogenesis, however, VEGF interactions in the retina have been studied extensively and remain a key therapeutic target in vascular disease. VEGF expression is driven by hypoxia because of retinal ischemia and stimulates angiogenesis by acting on tyrosine kinase VEGF-receptors present on vascular endothelial cells. VEGF is expressed by retinal pigment epithelial cells (RPE), Müller glia, and other ocular cell types [22]. It has been shown that VEGF and IL-6 levels are increased in the aqueous and vitreous of patients with CRVO, which was found to be proportional to the level of retinal ischemia and macular edema [24, 25]. Furthermore, there is a correlation between aqueous VEGF and iris neovascularization and vascular permeability in patients diagnosed with ischemic CRVO [26], with vascular permeability changes likely driving the outcome of macular edema.

Epidemiology

Out of 3654 participants clinically evaluated in the Blue Mountains Eye Study, clinical signs of RVO were found in 59 participants (1.6%) over a 10-year cumulative incidence, of which 15 (25%) were CRVO [2]. RVO was the fifth most prevalent form of unilateral blindness in the population studied. Prevalence of RVO in different age groups was found to be: 0.7% for <60 years; 1.2% for 60 to 69 years; 2.1% for 70 to 79 years; and 4.6% for >80 years of age. There was found to be no significantly increased probability for either gender's susceptibility to RVO. Visual acuity was most affected in patients with CRVO compared to BRVO, with a visual acuity of 20/200 or less in 60% of CRVO patients compared to 14% in BRVO.

The Beaver Dam Eye Study reported a CRVO incidence of 0.5% with a 15-year cumulative incidence [4], while a pooled study of the USA, Europe, Asia, and Australia projected that 16 million people worldwide may have unilateral RVO, with 2.5 million of those suffering from CRVO [3]. Non-ischemic CRVO is the most common sub-type of CRVO, with 81% of patients belonging to this classification [27].

Non-ischemic CRVO

Non-ischemic CRVO patients are characterized by sudden, unilateral blurred vision with a moderate loss of visual acuity (>20/200). Fundus imaging reveals mild venous tortuosity and dilatation, flame-shaped hemorrhages in all four quadrants, mostly in the periphery, as well as optic disc and macular edema. Cotton-wool spots may be evident, often in hypertensive patients, while transient retinal vessel sheathing may also be present [28, 29].

The occlusion site in non-ischemic CRVO is posterior to the lamina cribrosa and retrolaminar region. It has been suggested that the more posterior the occlusion site, the less severe the retinopathy due to the presence of more collateral vessels. Arteriosclerotic changes near to the central retinal vein, coupled with endothelial cell proliferation, induce narrowing of the central retinal vein lumen and cause stasis and thrombosis. It is also thought that nocturnal arterial hypotension may have an important part to play in precipitating CRVO by converting a partial thrombosis to a complete one due to reduced circulation during sleep [30]. This may explain why RVO symptoms are often noticed upon waking.

The central vein occlusion study group (CVOS) found that non-ischemic CRVO converted to ischemic CRVO in 15% of patients within the first 4-months of follow-up. After 3 years, a total of 34% of eyes were found to have converted to ischemic CRVO. It was also found that visual acuity recorded at the baseline is a reliable predictor of visual acuity outcome at 3 years. Patients with poor visual acuity (<20/200) were found to have an 80% chance of a visual acuity below 20/200 after 3 years, while 65% of patients with good visual acuity (>20/40) at baseline maintained visual acuity within the same range [31].

Ischemic CRVO

Ischemic CRVO is defined as a central retinal vein occlusion that causes reduced retinal perfusion, closure of capillaries, and retinal hypoxia (Fig. **2**). It is also marked by the presence of a relative afferent pupillary defect (RAPD), which is mild or absent in non-ischemic CRVO. As mentioned above, some patients change from non-ischemic to ischemic CRVO in a short timeframe or progressively. Compared to non-ischemic CRVO, ischemic CRVO has a marked decrease in vision, which is often noticed suddenly on waking. The site of occlusion is most likely in the lamina cribrosa region, or immediately posterior, and visual loss is often severe and lower than 20/200. Retinal hypoxia in ischemic CRVO likely leads to the release of VEGF and inflammatory mediators, which can cause macular edema, vitreous hemorrhage, and neovascular glaucoma. Vascular leakage and macular edema contribute to the significant loss of vision in ischemic CRVO patients.

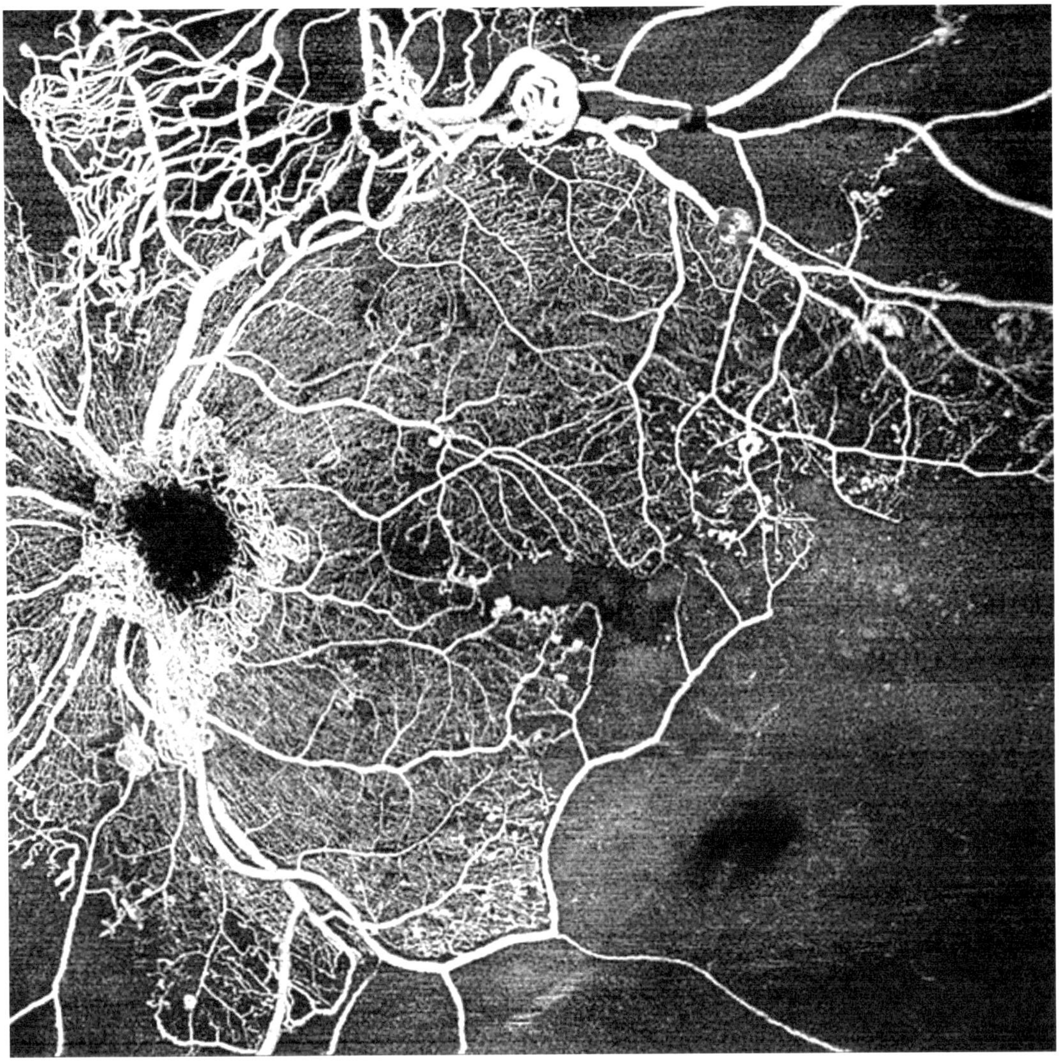

Fig. (2). OCT-A imaging of ischemic CRVO. A 63-year-old patient with CRVO presented with retinal ischemia, neovascularization, and arteriovenous shunts. This image was originally published in the Retina Image Bank® website. Jorge I. Soberanes M.D. Central Retinal Vein Occlusion by OCT Angiography. Retina Image Bank. 2022; 94589. © the American Society of Retina Specialists.

In ischemic CRVO, fundoscopy is marked by severe tortuosity and dilation of the central retinal vein, severe optic disc and macular edema, widespread blot and flame-shaped hemorrhages, and cotton-wool spots. Iris neovascularization (INV) develops in approximately 50% of eyes with ischemic CRVO and an elevated IOP can cause neovascular glaucoma, which occurs in one-third of the cases seen with iris neovascularization [28, 29]. The chances of retinal and optic disc neovascularization are proportional to the area of ischemia. Risk factors for INV include poor visual acuity, extensive retinal nonperfusion, and intraretinal hemorrhage.

Diagnosis of CRVO is straightforward, however, the main issue is differentiating between non-ischemic and ischemic CRVO. Functional testing such as electroretinography can help to determine between non-ischemic and ischemic CRVO [32]. Non-ischemic CRVO is relatively benign in comparison to ischemic CRVO, which can cause a severe loss in visual acuity, so the correct diagnosis and management of the condition are imperative for therapeutic intervention. Retinal capillary obliteration can help determine ischemic CRVO using FA, although this can be difficult to ascertain with poor quality angiograms [33], with >10-disc areas of capillary nonperfusion on FA considered ischemic CRVO. Patients with ischemic CRVO should be monitored regularly for early detection of iris neovascularization or neovascular glaucoma. If possible, patients should be continually monitored for over a year to check for significant ischemia and macular edema [34].

Hemiretinal Vein Occlusion (HRVO)

Hemi-retinal vein occlusions (HRVOs) are pathogenically like CRVOs; however, they only affect the superior or inferior regions of the retina and have a better prognosis (Fig. **3**). HRVO occurs when either the superior or inferior drainage is impaired and does not converge into the central retinal vein. HRVOs arise because of an anatomic variation in the vasculature at the optic nerve head, which is present in 20% of eyes. In these patients, the veins draining the inferior and superior regions merge posterior to the optic nerve head, and one of these veins is not subject to occlusion. Therefore, only one of the two trunks of the central retinal vein is causing a hemi-retinal vein occlusion. Historically, HRVO has been managed like BRVO with laser photocoagulation, however, it is not certain whether it should be treated as a BRVO, CRVO, or as its own entity, with anti-VEGF therapies [35].

There is a lack of clinical evidence specific to HRVO because of its past grouping with CRVO or BRVO. Only recently have the baseline and 12-month outcomes of VEGF inhibitor therapy in HRVO been compared to CRVO and BRVO [35]. In this study, it was reported that HRVO eyes that were previously untreated received VEGF inhibitors and had very good visual and anatomical outcomes.

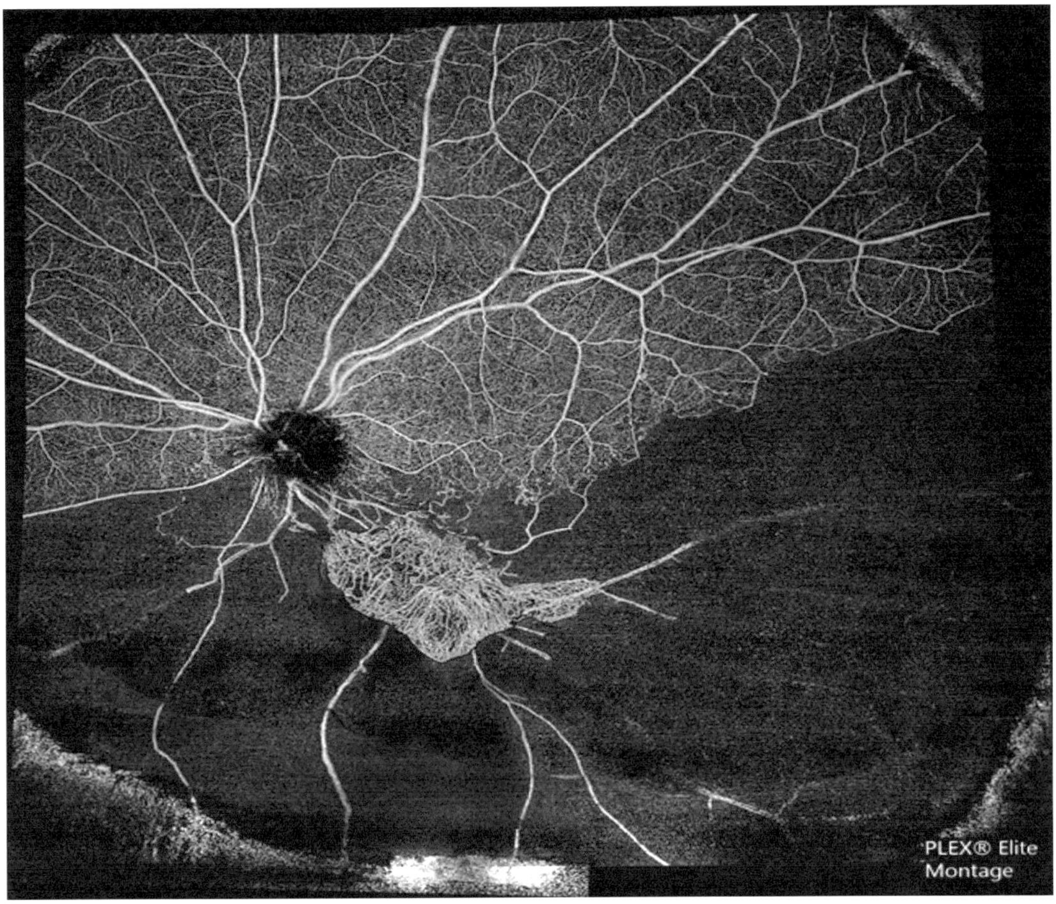

Fig. (3). Wide-field swept source OCT-A of Hemi-retinal Vein Occlusion (HRVO). OCT-A of a 59-year-old patient revealed extensive vessel loss in the inferior hemi quadrant with branching out neovascular frond inferior to the disc with terminal loops. This image was originally published on the Retina Image Bank® website. Sandeep Kumar, MBBS. The Barren Field. Retina Image Bank. 2022; 59123. © The American Society of Retina Specialists.

Etiology

Pathogenesis of HRVO is similar to CRVO and is also of the non-ischemic and ischemic types. However, clinical findings can be intermediate between CRVO and BRVO, and HRVO has often been misdiagnosed as a major BRVO [36]. Symptoms that arise in non-ischemic HRVO are like those described for non-ischemic CRVO. Visual loss in ischemic HRVO is more severe than in non-ischemic HRVO, as there is central vision loss due to the involvement of the macula. On occasion, both trunks can be involved due to an occlusion in the main trunk of the central retinal vein. It is also possible to have a non-ischemic pattern in one vein, and an ischemic occlusion in the other trunk [33]. Typically, each of the two trunks has drainage from one half of the retina (70% in non-ischemic and 74% in ischemic HRVO), however, there may be greater drainage from one trunk over the other [37].

The distinction between major BRVO and HRVO is important as major BRVO is often ischemic, while HRVO can be non-ischemic or ischemic, with the majority of HRVO cases presenting as the non-ischemic subtype. The occlusion site in major BRVO is at arteriovenous crossings, typically near the optic disc but rarely over it. On the other hand, HRVO occlusion is situated within the optic nerve. In HRVO edema is present in the relevant area of the optic disc, whereas the optic disc is fine in major BRVO unless the arteriovenous crossing affected is positioned in the optic disc. Collateral veins connecting the occluded vein with patent veins reveal the site of occlusion. In major BRVO, these are in the neural retina and not the optic disc, whereas in HRVO they are on the optic disc or in the optic nerve [33].

Epidemiology

In the Blue Mountains study, only 3 subjects (5.1%) out of 59 RVO patients were clinically described as HRVO. From published epidemiology studies, the prevalence of HRVO is estimated at <0.1%, while CRVO is 0.1 – 0.4% and BRVO is 0.6 – 1.1% [2 - 4].

Like CRVO, HRVO occurs mostly in elderly patients (90% are >50 years old) and ischemia is more common in the elderly with cardiovascular disease. In a series of 154 consecutive HRVO cases, 78% presented as non-ischemic, whereas 22% were ischemic HRVO [27]. Moreover, non-ischemic HRVO is likely to be even more prevalent as it may be asymptomatic.

Branch Retinal Vein Occlusion (BRVO)

German ophthalmologist Theodor von Leber in 1877 was the first to describe branch retinal vein occlusion. Yoshizo Koyanagi first described the link between BRVO and arteriovenous crossings in 1928, and it is now known that BRVOs occur at arteriovenous crossings in 99.9% of cases [38]. BRVO is often asymptomatic and is the most common form of retinal vein occlusion; it is three times more common than CRVO [4]. Arterial compression of the vein can induce thrombus formation by turbulent blood flow and is combined with vascular endothelial damage from systemic cardiovascular risk factors [6].

BRVO is more commonly observed in the temporal region of the retina when compared with the nasal region, with the superior quadrant affected more frequently affected than the inferior part of the temporal retina. This is likely due to the increased presence of arteriovenous crossings, which are more frequently seen in the superior-temporal quadrant than in any other region of the retina [39].

BRVO is typified in OCT-A imaging by the presence of cystoid macular edema, hyperreflectivity from retinal hemorrhages, and shadowing from the cystoid space and hemorrhages (Fig. **4**). The ellipsoid zone (EZ), which delineates the boundary between the inner and outer segments of the photoreceptors, may be disrupted and is a useful indicator for visual acuity prognosis [40]. BRVO can be categorized as either major BRVO or macular BRVO. Major BRVO is when greater than a quarter of the retina is affected, whereas macular BRVO is the term used when the macula is affected. As in other RVOs, the loss of vision in BRVO is caused by macular edema.

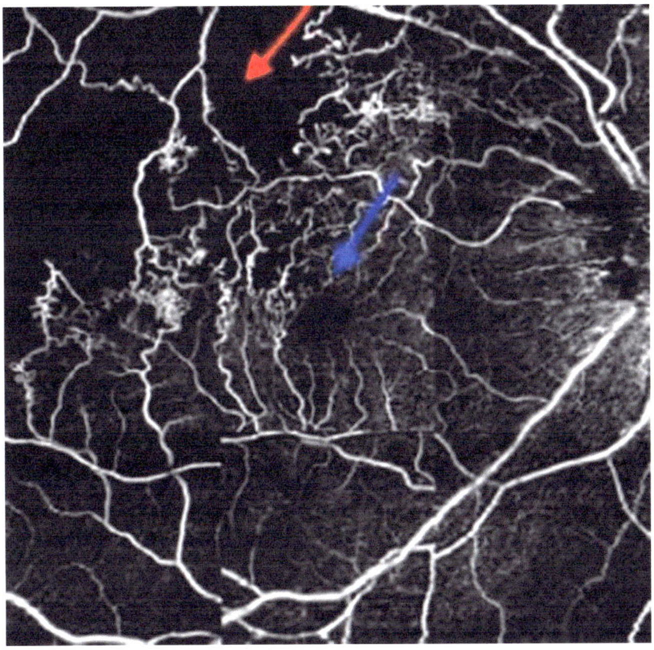

Fig. (4). OCT-A image of branch retinal vein occlusion (BRVO), arrowheads point to nonperfusion areas caused by superior BRVO. This image was originally published on the Retina Image Bank® website. Author - Manish Nagpal, M.D. Photographer - Gayathri Mohan. OCTA in a Branch Retinal Vein Occlusion. Retina Image Bank. 2019; 34186. © the American Society of Retina Specialists.

Etiology

BRVO, like other retinal vein occlusions, is more prevalent in the elderly and may be caused by hypertension, diabetic retinopathy, and hyperlipidemia [6]. For example, a significant link has been found between hypertension and both CRVO (odds ratio (OR) = 3.8) and BRVO (OR = 3.0) [19]. A history of smoking has also been included as a risk factor for BRVO [41]. The Eye Disease Case-control

Study Group found systemic hypertension was associated with 50% of BRVO cases, while cardiovascular disease, increased body mass index, and high serum levels of alpha 2-globulin were risk factors for BRVO, whereas the risk of BRVO decreased with higher levels of alcohol intake and high-density lipoprotein cholesterol [42].

Thrombus formation in BRVO can be caused by hypercoagulability from clotting disorders. BRVO is seen in sickle cell disease as well as other hematological disorders, while glaucoma and elevated IOP play no part in the pathogenesis of BRVO, unlike CRVO and HRVO [1].

Epidemiology

The Beaver Dam Eye Study found a prevalence and five-year incidence of 0.6% each for BRVO, and a 15-year cumulative risk of BRVO to be 1.8%, compared to 0.5% for CRVO [4]. Epidemiologic data from the Blue Mountain Eye Study identified that out of 59 patients with RVO, 41 (69.5%) were found to have BRVO [2]. A pooled analysis of population-based studies in the United States, Europe, Asia, and Australia with 49,869 subjects found an RVO prevalence of 0.52%; CRVO was 0.08% while BRVO was higher at 0.442%. A higher prevalence of BRVO was found in Asians (0.498%) and Hispanic (0.598%) populations when compared to white (0.282%), or black (0.353%) populations, although it was not statistically significant. No predilection for gender was found [1]. The risk of developing BRVO in the contralateral eye was found to be between 7 and 10% [43].

SEQUELAE AND MACULAR PERFUSION REPERCUSSIONS OF RVO; AN OCT-A EVALUATION

Angiography is used in the clinic to visualize the retinal vasculature and identify ischemic areas for prognosis and deciding treatment options for vascular disease. As discussed above, OCT-A can rapidly generate high-resolution images of the different vascular layers in the retina and the choroid. This includes the venules and veins of the superficial capillary plexus (SCP), which are in the ganglion cell layer (GCL) and drained by the central vein. The SCP vessels connect to the intermediate (ICP), and deep capillary plexuses (DCP), which drain blood at the level of the inner nuclear layer (INL). Here, we outline why OCT-A is gaining widespread clinical use in the monitoring and treatment of retinal ischemia, neovascularization, vitreous hemorrhage, and macular edema as a result of retinal vein occlusion.

FA and indocyanine green angiography (ICGA) are the current standard of care for visualizing vascular disease in the retina, which requires an intravenous injection of dyes and may not always generate clear images of the fovea and FAZ because of background fluorescence. FFA is commonly used to detect neovascularization in the retina; however, retinal pathology can become masked by retinal hemorrhages and leakage of fluorescein. FFA can visualize the leakage of fluorescein caused by the disruption of the blood-retina barrier, but it cannot image the deeper retinal capillary layers, such as the ICP and DCP, because of blocked fluorescence [44]. Moreover, these imaging modalities are not depth-resolved, so segmentation of different retinal layers is not routinely possible with FFA or ICGA [45]. FFA and ICGA can also be relatively expensive and time-consuming, and their likelihood to cause allergic reactions increases with use, while indocyanine green dye is also contraindicated in pregnancy and kidney disease [46, 47].

On the other hand, OCT-A is a non-invasive imaging method that can rapidly visualize the retinal vasculature at high resolution without the need for dyes. It can generate volumetric angiography images within ten seconds and, therefore, is preferential for frequent follow-up examinations and segmenting of the deeper vascular layers. OCT has revolutionized clinical ophthalmology because of its rapid, non-invasive assessment of the retina in cross-section. In OCT imaging, one-dimensional scans (a-scans) are captured at several depths to create a two-dimensional image (b-scan), which can generate a three-dimensional image (c-scan) with rapid acquisition of successive b-scans. OCT-A images are created by phase and/or amplitude differences of erythrocyte motion and vascular flow in consecutive OCT scans (b-scans), to volumetrically reconstruct the retinal vasculature. Therefore, the flow of blood is used as an intrinsic contrast medium to generate images in a non-invasive manner, allowing the SCP and DCP to be visualized in a series of b-scans. OCT is based on low-coherence interferometry – backscattered light from tissues in the eye is compared to a reference beam. The combination of reflected light from the eye and the reference light gives rise to an interference pattern, and the areas of tissue that reflect a lot of light create a greater interference pattern than less reflective areas, such as the vitreous gel. Three-dimensional angiograms generated by OCT-A can be viewed from the internal limiting membrane to the choroid, to identify the SCP, ICP, and DCP, as well as the choriocapillaris.

OCT-A image resolution is superior to FA and can be quantitively processed, which means vessel density, vessel length density, perfusion density, and FAZ size and shape, can be accurately measured. These parameters are critical to understanding the progression and treatment of RVOs [48, 49]. In comparison to FFA, OCT-A can image, and quantify FAZ changes that may be obscured by vascular leakage [50, 51]. Meanwhile, clinical trials often use central retinal thickness (CRT) from OCT as the primary endpoint. CRT is defined as the average retinal thickness between inner and outer borders in the central 1mm^2, and an increase in CRT correlates with a loss of retinal function, while a decrease implies functional improvement [52, 53].

In comparison to FFA, conventional OCT-A imaging is limited by the field of view and the inability to detect vascular leakage as it does not use a fluorescent dye to visualize blood flow. OCT scans typically range in size from 2 x 2mm to 12 x 12mm and the quality is reduced with a widened field of view as an equal number of OCT b-scans are collected for all scanning areas [45]. This can lead to difficulty detecting nonperfusion areas in peripheral regions, however, protocols to enlarge the field of view to 20 x 20mm have been developed [54], and there is increasing interest in wide-field OCT-A as a diagnostic tool. Montage imaging of OCT-A scans is one method to increase the field of view, which does not compromise image quality; however, it is time-consuming and labour-intensive. It also requires patient cooperation for multiple OCT scans [55]. Another alternative approach to increasing the field of view has been to use trial frames with a +20-diopter lens (Extended Field Imaging; EFI), between the OCT-A probe and the eye, to increase the light incidence angle and generate an imaging field expansion [56]. On average, EFI images were found to visualize an area 188.5% larger than those without EFI [57]. Another drawback of OCT is that software programs do not have normalized data to validate the clinically observed vasculature structures and whether they are abnormal or are down to variation between patients [12].

Currently available OCT devices are either spectral domain OCT (SD-OCT), with imaging speeds from 25,000 to 85,000 a-scans per second or swept-source OCT (SS-OCT) devices, which can reach a speed of >100,000 a-scans per second. The two systems differ in light source, optic components, and photodetection device. Compared to SD-OCT, SS-OCT generally has a faster acquisition time, and the point photodetector device is relatively simpler. For example, spectral domain devices use a broadband light source, whereas a swept-source light source has a wavelength focused at ~1µm that 'sweeps' within a limited band of wavelengths. In SD-OCT, the photodetector is a spectrometer that is comprised of a Fourier transform lens, a diffraction grating, and a detector array to determine the resolution. On the other hand, in SS-OCT, the sweep range of the tuneable laser determines the axial resolution. The wavelength of the light source is important for the visualization of ocular tissues; longer wavelengths can penetrate and visualize the choriocapillaris and choroid better, however, the resolution is decreased. When shorter wavelengths are used, signal attenuation can occur when there is RPE clumping or the presence of drusen [58]. Wide- and full-field swept-source OCT is becoming more available and offers a larger field of view with fast acquisition times and has significant potential, but it is yet to reach widespread commercial applicability.

Macular Nonperfusion/Retinal Ischemia

Nonperfusion areas are regions of the retina without perfused capillaries that cause ischemia. Retinal ischemia causes a cascade of cellular changes, including the overexpression of VEGF, which leads to neovascularization and increased vascular permeability. Impaired circulation in the retina also leads to vision loss as retinal cells, such as RGCs and photoreceptors, become dysfunctional and lose viability due to hypoxia and an altered metabolic state. Therefore, retinal ischemia is a sight-threatening consequence of CRVO, HRVO, and BRVO that must be accurately diagnosed for therapeutic intervention.

FFA has been the conventional approach for evaluating macular perfusion after RVO; it is used clinically to visualize the SCP to determine ischemia and changes in the perifoveal capillary network. This information is used for a prognostic evaluation according to the area of ischemia and macular involvement. However, recent studies have found that microvascular changes in RVO may not be fully represented in FFA as the axial resolution is not able to fully resolve the DCP, due to a lack of depth-resolved imaging. As discussed above, FFA is limited in its ability to image the ICP and DCP – this is primarily due to the fluorescein fluorescence from the choriocapillaris, and the scattering of light from the nerve fiber layer, and deeper retinal layers, which increase background fluorescence signal and mask the signal from the DCP. Importantly, it has been suggested that the DCP is more vulnerable to hemodynamic changes following RVO than the SCP, which means that imaging of the DCP is critical for a correct prognosis following RVO. There is consistent evidence showing that nonperfusion areas are more extensive in the DCP than the SCP [59 - 61], and these areas of nonperfusion are better visualized in OCT-A than in FFA [62]. Moreover, areas of nonperfusion have been found in the SCP and DCP of the contralateral eye in RVO patients, when compared to controls. This may be a hallmark of previous RVOs in these eyes [51]. Nonperfusion in both the SCP and DCP has also been reported to significantly correlate with nonperfusion of the peripheral retina [63]. Nonperfusion of the DCP may impact visual function as it nourishes the zone between the INL and the outer plexiform layer, which contains neuronal synapses that receive visual signals from photoreceptors [60]. As the post-mitotic retinal neurons cannot regenerate in adulthood, a loss in their viability leads to permanent vision loss.

The vascular density of the SCP and DCP can be calculated as a percent of the area and depth occupied by capillaries within a selected area of an OCT-A scan. This approach has been used to determine the extent of retinal ischemia and evaluate whether OCT-A can be used to distinguish between non-ischemic and ischemic CRVO. The detection of nonperfused areas may not indicate the complete absence of vascular flow, but instead, some of these regions may just fall under the threshold of detection for the OCT device [63]. One study found a statistically significant reduction in parafoveal and whole vascular density in both SCP and DCP of ischemic CRVO eyes in comparison to eyes with non-ischemic CRVO, however, foveal vascular density was found not to be significantly different [64].

Calculating the area of nonperfusion in the parafoveal region with OCT-A was found to be the most relevant factor that correlated with changes in visual acuity and macular sensitivity in microperimetry for RVO. It was also found to be more significant than the EZ continuity, which delineates the inner and outer segments of photoreceptors [65]. Measurement of the FAZ using OCT-A can also provide additional prognostic information in patients with CRVO. The FAZ size is increased in the DCP of eyes with RVO when compared to controls and the contralateral eye, and the FAZ of the SCP. The FAZ was found to be enlarged in the SCP and DCP of BRVO [51], as well as CRVO eyes [68]. A significant correlation was also found between visual acuity and FAZ area in CRVO patients that did not have macular edema [66].

Neovascularization

Neovascularization describes the proliferation of new, abnormal blood vessels that can impair vision when it occurs in the eye. Retinal vein occlusions can cause neovascularization by producing an overexpression of VEGF in retinal cells and the subsequent formation of new blood vessels. These new capillaries can leak blood or fluid into the retina or vitreous, which affects vision and may even cause retinal detachment. Several neovascular problems can arise in eyes that have CRVO, these include INV; angle neovascularization; neovascularization of optic disc (NVD); neovascularization elsewhere (NVE); neovascular glaucoma (NVG); and vitreous hemorrhage. After retinal ischemia, collateral vessels can form that traverse the nonperfusion area as a long vessel, or as a bunch of sinuous vessels. These collateral vessels can be traced to the DCP and are present in both CRVO and BRVO [60].

When compared to conventional FFA, OCT-A can improve the visualization of optic disc venous collaterals (OVCs) and NVDs in ischemic retinal disease [67]. OVCs may arise from the retinal capillary bed and develop from the existing retinal vascular network, and OCT-A was shown to delineate them better than FFA. It is clinically important to differentiate venous collaterals from neovascularization as collaterals may prevent worse visual outcomes, while neovascularization needs laser photocoagulation to halt any serious vision loss. OCT-A identified OVCs at the SCP level, however, neovascular vessels are prominent above the retina at the vitreous level. It was determined that OVCs are more 'looped' vessels, while new, abnormal vessels are a mesh of fine vessels. The longer wavelengths used in OCT-A enable better penetration through intraretinal hemorrhages, while there is also an absence of background fluorescence caused by fluorescein leakage at these sites. Therefore, OCT-A can be preferential for imaging microvascular abnormalities in the SCP and DCP following RVO, including neovascular fronds and changes in the FAZ.

Retinal neovascularization that occurs within 1 disc diameter is deemed to be NVD, whereas it is classified as NVE if it is further than 1 disc diameter away. NVE can be well visualized using OCT-A, primarily due to the absence of leakage and background fluorescence from fluorescein [68]. NVEs present as homogenous hyperreflective loops that breach the inner limiting membrane (ILM) and enter into the vitreous. OCT was used to define NVE development in three stages; I – disruption of the ILM; II – horizontal proliferation along the ILM; III – Breach of the posterior hyaloid and linear growth [69]. Importantly, this can allow tracking of vasculature changes over time and the response to therapeutic intervention with anti-angiogenic agents. According to one study, NVE was found in 41% of eyes with ischemic RVO using wide-field OCT-A and was defined as sea-fan and nodular-type vessels according to their morphology and localization. Meanwhile, standard clinical examination, including FA, only detected NVE in 10% of eyes from the same population. Most importantly, NVE with nodular-type vessels was identified in one case using wide-field OCT-A but was not detected using ultra-wide-field FFA [70]. This work highlighted that wide-field OCT-A may be an important method for the detection and characterization of neovascularization in patients with ischemic RVO.

Vitreous Hemorrhage and Anterior Segment Neovascularization

Another consequence of retinal neovascularization following RVO is vitreous hemorrhage, which can significantly impair vision. Vitreous hemorrhage occurs when blood enters the vitreous cavity, which is normally a transparent hydrophilic gel that maintains the structure and pressure within the eye (Fig. **5**). Vitreous hemorrhage can cause visual floaters and may present as the main symptom of undetected retinal vein occlusion. In one study, 29% of ischemic CRVO eyes (n=31) had vitreous hemorrhage associated with neovascularization [71]. In BRVO, vitreous hemorrhage was found to occur in 3.9% of cases [1].

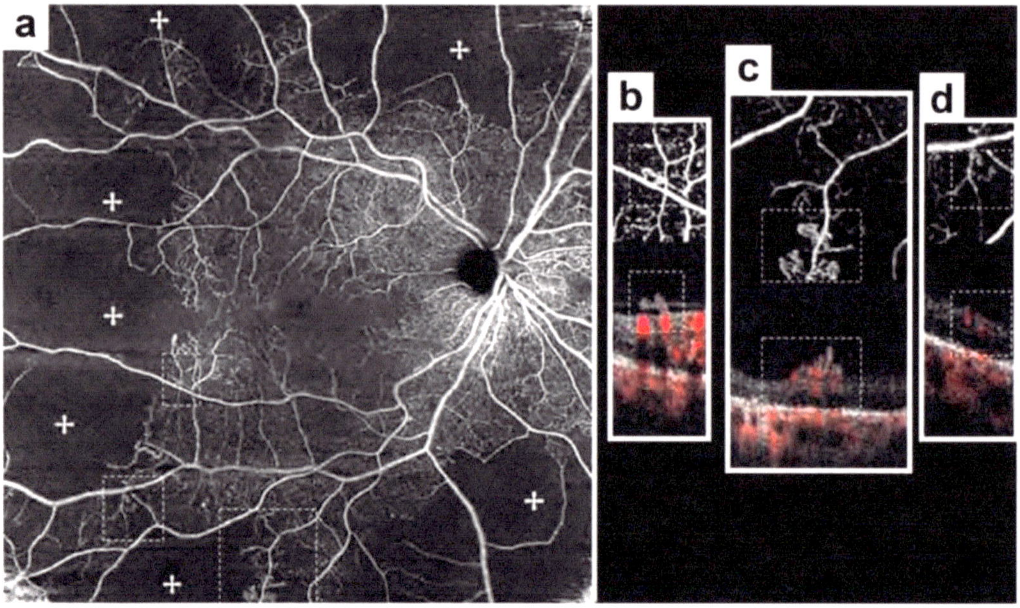

Fig. (5). Retinal nonperfusion and vitreous hemorrhage imaging by OCT-A. (**a**) SD-OCT-A (8 x 8mm) montage showing areas of nonperfusion (+). (**b** and **c**) neovascularization that is breaching the ILM and entering the vitreous. (**d**) Intraretinal neovascularization within the ILM. Image unchanged from Vaz-Pereira, S. *et al.,* 2020. [77] and is used under the Creative Commons Attribution 4.0 International License (https://creativecommons.org/licenses/by/4.0/).

Approximately 60% of patients with ischemic CRVO develop some form of anterior-segment neovascularization within 2 years of disease onset [72]. Retinal ischemia causes the elevation of VEGF and subsequent neovascularization; iris neovascularization develops in two-thirds of ischemic CRVO cases, and one-third of these patients also develop neovascular glaucoma. However, only 2% of BRVO patients develop INV. In one study, INV or angle neovascularization occurred in 58% of the eyes with CRVO [71], whereas another study reported 52% of eyes with ischemic CRVO having INV and 6% of eyes with non-ischemic CRVO having INV [73]. INV can be readily observed using slit-lamp microscopy and ICGA, as well as anterior segment OCT-A (AS-OCTA) [74]. AS-OCTA is limited by motion artifacts, but it is useful in the quantification and management of INV in a clinical setting.

Neovascularization that is caused by retinal ischemia from RVO can lead to glaucoma. Glaucoma is a group of disorders that cause progressive degeneration of the optic nerve and RGC loss at the optic nerve head. NVG is a secondary type of glaucoma that is caused by new blood vessel formation that affects the angle between the lens and the cornea. A fibrovascular membrane forms on the surface of the iris and the iridocorneal angle of the anterior chamber [32]. Closure of the angle by the membrane leads to obstruction of the aqueous outflow and the elevation of intraocular pressure, which causes glaucoma. Vision loss from glaucomatous change is irreversible and neovascular glaucoma typically leads to a poor visual prognosis, so early diagnosis is important to prevent extensive vision loss. NVG may arise within 2 weeks to 2 years after CRVO but typically appears after 3 months [75]. However, NVG rarely occurs in cases of BRVO [1]. OCT-A can be a promising approach to monitoring the progression of neovascularization in different ocular layers, including the anterior segment [76].

Macular Edema

The macula is the central area of the retina where light is focused to enable high acuity central vision. The fovea is a cone photoreceptor-rich region at the center of the macula that is present as a small depression in OCT imaging. Leaking of blood and fluids into the macula results in swelling, known as cystoid macula edema (CME) (Fig. **6**). CRVO and BRVO can both cause CME, which can lead to significant vision loss in patients and requires effective management and therapy to restore sight. The Central Vein Occlusion Study (CVOS) found that 21% of 728 eyes with CRVO had macular edema and a visual acuity lower than 20/50 [78]. Macular edema can occur in up to 90% of BRVO cases – the lack of blood flow to the macula causes an over-expression of endothelin-1, inflammatory cytokines, and VEGF, which causes vascular permeability and exudates that result in macular edema. Macular edema can be perfused or nonperfused, with visual outcomes better with perfused macular edema [79 - 81].

OCT imaging can generate cross-sectional, high-resolution views of the macula, which is vital for the diagnosis and monitoring of ischemic RVOs, as well as the progression of CME and response to treatment. OCT-A can visualize areas with edema in the outer plexiform layer that has arisen due to ischemia of interneurons within the inner nuclear and plexiform layers, in recent-onset CRVO [82]. Cystoid spaces in the SCP layer are more frequent in CRVO, while they are more common in the DCP in BRVO. In severe CME, OCT may also show sub-retinal fluid (SRF) underlying the neural retina. It has previously been shown that CME is more readily evident in OCT-A when compared to OCT and FA [61]. Cystoid areas have no reflectance, so they generate no signal in OCT. They are adjacent to nonperfusion areas, although nonperfusion areas do not always produce cystoid spaces [59]. Hyperreflective areas of cystoid edema in OCT are generated by the presence of lipids and hard exudates in the IRF. CME is typically restricted to the macula and resolves within ~4 months, however, chronic macular edema that lasts longer than 6-9 months can permanently damage photoreceptors and cause fibrosis.

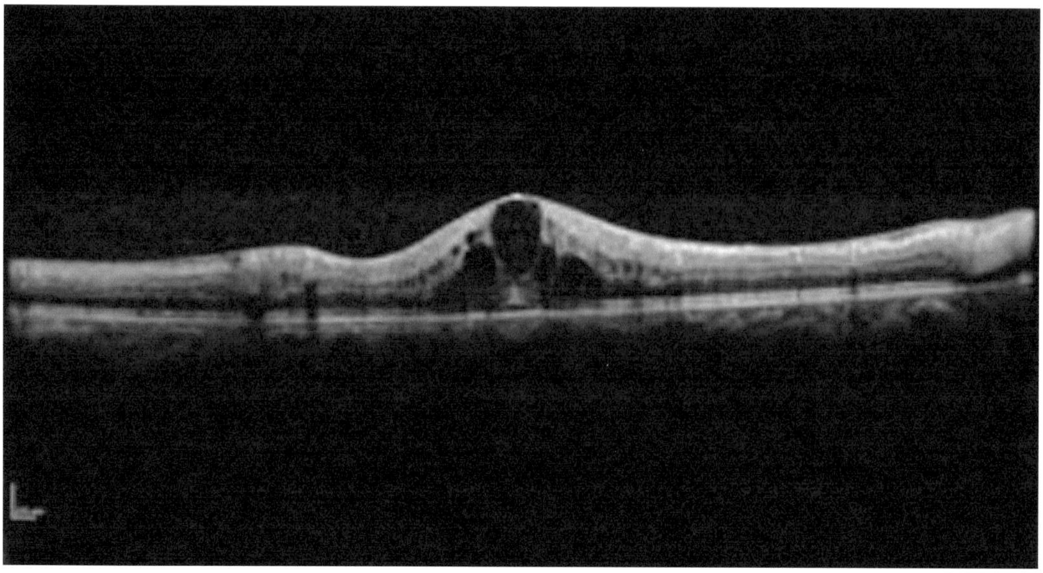

Fig. (6). OCT cross-sectional imaging of CRVO associated macular edema. Cystoid spaces lack reflectivity in retinal OCT images. This image was originally published in the Retina Image Bank® website. Jeffrey S. Heier, M.D. CRVO-associated Macular Edema. Retina Image Bank. 2012; 179. © The American Society of Retina Specialists.

SRF, which exists as a non-reflective cystoid space between the neural retina and the RPE, and the intra-retinal fluid (IRF), which is comprised of cystoid spaces situated within the neural retina, are hallmarks of acute CME. OCT is the best available method that enables the visualization of the SRF and IRF for the effective diagnosis, management, and therapeutic intervention for CME.

CURRENT STANDARD OF CARE & FUTURE THERAPEUTIC MODALITIES

There is no currently available therapy to restore photoreceptor viability in ischemic areas, however, there has been a revolution in the management of vascular disease with the advent of anti-VEGF therapeutics. In the case of non-ischemic CRVO diagnosis, initial follow-up should be within 6 weeks to monitor for any edema or ischemia. Ischemic CRVO patients should be seen monthly to identify the onset of anterior segment neovascularization, such as INV and NVG. The risk of INV is highest within the first 90 days [78]. There is no effective therapy for the prevention or reversing of CRVO, but OCT-A monitoring is key to visualizing the progression of CRVO sequelae and their treatment response. The therapies for CRVO and BRVO are aimed at vision-threatening sequelae, which include neovascularization and macular edema (Fig. **7**). Therapies for complications that arise from BRVO include anti-aggregative therapy and fibrinolysis, vitrectomy and sheathotomy, macular grid retinal laser therapy, intravitreal steroids, and intravitreal anti-VEGF approaches [1]. OCT-A is a valuable tool to monitor changes in retinal vascularization, vessel density, the foveal vascular zone, and the response to therapeutics such as anti-VEGF treatments, which can be accurately quantified using image processing.

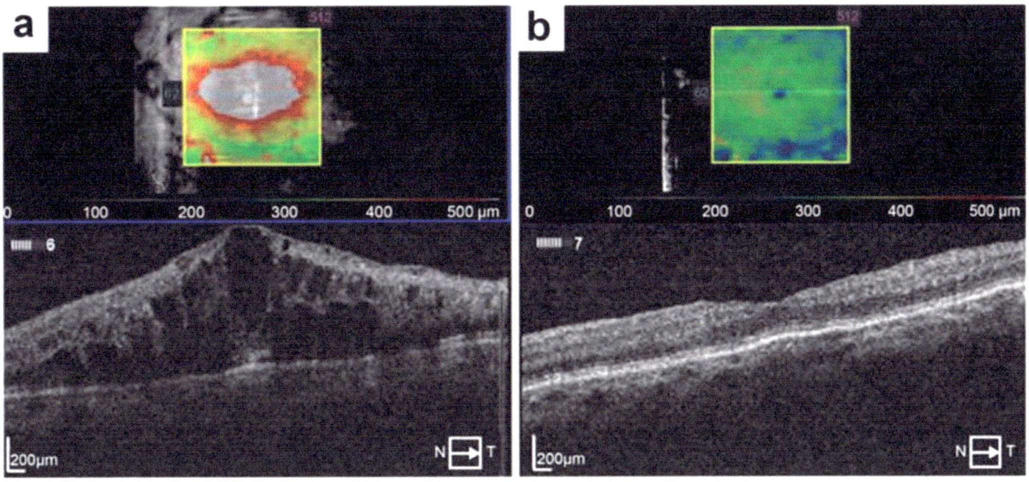

Fig. (7). OCT-A imaging of a CRVO patient treated with aflibercept (Eylea). (**a**) Before treatment with aflibercept, hyporeflective cystoid macular edema is evident. (**b**) Macular edema associated with CRVO was significantly reduced after treatment with aflibercept. This image was originally published on the Retina Image Bank® website. Theodore Leng, M.D. CRVO Treated With EYLEA. Retina Image Bank. 2017; 27403. © The American Society of Retina Specialists.

Anti-VEGF Therapeutics

In CRVO and BRVO, retinal ischemia causes an increase in VEGF expression and secretion, which leads to neovascularization, increased vascular permeability, and vasodilation. Targeting VEGF has been successful in limiting the progression of vision loss due to RVO by restricting neovascularization of the retina and the anterior segment. Anti-VEGF therapy has been proven to help reduce INV and angle neovascularization in NVG [83]. Several investigators have reported on the use of bevacizumab, ranibizumab, or aflibercept in INV and have shown a reduction or complete resolution of INV after a short period, typically less than a week [74, 84 - 86].

Most importantly, anti-VEGF therapy can effectively decrease macular edema. Intravitreal ranibizumab (Lucentis) and aflibercept (Eylea) are both FDA-approved for treating macular edema due to RVO. Ranibizumab (BRAVO and CRUISE trials) and aflibercept (GALILEO/COPERNICUS and VIBRANT trials) clinical trials have shown these drugs to be efficacious as a therapeutic approach to treat macular edema. Bevacizumab (Avastin) has been used off-label to treat macular edema in CRVO and BRVO. Ranibizumab is a recombinant, humanized monoclonal antibody fragment (Fab) which binds VEGF-A isoforms, while bevacizumab is a full-length, humanized monoclonal antibody that binds VEGF-A isoforms at a lower affinity than ranibizumab. Aflibercept is a recombinant fusion protein that is composed of the human VEGF receptor 1 and 2 extracellular domains fused to the Fc part of a human immunoglobulin (IgG1). It targets VEGF-A, VEGF-B, and placental growth factor (PIGF). Aflibercept has a higher binding affinity for VEGF-A over ranibizumab and bevacizumab. Susvimo, previously called Port Delivery System with ranibizumab, is a refillable eye implant indicated for the treatment of neovascular (wet) age-related macular degeneration. It is inserted into the eye with a one-time, outpatient procedure and may be used in the future as an anti-VEGF therapy with a reduced treatment burden in RVOs.

Anti-VEGF therapies have revolutionized retinal therapeutics and have had considerable success in the management of retinal vascular disease, such as macular edema from RVOs. The US patent for Lucentis (ranibizumab) expired in 2020, while patent coverage in the US for Eylea (aflibercept) will end in 2023, which has led to the emergence of potential biosimilars to treat retinal vascular disease. Biosimilars are drugs with comparable safety, efficacy, pharmacodynamic, and pharmacokinetic profiles to the innovator drug, such as ranibizumab. Razumab was the first biosimilar to ranibizumab and was approved for use in India in 2015, while Byooviz (SB110) was recently approved by the FDA in 2021. There are six other biosimilars in clinical trials, which are FYB 201 (Germany), Xlucane (Sweden), R-TPR-024 (India), SJP-0133 (Japan), LUBT010 (India), and CKD-701 (South Korea) [87].

Faricimab (Vabysmo) is a bi-specific monoclonal antibody that inhibits both VEGF-A and angiopoietin-2 (Ang-2) and is also administered by intravitreal injection. Faricimab received FDA regulatory approval for the treatment of retinal vascular diseases, such as wet age-related macular degeneration and diabetic macular edema, in January 2022, however, phase III clinical trials are ongoing for use in treating macular edema due to retinal vein occlusion [88]. The COMINO and BALATON trials are evaluating faricimab's efficacy and safety in patients with macular edema from CRVO and BRVO, in comparison with aflibercept.

Anti-VEGF Studies For CRVO

The CRUISE study evaluated 362 patients with CRVO, who received monthly injections of 0.3mg or 0.5mg ranibizumab, or sham injections, for 6 months. The primary endpoint was the mean change from baseline best-corrected visual acuity

(BCVA) after 6 months; the BVCA at baseline was 20/100, while the mean CRT at baseline was 685.2μm. The patients who received 0.3mg or 0.5mg ranibizumab had a mean change from baseline BCVA letter scores of 12.7 and 14.9 letters, respectively, when compared with 0.8 letters in the control group. An average gain of 9 letters was found only 7 days after the first injection, and after 6 months, significantly more ranibizumab-treated patients had BCVA of 20/40 or greater (0.3mg – 43.9%; 0.5mg = 46.9%) compared to the control group (20.8%). Furthermore, there was a significant reduction of the central foveal thickness from the baseline; a mean reduction of 434μm (0.3mg) and 452μm (0.5mg) was found in the ranibizumab treatment groups, while there was only a 168μm reduction in the control group. The median reduction in foveal thickness at 6 months was 94% and 97% in the 0.3mg and 0.5mg groups, respectively, compared to 24% in the sham group [89].

CRVO patients in the controlled phase III GALILEO and COPERNICUS studies received monthly injections of 2mg aflibercept or sham injections over 6 months. In the COPERNICUS study, 56.1% of patients dosed with 2mg aflibercept monthly gained at least 15 BVCA letters from the baseline, when compared with 12.3% of patients in the sham group [90, 91]. Similar results were seen in the primary endpoint of the GALILEO trial; 60.2% of patients dosed with aflibercept gained at least 15 BVCA letters from the baseline, while 22.1% of the sham group achieved the same. The aflibercept group gained 18 letters on average, whereas the main gain in the sham injections was only 3.3 letters, which was a secondary endpoint. Aflibercept was well tolerated, and serious adverse effects were more prevalent in the control group (13.5%) when compared to the experimental group (3.5%), which points to the intravitreal injection being responsible for adverse events [92]. The SCORE2 study compared aflibercept with bevacizumab for treating macular edema from CRVO, and bevacizumab was observed to be non-inferior to aflibercept in terms of visual acuity and retinal thickness improvements. After 6 months of either bevacizumab (1.25mg) or aflibercept (2.0mg) every 4 weeks, an average letter score from a baseline of 18.9 was measured in the aflibercept group, compared to 18.6 letters in the bevacizumab group [93].

Anti-VEGF Studies For BRVO

In the BRAVO study, patients with macular edema from BRVO were dosed monthly with 0.3mg or 0.5mg ranibizumab, or sham injections for 6 months. Patients in all groups were also subject to one rescue grid laser treatment if they had a gain of <5 letters on an ETDRS chart or <50μm improvement in central subfield thickness. After 6 months, the 0.3mg and 0.5mg ranibizumab groups gained an average of 16.6 and 18.3 letters, respectively. Only 18.7% and 19.8% of the 0.3mg and 0.5mg ranibizumab groups, respectively, required a rescue grid laser, whereas 54.5% of the sham group required a rescue laser. Overall, the BRAVO study showed that ranibizumab is efficacious and superior to grid laser in the treatment of macular edema due to BRVO.

The VIBRANT trial compared 2mg aflibercept to traditional grid laser therapy in patients with macular edema due to BRVO and with a BVCA of 20/40 to 20/230. Randomized patient groups received aflibercept every 4 weeks for 20 weeks, or a grid laser at baseline and a single rescue grid laser between weeks 12 to 20. The aflibercept group received further intravitreal injections of the drug every 8 weeks after week 24, while the grid laser group received sham injections. At week 24, the mean increase in BCVA was 17.0 in the aflibercept group and 6.9 in the grid laser group. Therefore, the VIBRANT study also confirmed that anti-VEGF injections, in this case, aflibercept, are more effective than grid laser as a therapeutic for macular edema from BRVO.

Laser Photocoagulation

Laser photocoagulation was the conventional therapeutic approach for BRVO, before the emergence of anti-VEGF therapies, as outlined by the BVOS [43]. Pan-retinal photocoagulation (PRP) inhibits neovascularization and is effective to treat open angle NVG when combined with anti-VEGF therapy [83]. The RPE layer absorbs the laser light, and the laser energy converts to thermal energy, denaturing the tissue protein and causing cell death and necrosis. Typically, between 1000 – 2000 micro-burns are used to cause scarring and hyperpigmentation, damaging the ischemic areas of the retina and lowering the VEGF levels. Patients with perfused macular edema and a visual acuity lower than 20/40, without any visual acuity improvements for 3 months, are considered for photocoagulation. Laser photocoagulation may also be used in the case of vitreous hemorrhage, in combination with pars plana vitrectomy.

Conventional Argon grid laser parameters are typically within the range of 0.1 seconds and 100μm diameter spot size with enough power to produce a very light burn (100mW). Macular grid laser is not advised for use in CRVO, as it has not been shown to improve visual acuity in patients, even though it reduces new blood vessel formation [94]. However, the CVOS study group advocated for the use of pan-retinal photocoagulation for INV once it has occurred [95]. The BVOS supported the use of grid laser photocoagulation for macular edema from BRVO [96], and sectoral PRP for retinal neovascularization [43].

Corticosteroids: Dexamethasone and Triamcinolone

The SCORE study compared intravitreal corticosteroid (triamcinolone acetonide) with observation only for the treatment of retinal vein occlusion. It showed that triamcinolone acetonide is effective in treating macular edema after CRVO when compared to the control group, however, it was not efficacious in the therapy of BRVO when compared to focal laser photocoagulation. CRVO patients (n=271) were included in the SCORE trial, and 1mg and 4mg doses of intravitreal triamcinolone acetonide were administered to evaluate its efficacy in macular edema from CRVO. The percentage of patients with a visual acuity letter score of >15 from baseline to 12 months was found to be 26.5% and 25.6% for 1mg and 4mg, respectively, while the observation-only group was 6.8%. Central retinal thickness measured by OCT was found to be reduced in all groups. The safety profile was superior in the 1mg triamcinolone group as the incidence rate of adverse events was higher for the 4mg group, particularly with elevated IOP and cataracts [97 - 99].

OZURDEX is a biodegradable dexamethasone implant made of lactic and glycolic acid that is administered through a small pars plana puncture with an applicator. It is FDA-approved for the treatment of macular edema following CRVO or BRVO and is often used as a second-line approach to treat eyes with chronic edema that have responded poorly to anti-VEGF injections (Fig. **8**).

In the GENEVA study, 1267 patients were allocated to sham injections or 0.35mg, and 0.7mg, single treatment dexamethasone implant groups. Average visual acuity was 20/80 in all groups and mean CRT was 550µm at baseline. After a single dose, the time to a >15-letter BVCA improvement was significantly lower in the dexamethasone groups compared with the sham control group. The percentage of eyes with a >15-letter improvement in BVCA was also significantly greater in both dexamethasone implant groups over the control between days 30 to 90. BVCA improvements with the dexamethasone implant were observed in both BRVO and CRVO patients. By day 60, the percentage of dexamethasone implant-treated eyes with IOP >25mmHg peaked at 16%, but by day 180, it was the same as the sham group and there was also no significant difference between the groups in the incidence of cataracts [100].

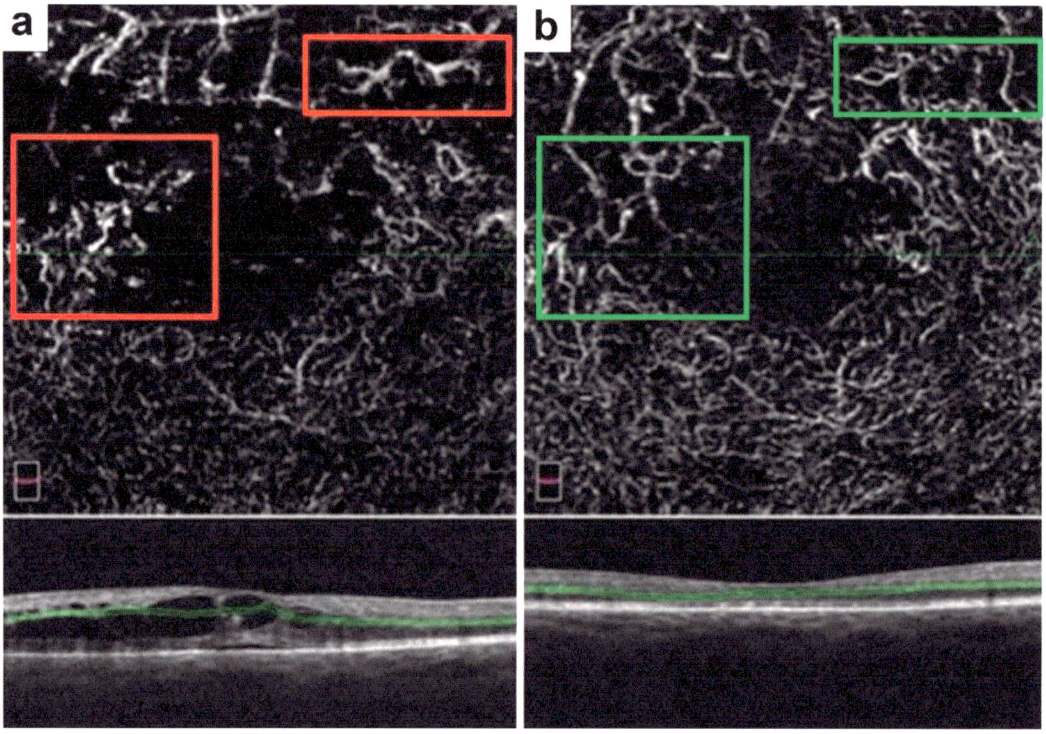

Fig. (8). OCT-A images of superior-temporal BRVO: deep retinal plexus before dexamethasone implant (**a**) showing telangiectatic vessels (red squares) and after dexamethasone implant (**b**), showing vessel caliber reduction (green squares). Image unchanged from Mastropasqua, R., *et al.,* 2017 [101] and is used under the Creative Commons Attribution 4.0 International License (https://creativecommons.org/licenses/by/4.0/).

CONCLUDING REMARKS

In summary, OCT-A is a remarkable tool to accurately diagnose retinal vein occlusions and monitor the changes in macular perfusion and RVO sequelae after therapeutic intervention, which expands on the capabilities of FFA imaging and the current standard of care for retinal vascular disease. For example, volumetric angiograms can be rapidly generated by OCT-A to visualize the SCP, ICP, DCP, and choriocapillaris. Importantly, OCT-A can provide high-resolution images of the DCP, which is particularly vulnerable to the hemodynamic changes that occur with RVOs.

The non-invasive nature of OCT means that the clinical course of RVO can be effectively monitored in patients with a relatively low level of compliance. OCT-A is also a valuable method to quantify clinic parameters such as vessel density and FAZ metrics to more clearly understand the pathological changes associated with RVO. With the onset of machine learning and artificial intelligence, there will also be new approaches to rapidly quantify these metrics and correlate the

OCT-A images with visual acuity changes and improvements from therapy. The small field of view limitation of OCT-A is currently being challenged with montage approaches and extended fields of view with positive diopter lenses in-between the eye and the OCT-A probe. Advances in OCT-A imaging are currently being researched and once they have gained wide clinical applicability, they will offer a larger field of view to rapidly incorporate the peripheral retina and its changes associated with RVO.

Anti-VEGF therapies have proven to be safe and efficacious for the treatment of neovascularization and macular edema secondary to RVO. Biosimilars and sustained release anti-VEGF therapeutics will help reduce the cost to the patient and usher in a new era of clinical ophthalmology that lowers the burden of retinal vascular disease. Dexamethasone implants are also efficacious as a second-line therapeutic approach if patients do not respond to anti-VEGF drugs. Future anti-VEGF therapeutics will aim to inhibit neovascularization with minimal surgical intervention, as monthly intravitreal injections are burdensome for the patient and clinical staff. This includes viral vectors, such as Adeno-associated viruses (AAVs), encoding secreted anti-VEGF therapeutics or bi-specific approaches targeting VEGF and angiopoietin-2, which have both been shown to be efficacious in the treatment of exudative age-related macular degeneration.

There is also research ongoing into the regeneration of retinal cell types that have lost viability due to retinal ischemia, or age-related degeneration. These include cell transplantation of retinal progenitor cells or *in vivo* reprogramming approaches, as it is well established that Müller glia cells in the zebrafish retina can re-populate damaged photoreceptors. Understanding the mechanisms behind retinal neurogenesis from glial cell types in lower-order vertebrates could pave the way to restoring vision lost to the most common retinal pathologies.

LIST OF ABBREVIATIONS

BCVA Best-corrected Visual Acuity

BRVO Branch Retinal Vein Occlusion

BVOS Branch Retinal Vein Occlusion Study

CME Cystoid Macular Edema

CRT Central Retinal Thickness

CRVO Central Retinal Vein Occlusion

CVOS Central Retinal Vein Occlusion Study

DCP Deep Capillary Plexus

ERG Electroretinogram

EZ Ellipsoid Zone

FFA	Fundus Fluorescein Angiography
FAZ	Foveal Avascular Zone
HRVO	Hemi-Retinal Vein Occlusion
ICGA	Indocyanine Green Angiography
ICP	Intermediate Capillary Plexus
IL	Interleukin
ILM	Inner Limiting Membrane
INL	Inner Nuclear Layer
INV	Iris Neovascularization
IOP	Intra-ocular Pressure
IRF	Intra-Retinal Fluid
NVD	Neovascularization of Optic Disc
NVE	Neovascularization Elsewhere
NVG	Neovascular Glaucoma
OCT	Optical Coherence Tomography
OCT-A	Optical Coherence Tomography Angiography
OR	Odds Ratio
PRP	Pan-retinal Photocoagulation
RAPD	Relative Afferent Pupillary Defect
RGC	Retinal Ganglion Cell
RPE	Retinal Pigment Epithelium
RVO	Retinal Vein Occlusion
SCP	Superficial Capillary Plexus
SRF	Sub-Retinal Fluid
VEGF	Vascular Endothelial Growth Factor.

ACKNOWLEDGMENTS

We express our deep appreciation to the technical staff of the Retina Specialists Unit at Oftalmologia Integral ABC (Nonprofit Medical and Surgical Organization) affiliated with the Postgraduate Division Studies at the National Autonomous University of Mexico.

DISCLAIMER

All the scientific comments issued in this chapter are solely the responsibility of the authors and not of the institutions with which they are affiliated.

REFERENCES

[1] Shahid H, Hossain P, Amoaku WM. The management of retinal vein occlusion: Is interventional ophthalmology the way forward? Br J Ophthalmol 2006; 90(5): 627-39. Available from: www.bjophthalmol.com
[http://dx.doi.org/10.1136/bjo.2005.068668] [PMID: 16622095]

[2] Mitchell P, Smith W, Chang A. Prevalence and associations of retinal vein occlusion in Australia. The Blue Mountains Eye Study. Arch Ophthalmol 1996; 114(10): 1243-7. Available from: https://jamanetwork.com/journals/jamaophthalmology/fullarticle/641845
[http://dx.doi.org/10.1001/archopht.1996.01100140443012] [PMID: 8859084]

[3] Rogers S, McIntosh RL, Cheung N, Lim L, Wang JJ, Mitchell P. The prevalence of retinal vein occlusion: pooled data from population studies from the united states, europe, asia, and australia. Ophthalmology 2010; 117(2): 313.

[4] Klein R, Klein BEK, Moss SE, Meuer SM, Gutman FA, Ferris FL. The epidemiology of retinal vein occlusion: The beaver dam eye study. Trans Am Ophthalmol Soc 2000; 98:133. 98: 133.

[5] Hayreh SS. Prevalent misconceptions about acute retinal vascular occlusive disorders. Prog Retin Eye Res 2005; 24(4): 493-519. Available from: https://www.sciencedirect.com/science/article/pii/S1350946204001016
[http://dx.doi.org/10.1016/j.preteyeres.2004.12.001] [PMID: 15845346]

[6] Karia N. Retinal vein occlusion: Pathophysiology and treatment options. Clin Ophthalmol 2010; 4: 809-16. Available from: https://pubmed.ncbi.nlm.nih.gov/20689798
[http://dx.doi.org/10.2147/OPTH.S7631] [PMID: 20689798]

[7] Huang D, Swanson EA, Lin CP, Schuman JS, Stinson WG, Chang W. Optical coherence tomography. Science 1979; 254(5035): 1178-81.
[http://dx.doi.org/10.1126/science.1957169]

[8] Wojtkowski M, Leitgeb R, Kowalczyk A, Bajraszewski T, Fercher AF. *In vivo* human retinal imaging by Fourier domain optical coherence tomography. J Biomed Opt 2002; 7(3): 457-63.
[http://dx.doi.org/10.1117/1.1482379] [PMID: 12175297]

[9] Wang L, Fu R, Xu C, Xu M. Methods and applications of full-filed optical coherence tomography: A review. J Biomed Opt 2022; 27: 5.
[http://dx.doi.org/10.1117/1.JBO.27.5.050901]

[10] von der Emde L, Saßmannshausen M, Morelle O, *et al.* Reliability of retinal layer annotation with a novel, high-resolution optical coherence tomography device: A comparative study. Bioengineering 2023; 10(4): 438.
[http://dx.doi.org/10.3390/bioengineering10040438] [PMID: 37106625]

[11] Schmidt-Erfurth U, Reiter GS, Riedl S, *et al.* AI-based monitoring of retinal fluid in disease activity and under therapy. Prog Retin Eye Res 2022; 86: 100972.
[http://dx.doi.org/10.1016/j.preteyeres.2021.100972] [PMID: 34166808]

[12] Singh RP, Tsai G, Banaee T, Conti FF. Optical coherence tomography angiography in eyes with retinal vein occlusion. J Ophthalmic Vis Res 2018; 13(3): 315-32. Available from: https://pubmed.ncbi.nlm.nih.gov/30090189
[http://dx.doi.org/10.4103/jovr.jovr_264_17] [PMID: 30090189]

[13] Balaratnasingam C, Inoue M, Ahn S, *et al.* Visual acuity is correlated with the area of the foveal avascular zone in diabetic retinopathy and retinal vein occlusion. Ophthalmology 2016; 123(11): 2352-67. Available from: http://www.aaojournal.org/article/S0161642016306571/fulltext
[http://dx.doi.org/10.1016/j.ophtha.2016.07.008] [PMID: 27523615]

[14] Rehak J, Rehak M. Branch retinal vein occlusion: pathogenesis, visual prognosis, and treatment modalities. Curr Eye Res 2008; 33(2): 111-31. Available from: https://pubmed.ncbi.nlm.nih.gov/18293182/

[http://dx.doi.org/10.1080/02713680701851902] [PMID: 18293182]

[15] Campochiaro PA, Hafiz G, Shah SM, *et al.* Ranibizumab for macular edema due to retinal vein occlusions: Implication of VEGF as a critical stimulator. Mol Ther 2008; 16(4): 791-9. Available from: https://pubmed.ncbi.nlm.nih.gov/18362932/ [http://dx.doi.org/10.1038/mt.2008.10] [PMID: 18362932]

[16] Koizumi H, Ferrara DC, Bruè C, Spaide RF. Central retinal vein occlusion case-control study. Am J Ophthalmol 2007; 144(6): 858-863.e1. Available from: https://pubmed.ncbi.nlm.nih.gov/17916319/ [http://dx.doi.org/10.1016/j.ajo.2007.07.036] [PMID: 17916319]

[17] The Eye Disease Case-Control Study Group. Risk factors for central retinal vein occlusion. Arch Ophthalmol 1996; 114(5): 545-54. [http://dx.doi.org/10.1001/archopht.1996.01100130537006] [PMID: 8619763]

[18] Cheung N, Klein R, Jie JW, Cotch MF, Islam AFM, Klein BEK. Traditional and novel cardiovascular risk factors for retinal vein occlusion: The multi-ethnic study of atherosclerosis. Invest Ophthalmol Vis Sci 2008; 49(10): 4297.

[19] O'Mahoney PRA, Wong DT, Ray JG. Retinal vein occlusion and traditional risk factors for atherosclerosis. Arch Ophthalmol 2008; 126(5): 692-9. Available from: https://pubmed.ncbi.nlm.nih.gov/18474782/ [http://dx.doi.org/10.1001/archopht.126.5.692] [PMID: 18474782]

[20] Hayreh SS, March W, Phelps CD. Ocular hypotony following retinal vein occlusion. Arch Ophthalmol 1978; 96(5): 827-33. Available from: https://jamanetwork.com/journals/jamaophthalmology/fullarticle/632586 [http://dx.doi.org/10.1001/archopht.1978.03910050433006] [PMID: 655920]

[21] David R, Zangwill L, Badarna M, Yassur Y. Epidemiology of retinal vein occlusion and its association with glaucoma and increased intraocular pressure. Ophthalmologica 1988; 197(2): 69-74. Available from: https://www.karger.com/Article/FullText/309923 [http://dx.doi.org/10.1159/000309923] [PMID: 3186211]

[22] Yoshimura T, Sonoda KH, Sugahara M, Mochizuki Y, Enaida H, Oshima Y. Comprehensive analysis of inflammatory immune mediators in vitreoretinal diseases. PLoS One 2009; 4(12): 8158.

[23] Funk M, Kriechbaum K, Prager F, *et al.* Intraocular concentrations of growth factors and cytokines in retinal vein occlusion and the effect of therapy with bevacizumab. Invest Ophthalmol Vis Sci 2009; 50(3): 1025-32. Available from: https://pubmed.ncbi.nlm.nih.gov/19060280/ [http://dx.doi.org/10.1167/iovs.08-2510] [PMID: 19060280]

[24] Noma H, Funatsu H, Mimura T, Harino S, Hori S. Vitreous levels of interleukin-6 and vascular endothelial growth factor in macular edema with central retinal vein occlusion. Ophthalmology 2009; 116(1): 87-93. Available from: https://pubmed.ncbi.nlm.nih.gov/19118700/ [http://dx.doi.org/10.1016/j.ophtha.2008.09.034] [PMID: 19118700]

[25] Noma H, Funatsu H, Mimura T, Harino S, Sone T, Hori S. Increase of vascular endothelial growth factor and interleukin-6 in the aqueous humour of patients with macular oedema and central retinal vein occlusion. Acta Ophthalmol 2010; 88(6): 646-51. Available from: https://pubmed.ncbi.nlm.nih.gov/19563372/ [http://dx.doi.org/10.1111/j.1755-3768.2009.01524.x] [PMID: 19563372]

[26] Boyd SR, Zachary I, Chakravarthy U, *et al.* Correlation of increased vascular endothelial growth factor with neovascularization and permeability in ischemic central vein occlusion. Arch Ophthalmol 2002; 120(12): 1644-50. Available from: https://pubmed.ncbi.nlm.nih.gov/12470137/ [http://dx.doi.org/10.1001/archopht.120.12.1644] [PMID: 12470137]

[27] Hayreh SS, Zimmerman MB, Podhajsky P. Incidence of various types of retinal vein occlusion and their recurrence and demographic characteristics. Am J Ophthalmol 1994; 117(4): 429-41. Available from: http://www.ajo.com/article/S0002939414700017/fulltext [http://dx.doi.org/10.1016/S0002-9394(14)70001-7] [PMID: 8154523]

[28] Hayreh SS. Classification of central retinal vein occlusion. Ophthalmology 1983; 90(5): 458-74. Available from: http://www.aaojournal.org/article/S0161642083345309/fulltext
[http://dx.doi.org/10.1016/S0161-6420(83)34530-9] [PMID: 6877778]

[29] Battaglia Parodi M, Bandello F. Branch retinal vein occlusion: classification and treatment. Ophthalmologica 2009; 223(5): 298-305. Available from: https://www.karger.com/Article/FullText/213640
[http://dx.doi.org/10.1159/000213640] [PMID: 19372724]

[30] Hayreh SS, Zimmerman MB, Podhajsky P, Alward WLM. Nocturnal arterial hypotension and its role in optic nerve head and ocular ischemic disorders. Am J Ophthalmol 1994; 117(5): 603-24. Available from: http://www.ajo.com/article/S0002939414700674/fulltext
[http://dx.doi.org/10.1016/S0002-9394(14)70067-4] [PMID: 8172267]

[31] Clarhson JC. Natural history and clinical management of central retinal vein occlusion. Arch Ophthalmol 1997; 115(4): 486-91. Available from: https://jamanetwork.com/journals/jamaophthalmology/fullarticle/642073
[http://dx.doi.org/10.1001/archopht.1997.01100150488006] [PMID: 9109757]

[32] Hayreh SS. Neovascular glaucoma. Prog Retin Eye Res 2007; 26(5): 470-85. Available from: https://pubmed.ncbi.nlm.nih.gov/17690002/
[http://dx.doi.org/10.1016/j.preteyeres.2007.06.001] [PMID: 17690002]

[33] Hayreh SS. Retinal vein occlusion. Indian J Ophthalmol 1994; 42(3): 109-32. Available from: https://www.ijo.in/article.asp?issn=0301-4738;year=1994;volume=42;issue=3;spage=109;epage=132;aulast=Hayreh
[PMID: 7829175]

[34] Stem MS, Talwar N, Comer GM, Stein JD. A longitudinal analysis of risk factors associated with central retinal vein occlusion. Ophthalmology 2013; 120(2): 362-70.
[http://dx.doi.org/10.1016/j.ophtha.2012.07.080]

[35] Hunt AR, Nguyen V, Arnold JJ, Mcallister IL, Mehta H, Invernizzi A. Hemiretinal vein occlusion 12-month outcomes are unique with vascular endothelial growth factor inhibitors: data from the Fight Retinal Blindness! Registry. Brit J Ophthal 2022; 107: 6. Available from: https://bjo.bmj.com/content/early/2022/01/24/bjophthalmol-2021-320482 (cited 2022 Jul 6)

[36] Hayreh SS, Hayreh MS. Hemi-central retinal vein occulsion. Pathogenesis, clinical features, and natural history. Arch Ophthalmol 1980; 98(9): 1600-9. Available from: https://jamanetwork.com/journals/jamaophthalmology/fullarticle/633523
[http://dx.doi.org/10.1001/archopht.1980.01020040452011] [PMID: 7425921]

[37] Hayreh SS, Rojas P, Podhajsky P, Montague P, Woolson RF. Ocular neovascularization with retinal vascular occlusion-III. Incidence of ocular neovascularization with retinal vein occlusion. Ophthalmology 1983; 90(5): 488-506. Available from: http://www.aaojournal.org/article/S0161642083345425/fulltext
[http://dx.doi.org/10.1016/S0161-6420(83)34542-5] [PMID: 6192376]

[38] Mirshahi A, Feltgen N, Hansen LL, Hattenbach LO. Retinal vascular occlusions: An interdisciplinary challenge. Dtsch Arztebl Int 2008; 105(26): 474-9. Available from: https://pubmed.ncbi.nlm.nih.gov/19626196

[39] Zhao J, Sastry SM, Sperduto RD, *et al.* Arteriovenous crossing patterns in branch retinal vein occlusion. Ophthalmology 1993; 100(3): 423-8. Available from: http://www.aaojournal.org/article/S0161642093316337/fulltext
[http://dx.doi.org/10.1016/S0161-6420(93)31633-7] [PMID: 8460014]

[40] Ota M, Tsujikawa A, Murakami T, *et al.* Association between integrity of foveal photoreceptor layer and visual acuity in branch retinal vein occlusion. Br J Ophthalmol 2007; 91(12): 1644-9. Available from: https://pubmed.ncbi.nlm.nih.gov/17504858/
[http://dx.doi.org/10.1136/bjo.2007.118497] [PMID: 17504858]

[41] Scott IU, Ip MS, VanVeldhuisen PC, *et al.* A randomized trial comparing the efficacy and safety of intravitreal triamcinolone with standard care to treat vision loss associated with macular Edema secondary to branch retinal vein occlusion: the Standard Care *vs* Corticosteroid for Retinal Vein Occlusion (SCORE) study report 6. Arch Ophthalmol 2009; 127(9): 1115-28. Available from: https://jamanetwork.com/journals/jamaophthalmology/fullarticle/423952 [http://dx.doi.org/10.1001/archophthalmol.2009.233] [PMID: 19752420]

[42] Sperduto RD, Yannuzzi LA, Sorenson JA, Sobel RS, Daly JR, DeRosa JT. Risk factors for branch retinal vein occlusion. Am J Ophthalmol 1993; 116(3): 286-96. Available from: http://www.ajo.com/article/S0002939414713455/fulltext [http://dx.doi.org/10.1016/S0002-9394(14)71345-5] [PMID: 8357052]

[43] Rosenberg NR. Argon laser scatter photocoagulation for prevention of neovascularization and vitreous hemorrhage in branch vein occlusion. A randomized clinical trial. Arch Ophthalmol 1986; 104(1): 34-41. Available from: https://jamanetwork.com/journals/jamaophthalmology/fullarticle/635855 [http://dx.doi.org/10.1001/archopht.1986.01050130044017] [PMID: 2417579]

[44] Spaide RF, Klancnik JM Jr, Cooney MJ. Retinal vascular layers imaged by fluorescein angiography and optical coherence tomography angiography. JAMA Ophthalmol 2015; 133(1): 45-50. Available from: https://jamanetwork.com/journals/jamaophthalmology/fullarticle/1910581 [http://dx.doi.org/10.1001/jamaophthalmol.2014.3616] [PMID: 25317632]

[45] de Carlo TE, Romano A, Waheed NK, Duker JS. A review of optical coherence tomography angiography (OCTA). Int J Retina Vitreous 2015; 1(1): 5. Available from: https://journalretinavitreous.biomedcentral.com/articles/10.1186/s40942-015-0005-8 [http://dx.doi.org/10.1186/s40942-015-0005-8] [PMID: 27847598]

[46] Kwiterovich KA, Maguire MG, Murphy RP, *et al.* Frequency of adverse systemic reactions after fluorescein angiography. Results of a prospective study. Ophthalmology 1991; 98(7): 1139-42. Available from: http://www.aaojournal.org/article/S0161642091321651/fulltext [http://dx.doi.org/10.1016/S0161-6420(91)32165-1] [PMID: 1891225]

[47] López-Sáez MP, Ordoqui E, Tornero P, *et al.* Fluorescein-induced allergic reaction. Ann Allergy Asthma Immunol 1998; 81(5): 428-30. Available from: http://www.annallergy.org/article/S1081120610631407/fulltext [http://dx.doi.org/10.1016/S1081-1206(10)63140-7] [PMID: 9860035]

[48] Spaide RF, Fujimoto JG, Waheed NK, Sadda SR, Staurenghi G. Optical coherence tomography angiography. Prog Retin Eye Res 2018; 64: 1-55. [http://dx.doi.org/10.1016/j.preteyeres.2017.11.003] [PMID: 29229445]

[49] Jia Y, Bailey ST, Hwang TS, *et al.* Quantitative optical coherence tomography angiography of vascular abnormalities in the living human eye. Proc Natl Acad Sci 2015; 112(18): E2395-402. Available from: www.pnas.org/cgi/doi/10.1073/pnas.1500185112 [http://dx.doi.org/10.1073/pnas.1500185112] [PMID: 25897021]

[50] Adhi M, Filho MAB, Louzada RN, *et al.* Retinal capillary network and foveal avascular zone in eyes with vein occlusion and fellow eyes analyzed with optical coherence tomography angiography. Invest Ophthalmol Vis Sci 2016; 57(9): OCT486-94. Available from: http://imagej.nih.gov/ij/ [http://dx.doi.org/10.1167/iovs.15-18907] [PMID: 27442342]

[51] Rispoli M, Savastano MC, Lumbroso B. Capillary network anomalies in branch retinal vein occlusion on optical coherence tomography angiography. Retina 2015; 35(11): 2332.

[52] Tadayoni R, Waldstein SM, Boscia F, *et al.* Sustained Benefits of Ranibizumab with or without Laser in Branch Retinal Vein Occlusion. Ophthalmology 2017; 124(12): 1778-87. Available from: https://pubmed.ncbi.nlm.nih.gov/28807635/ [http://dx.doi.org/10.1016/j.ophtha.2017.06.027] [PMID: 28807635]

[53] Larsen M, Waldstein SM, Boscia F, *et al.* Individualized Ranibizumab Regimen Driven by Stabilization Criteria for Central Retinal Vein Occlusion. Ophthalmology 2016; 123(5): 1101-11.

Available from: https://pubmed.ncbi.nlm.nih.gov/26896124/
[http://dx.doi.org/10.1016/j.ophtha.2016.01.011] [PMID: 26896124]

[54] Tan B, Chua J, Lin E, *et al.* Quantitative microvascular analysis with wide-field optical coherence tomography angiography in eyes with diabetic retinopathy. JAMA Netw Open 2020; 3(1): e1919469. Available from: https://jamanetwork.com/journals/jamanetworkopen/fullarticle/2758862
[http://dx.doi.org/10.1001/jamanetworkopen.2019.19469] [PMID: 31951275]

[55] Zhang Q, Rezaei KA, Saraf SS, Chu Z, Wang F, Wang RK. Ultra-wide optical coherence tomography angiography in diabetic retinopathy. Quant Imaging Med Surg 2018; 8(8): 743-53. Available from: https://pubmed.ncbi.nlm.nih.gov/30306055/
[http://dx.doi.org/10.21037/qims.2018.09.02] [PMID: 30306055]

[56] Uji A, Yoshimura N. Application of extended field imaging to optical coherence tomography. Ophthalmology 2015; 122(6): 1272-4. Available from: http://www.aaojournal.org/article/S0161642014012263/fulltext
[http://dx.doi.org/10.1016/j.ophtha.2014.12.035] [PMID: 25638010]

[57] Kimura M, Nozaki M, Yoshida M, Ogura Y. Wide-field optical coherence tomography angiography using extended field imaging technique to evaluate the nonperfusion area in retinal vein occlusion Clin Ophthalmol 2016; 10: 1291-5.
[http://dx.doi.org/10.2147/OPTH.S108630]

[58] OCT Technology: Will We Be "Swept" Away? Available from: https://www.reviewofophthalmology.com/article/oct-technology-will-we-be-swept-away (cited 2022 Jul 13)

[59] Kashani AH, Lee SY, Moshfeghi A, Durbin MK, Puliafito CA. Optical coherence tomography angiography of retinal venous occlusion. Retina 2015; 35(11): 2323-31. Available from: https://pubmed.ncbi.nlm.nih.gov/26457395/
[http://dx.doi.org/10.1097/IAE.0000000000000811] [PMID: 26457395]

[60] Coscas F, Glacet-Bernard A, Miere A, *et al.* Optical coherence tomography angiography in retinal vein occlusion: evaluation of superficial and deep capillary plexa. Am J Ophthalmol 2016; 161: 160-171.e2, 2. Available from: http://www.ajo.com/article/S0002939415006364/fulltext
[http://dx.doi.org/10.1016/j.ajo.2015.10.008] [PMID: 26476211]

[61] Suzuki N, Hirano Y, Yoshida M, *et al.* Microvascular abnormalities on optical coherence tomography angiography in macular edema associated with branch retinal vein occlusion. Am J Ophthalmol 2016; 161: 126-132.e1. Available from: https://pubmed.ncbi.nlm.nih.gov/26454243/
[http://dx.doi.org/10.1016/j.ajo.2015.09.038] [PMID: 26454243]

[62] Seknazi D, Coscas F, Sellam A, Rouimi F, Coscas G, Souied EH. Optical coherence tomography angiography in retinal vein occlusion: Correlations between macular vascular density, visual acuity, and peripheral nonperfusion area on fluorescein angiography. Retina 2018; 38(8): 1562.

[63] Tokayer J, Jia Y, Dhalla AH, Huang D. Blood flow velocity quantification using split-spectrum amplitude-decorrelation angiography with optical coherence tomography. Biomed Opt Express 2013; 4(10): 1909-24. Available from: https://pubmed.ncbi.nlm.nih.gov/24156053/
[http://dx.doi.org/10.1364/BOE.4.001909] [PMID: 24156053]

[64] Khodabandeh A, Shahraki K, Roohipoor R, *et al.* Quantitative measurement of vascular density and flow using optical coherence tomography angiography (OCTA) in patients with central retinal vein occlusion: Can OCTA help in distinguishing ischemic from non-ischemic type? Int J Retina Vitreous 2018; 4(1): 47. Available from: https://journalretinavitreous.biomedcentral.com/articles/10.1186/s40942-018-0152-9
[http://dx.doi.org/10.1186/s40942-018-0152-9] [PMID: 30607260]

[65] Kadomoto S, Muraoka Y, Ooto S, *et al.* Evaluation of macular ischemia in eyes with branch retinal vein occlusion: An optical coherence tomography angiography study. Retina 2018; 38(2): 272-82. Available from: https://pubmed.ncbi.nlm. nih.gov/28221256/
[http://dx.doi.org/10.1097/IAE.0000000000001541] [PMID: 28221256]

[66] Casselholmde Salles M, Kvanta A, Amrén U, Epstein D. Optical coherence tomography angiography in central retinal vein occlusion: Correlation between the foveal avascular zone and visual acuity. Invest Ophthalmol Vis Sci 2016; 57(9): OCT242-6. Available from: https://pubmed.ncbi.nlm.nih.gov/27409478/
[http://dx.doi.org/10.1167/iovs.15-18819] [PMID: 27409478]

[67] Singh A, Agarwal A, Mahajan S, *et al.* Morphological differences between optic disc collaterals and neovascularization on optical coherence tomography angiography. Graefes Arch Clin Exp Ophthalmol 2017; 255(4): 753-9. Available from: https://pubmed.ncbi.nlm.nih.gov/27942950/
[http://dx.doi.org/10.1007/s00417-016-3565-x] [PMID: 27942950]

[68] Sogawa K, Nagaoka T, Ishibazawa A, Takahashi A, Tani T, Yoshida A. En-face optical coherence tomography angiography of neovascularization elsewhere in hemicentral retinal vein occlusion. Int Med Case Rep J 2015; 8: 263.
[http://dx.doi.org/10.2147/IMCRJ.S93702]

[69] Lee CS, Lee AY, Sim DA, *et al.* Reevaluating the definition of intraretinal microvascular abnormalities and neovascularization elsewhere in diabetic retinopathy using optical coherence tomography and fluorescein angiography. Am J Ophthalmol 2015; 159(1): 101-110.e1. Available from: https://pubmed.ncbi.nlm.nih.gov/25284762/
[http://dx.doi.org/10.1016/j.ajo.2014.09.041] [PMID: 25284762]

[70] Huemer J, Khalid H, Wagner SK, Nicholson L, Fu DJ, Sim DA. Phenotyping of retinal neovascularization in ischemic retinal vein occlusion using wide field OCT angiography. Eye 2020; 35(10): 2812-9. Available from: https://www.nature.com/articles/s41433-020-01317-9

[71] DeCroos FC, Todorich B, Alshareef R, Khuthaila M, Fekrat S, Ho AC. Neovascular events in eyes with central retinal vein occlusion undergoing serial bevacizumab or ranibizumab intravitreal injections: A retrospective review. J Ophthalmic Vis Res 2014; 9(4): 461.

[72] Senthil S, Dada T, Das T, *et al.* Neovascular glaucoma : A review. Indian J Ophthalmol 2021; 69(3): 525-34.
[http://dx.doi.org/10.4103/ijo.IJO_1591_20] [PMID: 33595466]

[73] Hayreh SS, Zimmerman MB. Ocular neovascularization associated with central and hemicentral retinal vein occlusion. Retina 2012; 32(8): 1553-65. Available from: https://pubmed.ncbi.nlm.nih.gov/22495331/
[http://dx.doi.org/10.1097/IAE.0b013e318246912c] [PMID: 22495331]

[74] Shiozaki D, Sakimoto S, Shiraki A, Wakabayashi T, Fukushima Y, Oie Y. Observation of treated iris neovascularization by swept-source-based en-face anterior-segment optical coherence tomography angiography Scientific Reports 2019; 9(1): 1-6. Available from: https://www.nature.com/articles/s41598-019-46514-z
[http://dx.doi.org/10.1038/s41598-019-46514-z]

[75] Rodrigues GB, Abe RY, Zangalli C, *et al.* Neovascular glaucoma: A review. Int J Retina Vitreous 2016; 2(1): 26. Available from: https://journalretinavitreous.biomedcentral.com/articles/10.1186/s40942-016-0051-x
[http://dx.doi.org/10.1186/s40942-016-0051-x] [PMID: 27895936]

[76] Bellotti A, Labbé A, Fayol N, El Mahtoufi A, Baudouin C. Apport de l'OCT pour l'étude du glaucome néovasculaire. J Fr Ophtalmol 2007; 30(6): 586-91.
[http://dx.doi.org/10.1016/S0181-5512(07)89662-8] [PMID: 17646747]

[77] Vaz-Pereira S, Morais-Sarmento T, Marques RE. Optical coherence tomography features of neovascularization in proliferative diabetic retinopathy: A systematic review. Int J Retina Vitreous 2020; 6: 26.
[http://dx.doi.org/10.1186/s40942-020-00230-3]

[78] Baseline and early natural history report. the central vein occlusion study. Arch Ophthalmol 1993; 111(8): 1087-95. Available from: https://jamanetwork.com/journals/jamaophthalmology/

fullarticle/640325
[http://dx.doi.org/10.1001/archopht.1993.01090080083022] [PMID: 7688950]

[79] Finkelstein D. Ischemic macular edema. Recognition and favorable natural history in branch vein occlusion. Arch Ophthalmol 1992; 110(10): 1427-34. Available from: https://pubmed.ncbi.nlm.nih.gov/1417544/
[http://dx.doi.org/10.1001/archopht.1992.01080220089028] [PMID: 1417544]

[80] Fraenkl SA, Mozaffarieh M, Flammer J. Retinal vein occlusions: The potential impact of a dysregulation of the retinal veins. EPMA J 2010; 1(2): 253-61. Available from: https://pubmed.ncbi.nlm.nih.gov/21258633/
[http://dx.doi.org/10.1007/s13167-010-0025-2] [PMID: 21258633]

[81] Yamaguchi Y, Otani T, Kishi S. Serous macular detachment in branch retinal vein occlusion. Retina 2006; 26(9): 1029-33. Available from: https://pubmed.ncbi.nlm.nih.gov/17151490/
[http://dx.doi.org/10.1097/01.iae.0000254893.94013.16] [PMID: 17151490]

[82] Pichi F, Morara M, Veronese C, Lembo A, Nucci P, Ciardella AP. Perivenular whitening in central vein occlusion described by fundus autofluorescence and spectral domain optical coherence tomography. Retina 2012; 32(7): 1438-9. Available from: https://journals.lww.com/retinajournal/Fulltext/2012/07000/Perivenular_Whitening_in_Central_Vein_Occlusion.30.aspx
[http://dx.doi.org/10.1097/IAE.0b013e31825dd2a7] [PMID: 22722654]

[83] Ciftci S, Sakalar YB, Unlu K, Keklikci U, Caca I, Dogan E. Intravitreal bevacizumab combined with panretinal photocoagulation in the treatment of open angle neovascular glaucoma. Eur J Ophthalmol 2009; 19(6): 1028-33. Available from: https://journals.sagepub.com/doi/10.1177/112067210901900620
[http://dx.doi.org/10.1177/112067210901900620] [PMID: 19882572]

[84] Wakabayashi T, Oshima Y, Sakaguchi H, *et al.* Intravitreal bevacizumab to treat iris neovascularization and neovascular glaucoma secondary to ischemic retinal diseases in 41 consecutive cases. Ophthalmology 2008; 115(9): 1571-1580.e3, 1580.e1-1580.e3. Available from: http://www.aaojournal.org/article/S0161642008002030/fulltext
[http://dx.doi.org/10.1016/j.ophtha.2008.02.026] [PMID: 18440643]

[85] Ishibashi S, Tawara A, Sohma R, Kubota T, Toh N. Angiographic changes in iris and iridocorneal angle neovascularization after intravitreal bevacizumab injection. Arch Ophthalmol 2010; 128(12): 1539-45. Available from: https://jamanetwork.com/journals/jamaophthalmology/fullarticle/426569
[http://dx.doi.org/10.1001/archophthalmol.2010.282] [PMID: 21149776]

[86] Oshima Y, Sakaguchi H, Gomi F, Tano Y. Regression of iris neovascularization after intravitreal injection of bevacizumab in patients with proliferative diabetic retinopathy. Am J Ophthalmol 2006; 142(1): 155-157.e1. Available from: http://www.ajo.com/article/S0002939406002558/fulltext
[http://dx.doi.org/10.1016/j.ajo.2006.02.015] [PMID: 16815267]

[87] Kapur M, Nirula S, Naik MP. Future of anti-VEGF: Biosimilars and biobetters. Int J Retina Vitreous 2022; 8(1): 2. Available from: https://journalretinavitreous.biomedcentral.com/articles/10.1186/s40942-021-00343-3
[http://dx.doi.org/10.1186/s40942-021-00343-3] [PMID: 34983660]

[88] Shirley M. First Approval. Drugs 2022; 82(7): 825-30. Available from: https://link.springer.com/article/10.1007/s40265-022-01713-3

[89] Brown DM, Campochiaro PA, Singh RP, *et al.* Ranibizumab for macular edema following central retinal vein occlusion: six-month primary end point results of a phase III study. Ophthalmology 2010; 117(6): 1124-1133.e1. Available from: http://www.aaojournal.org/article/S0161642010001867/fulltext
[http://dx.doi.org/10.1016/j.ophtha.2010.02.022] [PMID: 20381871]

[90] Brown DM, Heier JS, Clark WL, *et al.* Intravitreal aflibercept injection for macular edema secondary to central retinal vein occlusion: 1-year results from the phase 3 COPERNICUS study. Am J

Ophthalmol 2013; 155(3): 429-437.e7. Available from: http://www.ajo.com/article/S0002939412006824/fulltext [http://dx.doi.org/10.1016/j.ajo.2012.09.026] [PMID: 23218699]

[91] Heier JS, Clark WL, Boyer DS, *et al.* Intravitreal aflibercept injection for macular edema due to central retinal vein occlusion: Two-year results from the COPERNICUS study. Ophthalmology 2014; 121(7): 1414-1420.e1. Available from: http://www.aaojournal.org/article/S0161642014000712/fulltext [http://dx.doi.org/10.1016/j.ophtha.2014.01.027] [PMID: 24679444]

[92] Korobelnik JF, Holz FG, Roider J, *et al.* Intravitreal aflibercept injection for macular edema resulting from central retinal vein occlusion. Ophthalmology 2014; 121(1): 202-8. Available from: https://pubmed.ncbi.nlm.nih.gov/24084497/ [http://dx.doi.org/10.1016/j.ophtha.2013.08.012] [PMID: 24084497]

[93] Scott IU, VanVeldhuisen PC, Ip MS, *et al.* Effect of bevacizumab *vs* aflibercept on visual acuity among patients with macular edema due to central retinal vein occlusion. JAMA 2017; 317(20): 2072-87. Available from: https://pubmed.ncbi.nlm.nih.gov/28492910/ [http://dx.doi.org/10.1001/jama.2017.4568] [PMID: 28492910]

[94] Ciardella AP, Morara M, Pichi F, Alkabes M, Romano S, Nucci P. Management of macular edema secondary to retinal vein occlusions. Exp Rev Ophthal 2014; 6(5): 557-64. Available from: https://www.tandfonline.com/doi/abs/10.1586/eop.11.59

[95] A randomized clinical trial of early panretinal photocoagulation for ischemic central vein occlusion. The Central Vein Occlusion Study Group N report. Ophthalmology 1995; 102(10): 1434-44. Available from: http://www.aaojournal.org/article/S0161642095308482/fulltext [http://dx.doi.org/10.1016/S0161-6420(95)30848-2] [PMID: 9097789]

[96] Group TBVOS. Argon laser photocoagulation for macular edema in branch vein occlusion. Am J Ophthalmol 1984; 98(3): 271-82. Available from: http://www.ajo.com/article/0002939484903167/fulltext [http://dx.doi.org/10.1016/0002-9394(84)90316-7] [PMID: 6383055]

[97] Ip MS, Oden NL, Scott IU, *et al.* SCORE Study report 3: Study design and baseline characteristics. Ophthalmology 2009; 116(9): 1770-1777.e1. Available from: http://www.aaojournal.org/article/S0161642009002863/fulltext [http://dx.doi.org/10.1016/j.ophtha.2009.03.022] [PMID: 19619896]

[98] Ip MS, Scott IU, VanVeldhuisen PC, *et al.* A randomized trial comparing the efficacy and safety of intravitreal triamcinolone with observation to treat vision loss associated with macular edema secondary to central retinal vein occlusion: the Standard Care *vs* Corticosteroid for Retinal Vein Occlusion (SCORE) study report 5. Arch Ophthalmol 2009; 127(9): 1101-14. Available from: https://pubmed.ncbi.nlm.nih.gov/19752419/ [http://dx.doi.org/10.1001/archophthalmol.2009.234] [PMID: 19752419]

[99] Scott IU, Ip MS, VanVeldhuisen PC, Oden NL, Blodi BA, Fisher M. A randomized trial comparing the efficacy and safety of intravitreal triamcinolone with standard care to treat vision loss associated with macular edema secondary to branch retinal vein occlusion: The standard care *vs* corticosteroid for retinal vein occlusion (SCORE) study report 6. Archophthal 2009; 127(9): 1115.

[100] Haller JA, Bandello F, Belfort R Jr, *et al.* Randomized, sham-controlled trial of dexamethasone intravitreal implant in patients with macular edema due to retinal vein occlusion. Ophthalmology 2010; 117(6): 1134-1146.e3. Available from: https://pubmed.ncbi.nlm.nih.gov/20417567/ [http://dx.doi.org/10.1016/j.ophtha.2010.03.032] [PMID: 20417567]

[101] Mastropasqua R, Toto L, Di Antonio L, Borrelli E, Senatore A, Di Nicola M. Optical coherence tomography angiography microvascular findings in macular edema due to central and branch retinal vein occlusions Scien Rep 2017; 7(1): 1-15. Available from: https://www.nature.com/articles/srep40763

CHAPTER 2

Optical Coherence Tomography Angiography Findings and Evaluation in Regional and Diffuse Retinal Infarction

Jose A. Roca-Fernandez, MD[1,2,*], Nathaly V. Huaman-Mendez, MD[2] and Caleb Llacctarimay, MD[3]

[1] *Cayetano Heredia University, Lima, Peru*

[2] *Retina Division, Ricardo Palma Clinic, Lima, Peru*

[3] *Hospital Nacional Sergio E. Bernales, Lima, Peru*

Abstract: Optical Coherence Tomography- Angiography (OCT-A) can separately detect the superficial vascular plexus and the deep vascular plexus. Paracentral acute middle maculopathy (PAMM) is an idiopathic or secondary entity to a local retinal vascular or systemic disease, characterized by capillary vascular occlusions. Some authors recognize it as a variant of acute macular neuroretinopathy (AMN). In general, the most frequent findings in the acute phase are a slight decrease in deep capillary plexus (DCP) perfusion, and hyperreflectivity of the middle layer; in the chronic phase, the findings are DCP hypoperfusion and hyporeflectivity of the middle layer.

Keywords: Retinal infarction, Paracentral acute middle maculopathy, PAMM, Vascular occlusion, Superficial capillary plexus, Deep capillary plexus, OCT-angiography.

INTRODUCTION

Classical histological publications highlight that there are two parallel vascular networks at the level of the internal retina, the superficial vascular plexus and the deep vascular plexus; the superficial vascular plexus consist of 75 microns vessels located between the nerve fiber layer (NFL) and the ganglion cell layer (GCL), it originates directly from arterioles and is the source of origin of the venula; the deep vascular plexus is represented by a dense and complex system of smaller

* **Corresponding author Jose A. Roca-Fernandez, MD:** Cayetano Heredia University, Lima, Peru; Retina Division, Ricardo Palma Clinic, Lima, Peru; Tel: +5112246593; Fax: +5112241603; ORCID ID: 0000 0002 9619 9178; E-mail: jaroca62@gmail.com

Miguel A. Quiroz-Reyes and Virgilio Lima-Gomez (Eds.)

vessels (20 microns) into the outer plexiform layer (OPL). Both networks are interconnected through small vessels of vertical course.

Optical Coherence Tomography- Angiography (OCT-A) can separately detect the superficial vascular plexus in the ganglion cell layer and the deep vascular plexus in the outer plexiform layer. These two networks have different aspects, which are not appreciated with standard angiography.

In healthy eyes, the superficial vascular plexus consists of larger vessels that end in the foveal avascular zone (FAZ). Deep vessels show an interconnected network of smaller dense vessels.

OCT-A allows identify four capillary networks/plexuses within the posterior pole. The superficial system is located predominantly within the GCL, known as the superficial capillary plexus (SCP), and to a lesser extent within the NFL, where it is most prominent around the optic nerve and is known as the radial peripapillary plexus. The deep system consists of an intermedia capillary plexus (ICP) within the inner portion of the inner nuclear layer (INL) bordering the inner plexiform layer (IPL) and a deep capillary plexus (DCP) within the outer portion of the inner nuclear layer (INL) bordering the outer plexiform layer (OPL).

Paracentral acute middle maculopathy (PAMM) is an idiopathic or secondary entity to a local retinal vascular or systemic disease, characterized by capillary vascular occlusions. There are reports associating it with different retinal vascular diseases, including diabetic retinopathy, retinal artery occlusion, central retinal vein occlusion, sickle cell retinopathy, Purtscher's retinopathy, hypertensive retinopathy, post upper respiratory tract infection, Covid-19 infection, among others, supporting ischemic pathogenesis.

Some authors recognize it as a variant of acute macular neuroretinopathy (AMN). Sarraf *et al.* have defined two forms of AMN, type 1 or PAMM, characterized by SD-OCT findings at the level of the inner nuclear layer (INL), and AMN type 2, which is associated with outermost layers of the retina abnormalities in the macular area. The mean age of patients with PAMM is 59 years and is described predominantly in men, while patients with traditional AMN lesions had a mean age of 33 years and tended to be women [1]. However, other authors consider that they are two distinct disorders with some overlapping characteristics.

In the fundus, compared to cotton-wool spots, the retinal whitening associated with PAMM lesions is markedly different, with a duller, less opaque grayish-white color, deeper in the retina, and without following the distribution of the nerve fiber layer.

OCT-A is recorded in conjunction with OCT-B scans, from the same location, allowing simultaneous visualization of structure and blood flow. Optical coherence tomography allows to evidence hyperreflective lesions in the form of an INL band, characteristic of PAMM in the acute phase, that eventually resolve in weeks, giving INL thinning, indicative of old PAMM lesions or old INL infarction. OCT-A during this chronic phase usually demonstrates loss of flow within the DCP, which can be self-limiting due to the mechanism of vascular reperfusion. [2].

With the advent of OCT-A, PAMM has emerged as a vascular pathology, however, it is important to complement the study of this "new" pathology with multimodal imaging and Spectral Domain OCT (SD-OCT).

While it is true that OCT-A studies have shown that both PAMM and AMN lesions are associated with capillary vascular occlusions, the affected primary capillary plexus remains controversial, and possibilities include superficial (SCP), intermediate (ICP), and deep capillary plexuses (DCP), as well as choriocapillaris.

Chu S and col. found that PAMM is associated with reduced blood flow at the level of SCP and DCP, ICP alone, or ICP and DCP. While AMN has been associated with occlusion of the deep capillary plexus (DCP) or the choriocapillaris [2].

PAMM lesions can be focal or diffuse; the focal lesions are related to perfusion preservation of the deep capillary plexus; the diffuse lesions, are seen in central retinal artery occlusion (CRAO), where there is a severe DCP lack of perfusion in the acute and chronic cases [3, 6]. The mechanism of ischemia and reperfusion explains the immediate microcirculation restoration observed in some of the focal lesions, however, in obstruction of large vessels, capillary reperfusion may not occur [4].

In general, the most frequent findings in the acute phase are a slight decrease in DCP perfusion, and focal or multifocal or diffuse hyperreflectivity of the middle layer; in the chronic phase, the findings are DCP hypoperfusion, and hyporeflectivity of the middle layer due to the development of atrophy.

In addition, Sridhar *et al.* proposed a classification for PAMM based on the patterns seen in en-face OCT and the presumed pathophysiological mechanism. The following three patterns were described: arteriolar, globular, and fern [5]. The arteriolar pattern showed band-like hyperreflectivity that corresponds to the distribution of a large retinal arteriole and is caused by a transient arteriole or true arteriolar occlusion. The globular pattern showed a focal ovoid patch or multifocal ovoid patches of hyperreflectivity of the middle retina caused by distal or capillary pericapillary ischemia; and finally, the fern pattern (Fig. **3**) was observed in the context of a central retinal vein occlusion with parafoveal multifocal hyperreflectivity of the middle retina due to perivenular ischemia, with periarterial preservation. A combination of patterns is possible [7].

CLINICAL ILLUSTRATIVE CASE

Female 39 years old. No pathological history. Episodes of amaurosis and photopsias in the right eye. Visual field with the presence of central scotoma (Figs. **1** - **4**).

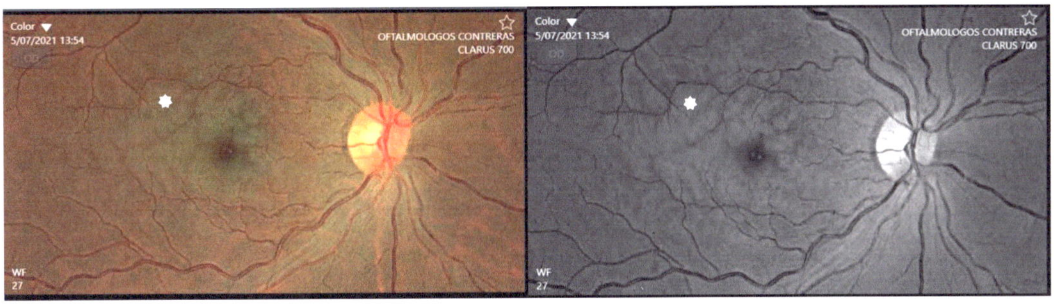

Fig. (1). Color and red-free retinography: Grayish-white lesions are observed deep in the retina and without following the distribution of the nerve fiber layer (asterisks). Oftalmologos Contreras – Lima, Peru.

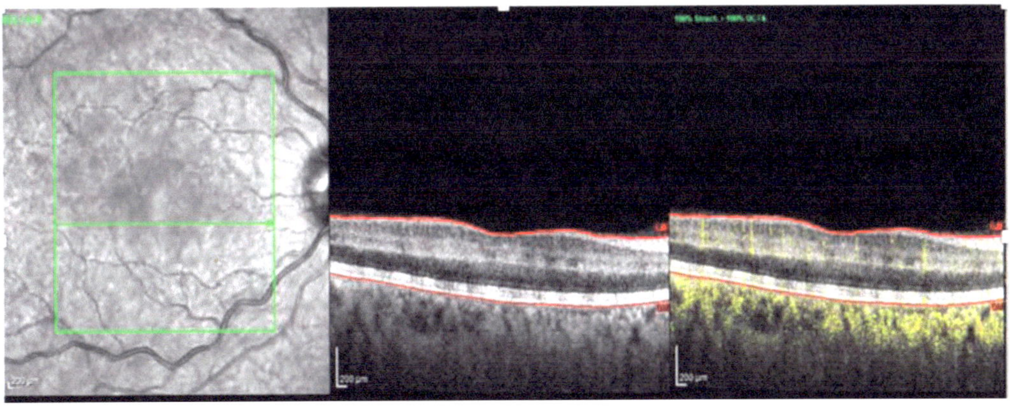

Fig. (2). Hyperreflectivity of the inner nuclear layer and external plexiform with flow projection; projection artifacts emitted from the superficial blood vessels to the deeper layers are evident.

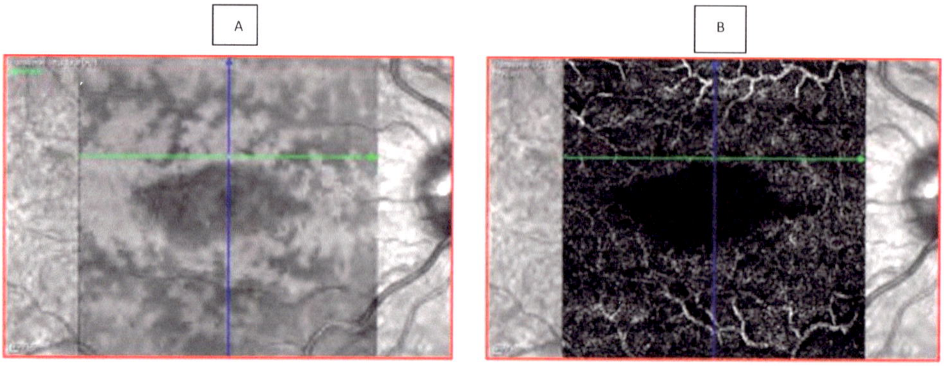

Fig. (3). En-face OCT perivenular hyperreflectivity at the level of the inner nuclear layer (**A**). OCT angiography demonstrated decreased capillary flow in the deep capillary plexus (**B**).

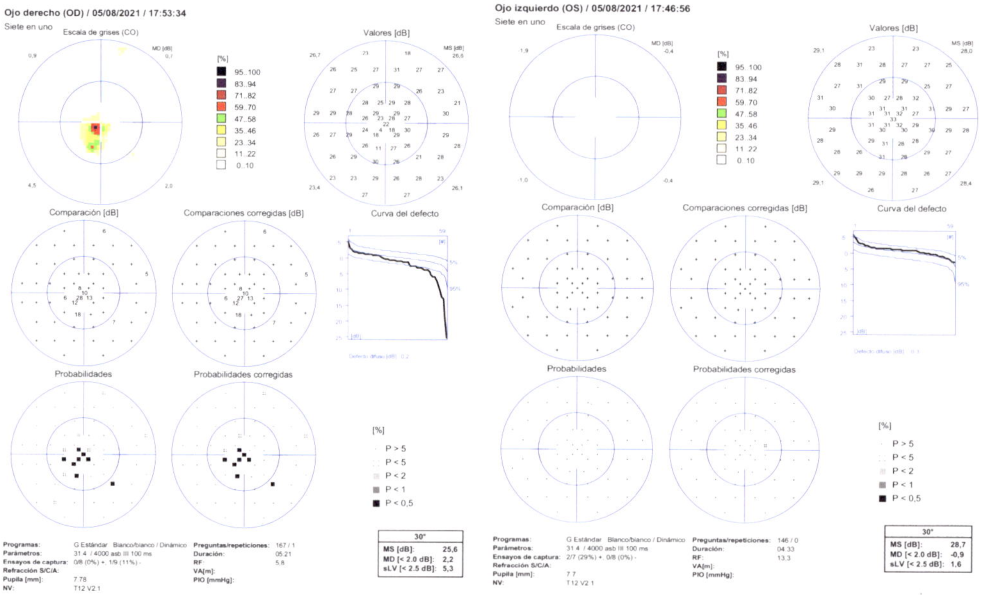

Fig. (4). Computerized visual field evidences the presence of central scotoma in the right eye. Left eye without alterations.

OCT-A allows us to explore vascular occlusions, however, the two main confounding factors in all the studies are the projection artifacts emitted from the superficial blood vessels to the deeper layers, and the attenuation of the OCT signal by artifacts below the hyperreflective lesions in the INL/ONL [2].

Chu *et al.* conducted a study in which, to better delineate the capillary plexuses, they used a version of resolved projection (RP)-OCT-A, which is an algorithm developed by Zhang *et al.*, which reduces projection artifacts while preserving the continuity of the intermedia and deep capillary plexuses. Their data show a wide range of anomalies in PAMM, they conclude that the location of the pathology begins in the ICP with secondary changes in the DCP [2].

Another factor to consider is segmentation, as it can affect the appearance of the SCP and DCP. In most normal eyes, standard segmentation provides accurate images. In cases of severe INL thinning, manual segmentation can help achieve a more accurate analysis of the DCP. The SCP can be placed between the inner limiting membrane and the inner plexiform layer. The DCP can be placed between the inner plexiform layer and the outer plexiform layer [3].

In addition, OCT-A allows to calculate the vessel density of the superficial and deep capillary plexuses. An objective vessel density can be calculated to quantify the degree of ischemia. While paracentral acute middle maculopathy lesions may maintain perfusion, old PAMM lesions lead to deep (and intermediate) capillary plexus loss.

CONCLUDING REMARKS

While acute focal lesions of PAMM can maintain perfusion, older PAMM lesions develop a corresponding loss of flow within the DCP (and intermediate capillary plexus).

Diffuse lesions of PAMM that occur in the context of CRAO lead to a severe lack of perfusion of DCP in acute and chronic cases.

Ischemia-reperfusion injury may be responsible for the pathogenesis of some focal PAMM lesions. Preservation of the deep vasculature has been associated with better visual outcomes.

It is important to develop techniques to overcome the limitations of OCT angiography, and, thus, facilitate the precise analysis of the flow in the macular capillaries.

No specific findings are found in the different vascular pathologies; it was seen in case studies that the same pathology could have different degrees of affection and limitation of the ischemic zone, depending on the degree of severity of the pathology.

REFERENCES

[1] Rishi P, Shah A, Chendilnathan C, Kumari S. OCT angiography features of paracentral acute middle maculopathy. Indian J Ophthalmol 2019; 67(3): 417-9. [http://dx.doi.org/10.4103/ijo.IJO_1249_18] [PMID: 30777975]

[2] Chu S, Nesper PL, Soetikno BT, Bakri SJ, Fawzi AA. Projection-resolved oct angiography of microvascular changes in paracentral acute middle maculopathy and acute macular neuroretinopathy. Invest Ophthalmol Vis Sci 2018; 59(7): 2913-22. [http://dx.doi.org/10.1167/iovs.18-24112] [PMID: 30025133]

[3] Nemiroff J, Phasukkijwatana N, Sarraf D. Optical coherence tomography angiography of deep capillary ischemia. Dev Ophthalmol 2016; 56: 139-45. [http://dx.doi.org/10.1159/000442806] [PMID: 27022753]

[4] Nemiroff J, Kuehlewein L, Rahimy E, *et al.* Assessing deep retinal capillary ischemia in paracentral acute middle maculopathy by optical coherence tomography angiography. Am J Ophthalmol 2016; 162: 121-132.e1. [http://dx.doi.org/10.1016/j.ajo.2015.10.026] [PMID: 26562176]

[5] Sridhar J, Shahlaee A, Rahimy E, *et al.* Optical coherence tomography angiography and en face optical coherence tomography features of paracentral acute middle maculopathy. Am J Ophthalmol 2015; 160(6): 1259-1268.e2. [http://dx.doi.org/10.1016/j.ajo.2015.09.016] [PMID: 26386158]

[6] Dansingani KK, Inoue M, Engelbert M, Freund KB. Optical coherence tomographic angiography shows reduced deep capillary flow in paracentral acute middle maculopathy. Eye 2015; 29(12): 1620-4. [http://dx.doi.org/10.1038/eye.2015.180] [PMID: 26381094]

[7] Ruiz Moreno JM, Ruiz Medrano J, Flores Moreno I. Optical coherence tomography angiography. MedSurg Ret Man 2017; 27-30.

CHAPTER 3

The Role of Macular Perfusion as a Contributing Factor in the Pathogenesis of Myopic Macular Traction Maculopathy

Miguel A. Quiroz-Reyes, MD[1,*], **Erick A. Quiroz-Gonzalez**[1,2], **Margarita Montano**[1], **Miguel A. Quiroz-Gonzalez**[1], **Sanjay Marasini**[3] and **Virgilio Lima-Gomez, MD**[4]

[1] *Oftalmologia Integral ABC, Retina Department, Medical and Surgical Assistance Institution (Nonprofit Organization), Affiliated with the Postgraduate Studies Division, National Autonomous University of Mexico, Mexico City, Mexico*

[2] *Institute of Ophthalmology, Fundacion Conde de Valenciana, Private Assistance Institution (Nonprofit Organization), Mexico City, Mexico*

[3] *Department of Ophthalmology, The University of Auckland, Auckland, New Zealand*

[4] *Ophthalmology Service, Hospital Juarez de Mexico, Public Assistance Institution (Nonprofit Organization), Mexico City, Mexico*

Abstract: Recently, qualitative and quantitative perfusional evaluations of vessel density (VD) and choriocapillaris flow patterns at the macular level have changed the evaluation spectrum and management of different macular pathologies. Published data on long-term macular perfusional findings and quantitative VD and flow evaluation (perfusion indices) in patients at different stages of successfully operated myopic traction maculopathy (MTM) compared with the corresponding values in normal control subjects are limited. This chapter describes the role of macular perfusion as a contributing factor to the pathogenesis of MTM.

The primary outcome measure included the long-term structural and perfusional macular status across groups. Forty-six eyes of 34 patients were included in the study group. The axial length was 29.89±1.67 mm. The postoperative follow-up period was 43±26.77 months. The preoperative BCVA was 1.29±0.54 logMAR, and the postoperative BCVA was 0.60±0.52 logMAR ($P<0.05$). The difference in perfusion indices across groups was statistically significant ($p<0.005$). Surgically resolved MTM eyes generally had a larger superficial foveal avascular zone area, lower vessel density, smaller choriocapillaris flow area (CFA), thinner central subfoveal thickness (CSFT),

* **Corresponding author Miguel A. Quiroz-Reyes, MD:** Oftalmologia Integral ABC, Retina Department, Medical and Surgical Assistance Institution (Nonprofit Organization), Affiliated with the Postgraduate Studies Division, National Autonomous University of Mexico, Mexico City, Mexico; Tel: +525 5217 2732; Fax: +525 55 1664 7180; E-mail: drquiroz@prodigy.net.mx and drquirozreyes7@gmail.com

and more macular defects. Better functional, structural, and perfusion index outcomes were observed in highly myopic eyes that underwent early surgery.

Keywords: Autologous retina grafting, Choriocapillaris flow area, Choriocapillaris subfoveal plexus, Deep vascular plexus, Foveal avascular zone, Foveoretinal detachment, High myopia, Myopic foveoschisis, Myopic macular degeneration, Myopic macular hole, Myopic macular hole-associated retinal detachment, Myopic traction maculopathy, Perfusion indices, Superficial vascular plexus, Vessel density.

INTRODUCTION

High myopia is a major cause of legal blindness in industrialized countries, and its prevalence has steadily increased over the last few decades. There is a myopia epidemic in East and Southeast Asia, with an estimated prevalence of 80–90% of the total population, of which approximately 10-20% of cases involve high myopia alone [1]. In the United States, it affects nearly 2% of the general population aged between 12 and 54 years [2]. Pathological myopia is the fifth leading cause of low vision or blindness in Japan, and the second leading cause among people older than 40 years of age in China [3].

Macular changes in patients with high myopia (spherical equivalent of -6.0 diopters or axial length greater than 26.5 mm) are characterized by retinal atrophy, ruptures in Bruch's membrane, and sclerotic thinning. Pathological myopia (PM) can be complicated by posterior staphyloma (PS) and macular atrophy [4]. In its early stages, myopic traction maculopathy (MTM), also called myopic foveoschisis (MF), is a schisis-like thickening of the retina. It has recently been described as tractional elongation of the Henle nerve fiber layer in eyes with high myopia and PS, rather than splitting of the retina [5, 6]. MF is more common in females [7, 8].

Scleral alterations have been proposed as the driving force of posterior segment pathologies. Scleral thinning and localized ectasia due to a reduction in the thickness of individual collagen fibers have been observed in myopic eyes [9, 10]. MF is a relatively new term that was first described by Panozzo and Mercanti [7] using optical coherence tomography (OCT) in terms of subtle macular changes, such as epiretinal membrane (ERM), vitreomacular traction (VMT), macular or foveal retinoschisis, retinal thickening, lamellar or partial-thickness macular hole, full-thickness myopic macular hole (MH) with or without retinal detachment, and PS. These scleral pathological alterations and subsequent increases in axial length may contribute to foveomacular retinoschisis, which exacerbates preexisting VMT. VMT is considered the cause of traction-related vitreoretinal interface abnormalities such as ERMs, posterior cortex hyaloid remnants, and retinal vessel rigidity [5]. In addition, enhanced-depth OCT imaging has revealed choroidal thinning in the macular region to be the consequence of age-related degenerative changes [11, 12].

The most recent MTM classification and its corresponding staging were proposed by Parolini *et al.* [13, 14]. This system describes the evolution of four retinal stages (1–4) and three foveal stages (a–c). Stages 1 and 2 represent the earliest stages of MTM, while stages 3 and 4 are associated with macular hole and retinal detachment, respectively. Progression in the stages was correlated with a decrease in the best-corrected visual acuity (BVCA) [14]. The pathological significance of MTM is important to determine when to surgically treat these patients but is most critical for deciding when to treat the fellow eye [15]. MF, as the earliest stage of MTM, is defined as tractional elongation of the Henle nerve fiber layer and is present in approximately 9-34% of patients with PM [7, 16, 17]. The natural evolution of highly myopic eyes with macular or foveal retinoschisis and foveoretinal detachment (FRD) involves the development of MHs [18 - 20].

In some patients, early stage MTM remains stable for several years. However, in others, it progresses to FRD and MH, with subsequent visual impairment [5]. Tractional forces, when combined with PS, are important causes of these consequences [21]. The specific cause of foveoschisis is not yet fully understood. However, a few proposed mechanisms for its pathogenesis include axial traction generated by progressive elongation of the eyeball and subsequent stretching forces developing in the posterior retina. The premacular vitreous cortex with tangential traction may be secondary to the rigidity of the internal limiting membrane (ILM) and retinal vessels. All these degenerative changes may occur within the context of PS [5, 22, 23].

Current options for the treatment of MTM at different stages include a three-port pars plana vitrectomy (PPV) technique with modified fovea-saved ILM or without ILM peeling, foveal-sparing ILM, inverted-flap ILM peeling, inverting multi-layer ILM flap techniques, free-autologous ILM transplantation, and autologous retina grafting techniques with silicone oil or gas tamponade. Macular buckling has also been attempted with favorable results [15, 24 - 27]. The identification of the early stages is a major factor in deciding the management strategy. Vitrectomy with the release of vitreoretinal traction yields good results and visual recovery. However, some patients require multiple interventions to achieve anatomical and functional success. Early stage symptomatic MTM, such as foveoschisis, may progress to myopic FRD, partial-thickness MH and/or full-thickness MH without retinal detachment, and macular hole retinal detachment (MHRD) within the natural course of the disease [5, 15].

The exact timing of macular surgery during different stages of MTM continues to be a controversial topic [11, 12], and there have been different surgical indications with variable anatomical and functional results [8, 25, 28, 29]. Recently, qualitative and quantitative perfusional evaluations of vessel density (VD) and choriocapillaris flow patterns at the macular level have changed the evaluation spectrum and management of different macular pathologies [30 - 33]. However, there are limited published data on long-term macular perfusional findings and quantitative VD and flow evaluation (perfusion indices) for patients at different stages of MTM who underwent successful macular surgery compared with normal control subjects. In this chapter, we selected surgical cases that met the criteria designed to minimize possible confounding variables. The aim of this chapter was to compare the quantitative data on macular microcirculation in the normal myopic group (Fig. **1a** to **b3**), control emmetropic group (Fig. **1c** to **d3**), and operated eyes in which the different stages of MTM resolved completely after macular surgery.

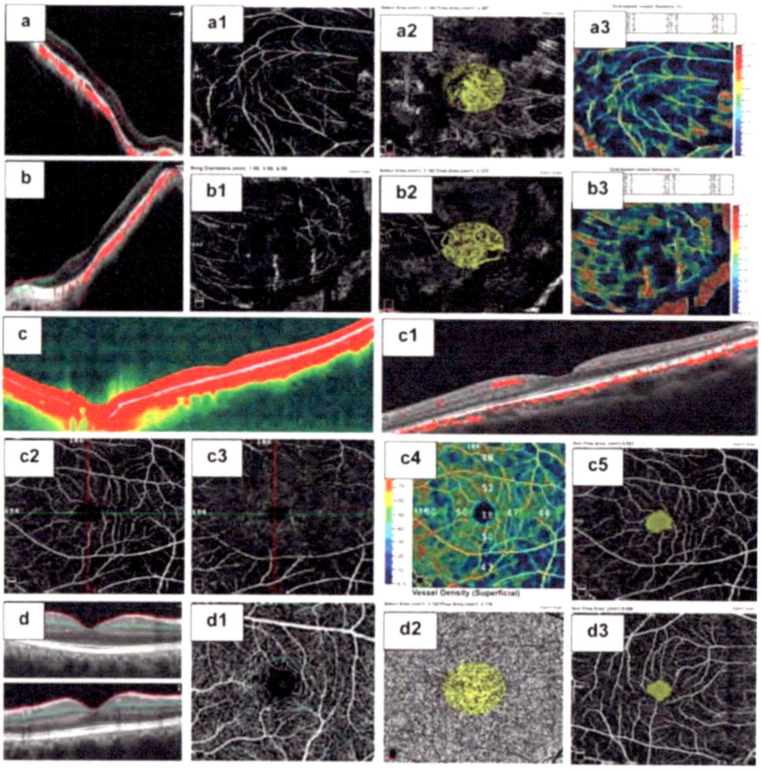

Fig. (1). ***Normal control groups.*** (**a**) Horizontal b scan of a highly myopic eye with automated red and green segmentation lines; the posterior hyaloid membrane is still attached. (a1) Image depicts a quantitative deep vascular plexus (DVP) slab with the ETDRS-like sectors grid overlay. (a2) Image depicts a normal quantified area of choroidal flow with an irregular but normal perfusion index at the selected subfoveal choriocapillaris. (a3) The color overlays on the OCTA angiography image indicate a normal vessel density value in the key to the right. (**b**) Horizontal segmented SD-OCT in highly myopic eyes with normal biomarkers. (b1) Image shows the slab of the superficial vascular plexus (SVP). (b2) Image depicting a normal area of choroidal flow at the subfoveal selected area. (b3) Image indicates a normal vessel density value in the key to the right. (**c**) Enhanced HD line 12 mm horizontal B scan designed to depict more detail in the vitreoretinal interface with brighter colors in a normal eye. (c1) Corresponding horizontal B scan with red dots indicating intraretinal and choriocapillaris vascular flow. (c2) and (c3) correspond to the normal SVP and DVP. (c4) The color overlays on the OCTA angiography image indicate a normal vessel density value in the key to the left. (c5) Image depicts a normal foveal avascular zone (FAZ) of 0.551 mm^2. (**d**) Image showing a crossline automated segmented green and red SD-OCT with normal biomarkers. (d1) Image depicts a normal SVP slab with a normal well-defined pericapillary network. (d2) Image shows a normal choriocapillaris flow area. (d3) Image shows a normal FAZ of 0.456 mm^2.

PREOPERATIVE EXAMINATION IN HIGHLY MYOPIC EYES

In the corresponding section of Chapter 7 (Part 1), we describe a detailed examination plan for symptomatic, highly myopic patients. In brief, preoperative assessments, including BCVA measurements, an Amsler grid test, slit-lamp fundoscopy using a panfundoscopic contact lens, and indirect ophthalmoscopy, should be conducted. Multiple cross-sectional structural evaluation images of the macular region should be acquired along the horizontal plane and along the crossline horizontal and vertical planes through the foveal center using spectral-domain (SD)-optical coherent tomography (OCT) and swept-source (SS)-OCT; the devices that we regularly use in our practice are the RTVue-XR platform SD-OCT (Optovue, Inc., Fremont, CA, USA) and a swept-source DRI OCT Triton device (Topcon Medical Systems, Inc., Oakland, CA, USA). Axial lengths should always be measured using partial coherence laser interferometry, preferably with the Zeiss IOL Master 700 (Carl Zeiss Meditec AG, Oberkochen, Germany). The presence of PS in highly myopic eyes should be confirmed using B-scan ultrasonography (US A and B, Quantel Medical, Du Bois Loli, Auvergne, France) and indirect ophthalmoscopy. Please refer to the corresponding section in chapter 9 (Part 1) for additional details on the preoperative microstructural evaluation and postoperative structural evaluation of highly myopic eyes.

Microstructural SD-OCT Findings and Corresponding Simplified MTM Classification

The most recent MTM classification [13, 14] has been complemented and simplified in the following descriptions of MTM staging for didactic purposes:

Stage 1 (Myopic Foveoschisis; MF)

This included eyes with macular thickening due to internal or external foveoschisis or hyporeflective splitting between the thin and faintly reflective outer and thicker, more reflective inner retina with column-like formations across the hyporeflective space, as described by Benhamou *et al.* [34], but without FRD as the main characteristic. These eyes can exhibit posterior hyaloid remnants or epiretinal macular membranes (Fig. **2a** to **e**).

Stage 2 (Foveal Retinal Detachment; FRD)

Eyes that exhibited evidence of foveal or extrafoveal macular detachment as a main structural tomographic characteristic with internal and/or external MF and posterior cortical vitreous remnants and/or the presence of epiretinal macular membranes (ERMs) (Fig. **2f** to **q**).

Stage 3 (Myopic Macular Hole; MH)

Eyes with tomographic evidence of a full-thickness macular hole as the main tomographic sign but without tomographic evidence of macular detachment (Fig. **2r** to **x**).

Stage 4 (Macular Hole Retinal Detachment; MHRD)

This stage includes eyes with posterior pole rhegmatogenous retinal detachment associated with an MH, such as MHRD; the extension of extramacular retinal detachment is defined by the number of retinal quadrants involved (Fig. **2y** and **z**).

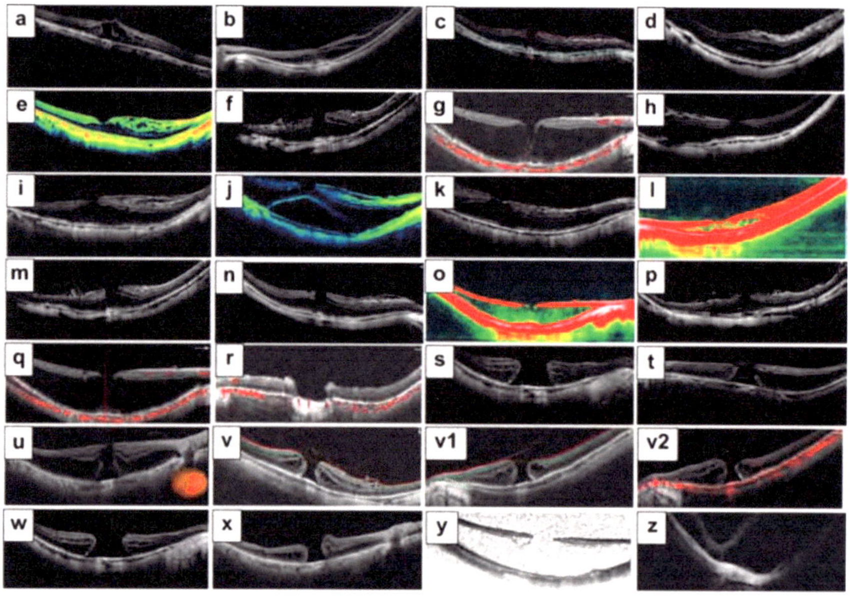

Fig. (2). Stages of MTM. (**a**) Image shows a high-definition (HD) 9 mm horizontal B scan of myopic foveoschisis (MF). (**b**) Image depicts MF with schisis-like retinal thickening of the macula. (**c**) Image shows complex MF. (**d**) Image shows MF with foveal thinning and an epiretinal membrane (ERM) on the nasal side. (**e**) Image depicts very elevated MF with tractional elongation of the Henle nerve fiber layer. (**f**) Image shows an HD 9 mm horizontal B scan in brighter color with MF. (**g**) Image depicts focal foveal retinal detachment (FRD) with associated traction and schisis-like foveal thickening. (**h**) Image shows FRD with macular detachment and inner layer schisis. (**i**) Image depicts macular FRD with an ERM and schisis-like thickening on the nasal side. (**j**) Image depicts color SD-OCT of a distinct FRD with thinning of the foveal inner layer. (**k**) Image depicts a superficial partial-thickness macular hole with schisis-like macular thickening. (**l**) Automated red and blue segmentation lines on a horizontal B scan of a partial-thickness MH. (**m**) Image shows a partial-thickness MH and posterior hyaloid remnants on the nasal side. (**n**) Image depicts a partial-thickness MH with ERM proliferation. (**o**) Image depicts a 9 mm horizontal scan in brighter color with dehiscence of the inner foveocentral layer and partial-thickness MH. (**p**) Complex image with a partial-thickness MH and ERM. (**q**) Highly elevated MF with a superficial MH. (**r**) Horizontal B scan with a full-thickness MH. (**s**) Image depicts a full MH with retinal thickness around the border. (**t**) Image shows an irregular full-thickness MH with a schisis-like thickening. (**u**) Enhanced HD line 12 mm image of a very elevated MF with a full-thickness MH, the corresponding color photo is shown at the right bottom. (**v**) to (**v3**) correspond to red and green segmentation line images of the full-thickness MH with traction and schisis-like thickening, red dots corresponding to the retina and choroidal vessels. (**w**) Full-thickness MH with an outer and inner layer schisis-like thickening. (**x**) Image depicts a full-thickness irregular MH. (**y**) Image depicts a retinal detachment associated with an MH. (**z**) Deep posterior staphyloma and retinal detachment associated with an MH.

Macular Surgery in Highly Myopic Eyes at Different MTM Stages

To review some of the detailed macular surgical techniques described in the early stages of MTM (MF/FRD), please refer to the corresponding section in chapter 7, Part 1 of this book. In the advanced stages of MH, modified ILM peeling techniques are recommended according to the surgeon's experience, including inverted-flap ILM peeling and free-autologous ILM transplantation techniques. In cases of MHRD, before staining the superficial macular structures or ILM, an air-gas exchange should be performed. Once the macula is attached under air, it is recommended that the macular hole be sealed with sodium hyaluronate for superficial macular revision and removal of macular posterior cortical remnants or the ILM to prevent the staining adjuvant from passing through the macular hole to preserve the retinal pigment epithelium (RPE). The technique recommended for patients with myopic MH and MHRD without a history of limitorrhexis consists of the construction of an ILM flap that is bent over the hole. The flap is then fixed with viscoelastic gas or silicon according to the surgeon's preferred technique. For patients with previous limitorrhexis, a modified free extramacular ILM flap self-transplantation fixed with viscoelastic and non-expandable bubbles consisting of a 20% sulfur hexafluoride mixture, a 15% non-expandable perfluoropropane gas mixture, or standard lighter-than-water 5,700 centistokes (cSt) silicone oil as a long-acting tamponade is recommended. Autologous neurosensory retinal grafting techniques for the MHRD surgical approach are not described in this chapter.

Methodology and Chapter Design

Preoperative Eye Characteristics

To analyze the long-term structural and perfusional outcomes of this type of vitreoretinal pathology in highly myopic patients, the authors applied their experiences from a selected group of operated eyes and further clarified these outcomes using examples of surgical cases. Additionally, the corresponding summary of the statistical evaluation is provided in this chapter as a supplemental material.

The surgery group included consecutively enrolled patients who underwent vitrectomy with successful and uncomplicated macular surgery using different ILM techniques for symptomatic MTM. The disease was staged according to the descriptions of previous stages.

The previously described surgical technique was performed by a single experienced surgeon. All the selected eyes had an axial length of >26.5 mm with no evidence of patchy foveal-affected chorioretinal atrophy, diffuse macular chorioretinal atrophy, or quiescent or active myopic choroidal neovascularization according to the amyloid. Tau, Neurodegeneration (ATN) Classification [35]. The diagnosis of different stages of MTM should be confirmed using spectral-domain OCT (SD-OCT) findings. Only eyes with posterior staphyloma determined by fundus examination and B-scan ultrasonography were analyzed. Eyes with patchy or diffuse chorioretinal atrophy affecting the center of the macula, active or involuted fibrous myopic choroidal pathological neovascularization, and Fuchs' spots affecting the fovea were not included. All eyes were followed up for more than six months and examined between four and 12 months until the last follow-up visit. Only patients who completed a postoperative follow-up period of at least six months and a long-term OCT-A postoperative perfusional evaluation at the last follow-up visit were included in the statistical analysis.

Functional findings in terms of BCVA are summarized in Fig. (3).

Perfusional Imaging Evaluation in MTM

The recommended postoperative perfusional imaging evaluation technique is as follows: Postoperative perfusional and quantitative VD and choroidal flow evaluations (perfusion indices) were performed using an OCT angiography device (RTVue XR OCT Avanti with AngioVue Software; OptoVue, Inc., Fremont, CA, USA). The AngioVue OCT angiography system is used for imaging, which uses a split-spectrum amplitude-decorrelation angiography software algorithm and acquires 70,000 A-scans/s to compose OCT angiography volumes consisting of 304 × 304 A-scans, achieving high axial resolution at depths of up to 5 μm and minimizing motion artifacts. Each OCT angiography cube scan consisted of 304 × 304 A-scans within a 3 mm × 3 mm square centered on the fovea, which yielded 304 B-scans. Each B-scan output displays an average of at least two scans. The AngioVue software includes a built-in projection artifact removal algorithm and has four default en face retinal imaging settings for automatic segmentation of the superficial vascular plexus (SVP), deep vascular plexus

(DVP), outer retinal layer, and choriocapillaris flow area (CFA). Auto-segmentation errors were corrected by automated adjustment of the contour and location of each segmentation line. The quality of the OCT angiography images was assessed using the signal strength index (SSI).

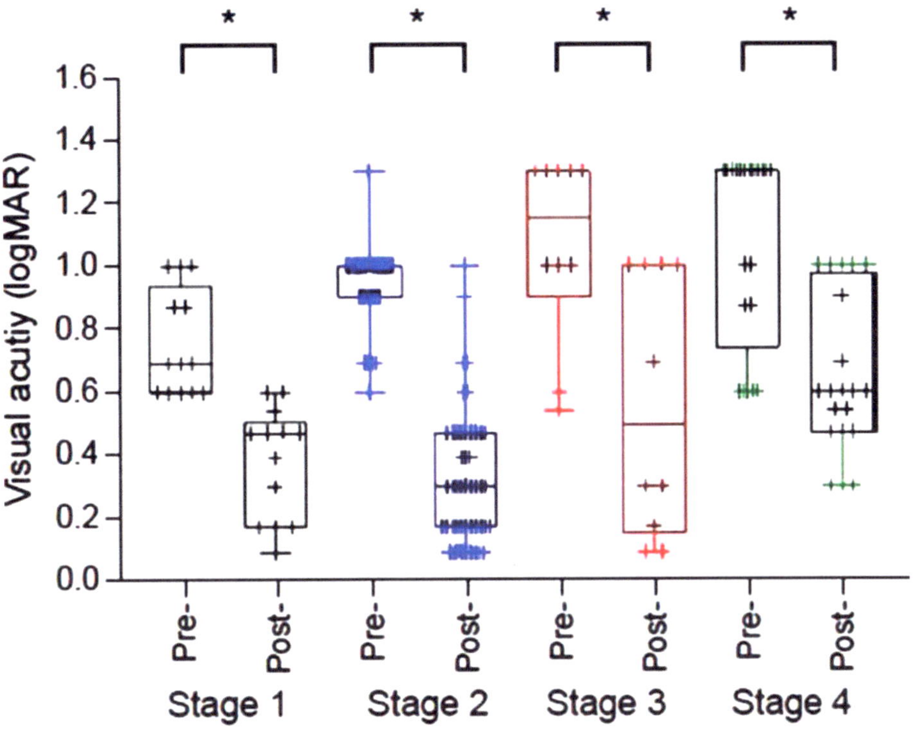

Fig. (3). Functional findings in terms of BCVA.

The foveal avascular zone (FAZ) area in the SVP slab was evaluated by analyzing en-face images saved as PNG files in the AngioVue system. Each FAZ area was automatically outlined following AngioAnalytics with angiometrics in the AngioVue software system to facilitate measurements. Only scans with more than 46 SSI were included. Projection artifacts were automatically excluded by digital outlining of the FAZ in the SVP. The superficial FAZ area was quantitatively calculated. A built-in tool in the AngioVue system measures the VD [36, 37], automatically generating a quantitative evaluation of the SVP and DVP. The built-in automated software processes the image-information, generating sets of VD and flow index (perfusion indices) for four en face sections of the retina. The defined perfusion indices were represented by VD as the proportion of the vessel area with blood flow over the total measured area, and whole-macula VD and CFA as density values within a 3 mm × 3 mm square and a 1-mm-diameter circle automatically selected in the foveal area, respectively.

Postoperative Structural and Perfusional Findings in MTM

A microstructural analysis of the SD-OCT findings was conducted based on the International Nomenclature for Optical Coherence Tomography (INOCT) Panel [38]. The results of the functional, structural, and perfusional outcomes across the treatment groups and different stages of the disease are summarized in Supplemental Table **4**. Briefly, perfusion analysis showed that the superficial FAZ area in the control emmetropic groups was significantly smaller than that in all other groups ($p < 0.0001$). The superficial foveal VD in the emmetropic group differed only from stage 3 to 4 of the disease ($p < 0.0001$). Deep foveal VD differed only between the emmetropic and stage 3 disease groups ($p = 0.0058$). Similarly, CFA was significantly larger in the emmetropic group ($p < 0.0001$). Decreased superficial foveal VD was correlated with poor visual outcomes in stage 4 disease ($p = 0.014$). Similarly, a smaller CFA was associated with poorer visual outcomes ($p = 0.048$) in stage 3 disease. Additionally, CSFT tended to correlate negatively with the final BCVA (Supplemental Table **4**).

Representative Surgical Cases

Surgical Case 1

A 47-year-old symptomatic man complained of progressive visual loss and distortion in his left eye that had persisted for 11 months. His BCVA at the first examination was 20/200 (logMAR 1.00) with a refractive defect of $-22+3.00 \times 20$ and applanation ocular tension of 14 mmHg. The axial length was 31.21 mm with PS, and the 12 mm high-definition (HD) SD-OCT findings (Fig. **4a**) complemented with segmented SD-OCT scans were consistent with a full-thickness MH with residual vitreous traction at the borders of the MH, schisis-like macular thickening around the hole, no evidence of macular detachment and thinning of the RPE, and peripapillary chorioretinal atrophy (Fig. **4b**) and thinning of the superficial layers of the retina (Fig. **4c**). The patient underwent an uneventful gas pars plana vitrectomy (PPV) with the ILM inverted technique with a closed MH, satisfactory postoperative evolution, and a well-recovered foveal profile with some postoperative thinning of the inner layers of the retina (Fig. **4d**). The comparative preoperative (Fig. **4e**) and postoperative perfusion indices in the SVP slabs were different with perfusion deterioration after surgery in the different macular subfields (Fig. **4f**). Better FAZ area characteristics were observed in the postoperative evaluation than those in the preoperative evaluation (Fig. **4g** and **4h**). The preoperative choroidal perfusion indices (Fig. **4i**) were lower than the long-term postoperative choroidal perfusion indices (Fig. **4j**).

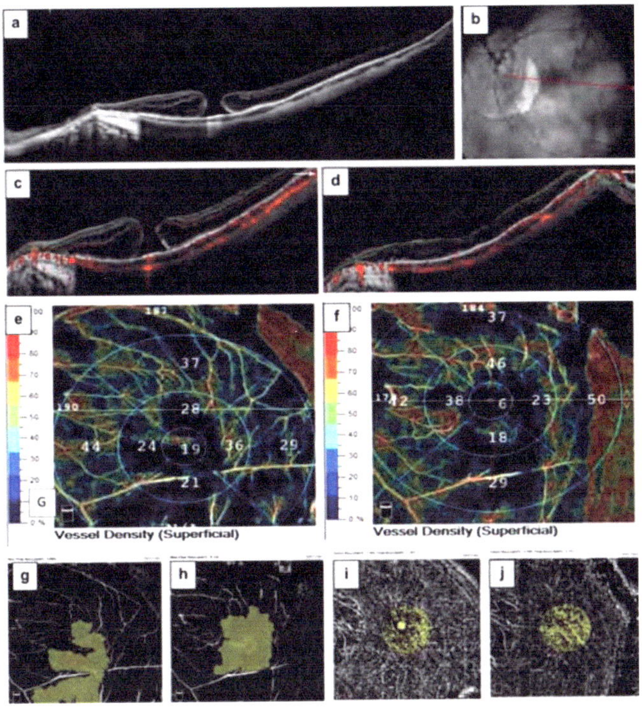

Fig. (4). ***Surgical case 1.*** (**a**) Image of a high-definition 12 mm horizontal B scan in a case of a full-thickness macular hole (MH). (**b**) En face image of the posterior pole of this case. Peripapillary chorioretinal atrophy is depicted along with diffuse retinal pigment epithelium. Red and green segmentation lines are depicted. (**c**) Horizontal cross-sectional b scan depicts a full-thickness MH and persistent vitreoretinal traction at the edges of the hole. (**d**) Long-term postoperative cross-sectional b scan of the corresponding macula with the MH closed; there is diffuse retinal thinning of the inner layers of the retina. (**e**) Preoperative perfusion evaluation at the SVP with the perfusion index values in the different subfields of the macula in the key to the left. (**f**) Comparative postoperative lower perfusion values at SVP. (**g**) Preoperative FAZ area. (**h**) Long-term postoperative FAZ area. (**i**) Preoperative choroidal perfusion indices. (**j**) Comparative long-term postoperative choroidal perfusion indices.

Surgical Case 2

A 39-year-old symptomatic woman complained of metamorphopsia and progressive visual loss in her right eye for seven months. Her preoperative right eye visual acuity was 20/160 (logMAR 0.90) with a refractive defect of -20+2.00 × 170 and applanation ocular tension of 11 mmHg. The right eye had an axial length of 28.71 mm with PS, and the preoperative HD SD-OCT findings were consistent with schisis-like macular thickening and the absence of central subretinal macular fluid (SRF) (Fig. **5a-c**). Macular surgery was performed using the modified foveal-sparing ILM peeling technique using BBG dye as an adjuvant to precisely identify the ILM and complete a modified foveal-sparing ILM technique, air-fluid exchange, and a nonexpandable 15% perfluoropropane gas mixture. After the 33-month follow-up, the foveomacular region remained attached (Fig. **5d** to **g**), with a final BCVA of 20/40 (logMAR 0.30), and extrafoveal nasal residual ERM remnants were observed (Fig. **5g**). Furthermore, some recognizable SD-OCT biomarkers, such as an irregular foveal contour and internal and external neuroretinal lines without total restoration of the central subfoveal ellipsoid, were observed, such as at the IS/OS line and the external limiting membrane (Fig. **5f** and **g**). The long-term postoperative perfusion evaluation was abnormal, with an enlarged and irregular FAZ (Fig. **5h**), which was lower than the normal perfusion indices on the SVP (Fig. **5i**) and DVP (Fig. **5j**). The choriocapillaris flow area was considered to be within the range (Fig. **5k**), with VD perfusion index values that were lower than normal (Fig. **5l**).

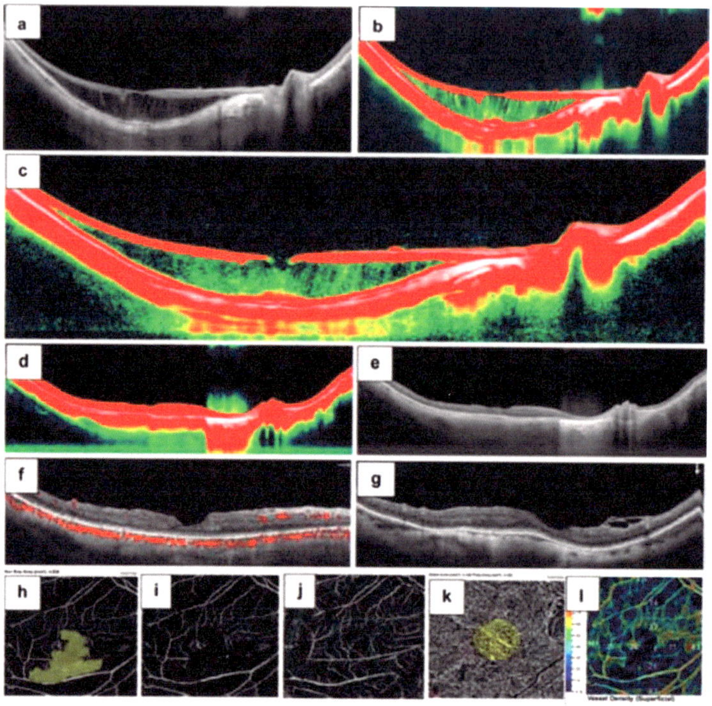

Fig. (5). ***Surgical case 2.*** A 39-year-old symptomatic woman complained of metamorphopsia and progressive visual loss in her right eye over seven months. Her preoperative right eye visual acuity was 20/160 (logMAR 0.90) with a refractive defect of -20.00+2.00 × 170 and an applanation ocular tension of 11 mmHg. The right eye had an axial length of 28.71 mm with PS. (**a**) Image shows a high-definition 12 mm horizontal B scan with schisis-like macular thickening and tractional elongation of the Henle nerve fiber layer. (**b**) Image corresponds to HD in brighter color. (**c**) Image of the corresponding eye two months later with dehiscence of the thin fovea. The patient underwent macular surgery with a modified foveal-sparing ILM-peeling technique using BBG dye as an adjuvant to precisely identify the ILM and complete a modified foveal-sparing ILM technique and a nonexpandable 15% perfluoropropane gas mixture. (**d**) and (**e**) Images depict that the foveomacular region remained attached after 33 months with a final BCVA of 20/40 (logMAR 0.30). (**f**) Image shows a horizontal B scan with an irregular foveal profile, well-defined ellipsoid zone and external limiting membrane line. (**g**) Image shows the corresponding vertical B scan with extrafoveal nasal and residual ERM remnants. The long-term postoperative perfusion evaluation was abnormal with an enlarged and irregular FAZ (image (**h**) and lower-than-normal perfusion indices on the SVP (image (**i**) and DVP (image (**j**). The choriocapillaris flow area was considered within range (Fig. **5** (**k**) with a VD perfusion index value lower than the mean (Fig. **5** (**l**). Modified figure adapted from [64] and is used under the Creative Commons Attribution 4.0 International License (https://creativecommons.org/licenses/by/4.0/).

Surgical Case 3

A 62-year-old symptomatic woman presented with aggravated metamorphopsia, progressive drop in central vision, and high myopia. She had PS in both eyes. The right eye, which had an axial length of 29.12 mm, underwent macular surgery because of a 9-month history of symptomatic myopic FRD (Fig. **6a**). The preoperative BCVA was 20/200 (logMAR 01.00); this eye underwent a three-port 25-G pars plana vitrectomy and nonfoveal ILM peeling with the foveal-sparing technique (Fig. **6b**), and fluid-air-gas exchange was performed with 15% C_3F_8 tamponade. After a 39-month longitudinal follow-up, the operated eye showed a postoperative BCVA of 20/25 (logMAR 0.10), abnormal postoperative perfusion indices (Fig. **6c** and **d**) with no evidence of recurrent FRD or progression to MH on SS and SD-OCT (Fig. **6e**), heterogeneous thin RPE on the superficial aspect of the en face of a heterogeneous thin RPE (Fig. **6f**), and the eye showed irregular and enlarged FAZ (Fig. **6g**), and normal choriocapillaris flow (Fig. **6h**). Some postoperative dissociated optic nerve fiber layer (DONFL) defects were detected without repercussions on the final vision in the HD (enhanced with a brighter color) 12 mm scan (Fig. **6i**). The perfusion indices at the SVP (Fig. **6j**) and DVP (Fig. **6k**) were below the mean.

Surgical Case 4

A 41-year-old man with five months of disabling metamorphopsia, high myopia, and moderate PS underwent 25-G three-port PPV and macular surgery on the phakic right eye due to a full-thickness MH (Fig. **7a**). This eye underwent vitreous and macular surgery consisting of a modified BBG dye-assisted ILM peeling technique (inverted flap) and 15% C_3F_8 long-acting nonexpandable gas tamponade. The preoperative BCVA was 20/400 (logMAR 1.30) and the axial length was 29.90 mm. After a 25-month follow-up, the final postoperative BCVA was 20/60 (logMAR 0.48) and showed a normal macular profile and SD-OCT biomarkers such as internal and external retinal OCT layers, subfoveal IS/OS, ELM line, and a well-preserved RPE layer (Fig. **7b** and **c**). The perfusion evaluation was abnormal in both plexuses (Fig. **7d** and **e**). The perfusion evaluation was abnormal in both plexuses (Fig. **7d** and **e**), with perfusion indices lower than normal (Fig. **7f**). The choriocapillaris flow was deficient (Fig. **7g**), with an abnormal and enlarged FAZ (Fig. **7h**). The VD perfusion index values at the SVP were lower than normal values (Fig. **7i**).

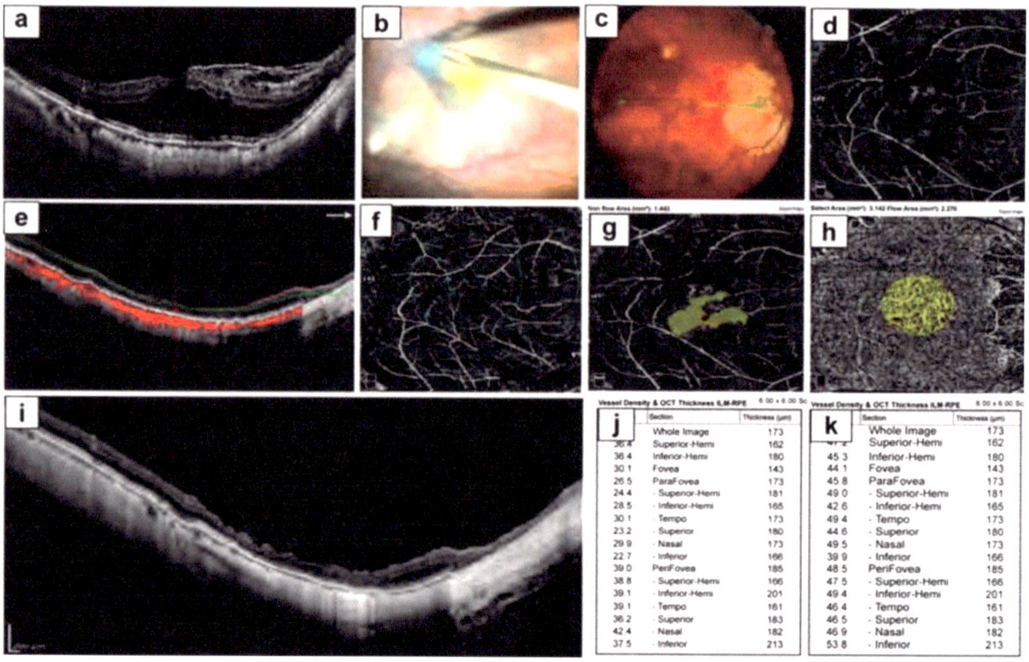

Fig. (6). ***Surgical case 3.*** A 62-year-old symptomatic woman presented with aggravating metamorphopsia, a progressive drop in central vision, and high myopia. She had PS in both eyes; the right eye with an axial length of 29.12 mm underwent surgery because of a 9-month history of symptomatic myopic FRD (Fig. **6** (**a**). The preoperative BCVA was 20/200 (logMAR 01.00); this eye underwent a three-port 25-G pars plana vitrectomy and nonfoveal ILM peeling with the foveal-sparing technique (Fig. **6b**), and fluid-air-gas exchange was performed with 15% C_3F_8 tamponade. (**c**) and (**d**) Images depict the superficial vascular plexus and deep vascular plexus with lower-than-mean perfusion indices. The operated eye showed a postoperative BCVA of 20/25 (logMAR 0.10). (**e**) Image depicts an automated red and blue segmentation line horizontal B scan with diffuse thinning of the superficial retinal layers and with no evidence of recurrent FRD or progression to MH. The red dots represent choroidal flow. (**f**) Image depicts the en face superficial aspect of the retina showing a heterogeneous thin RPE. (**g**) Image depicts an irregular and enlarged FAZ of 1.443 mm^2. (**h**) Image shows a normal choriocapillaris flow of 2.270 mm^2 (Fig. **6h**). (**i**) HD SS-OCT image enhanced with a brighter color 12 mm horizontal B scan depicting some postoperative DONFL defects, with no evidence of posterior hyaloid remnants detected. (**j**) and (**k**) Images depict perfusion index values of the SVP and DVP at the different submacular regions below the mean value. Modified figure adapted from [15] and is used under the Creative Commons Attribution 4.0 International License (https://creativecommons.org/licenses/by/4.0/).

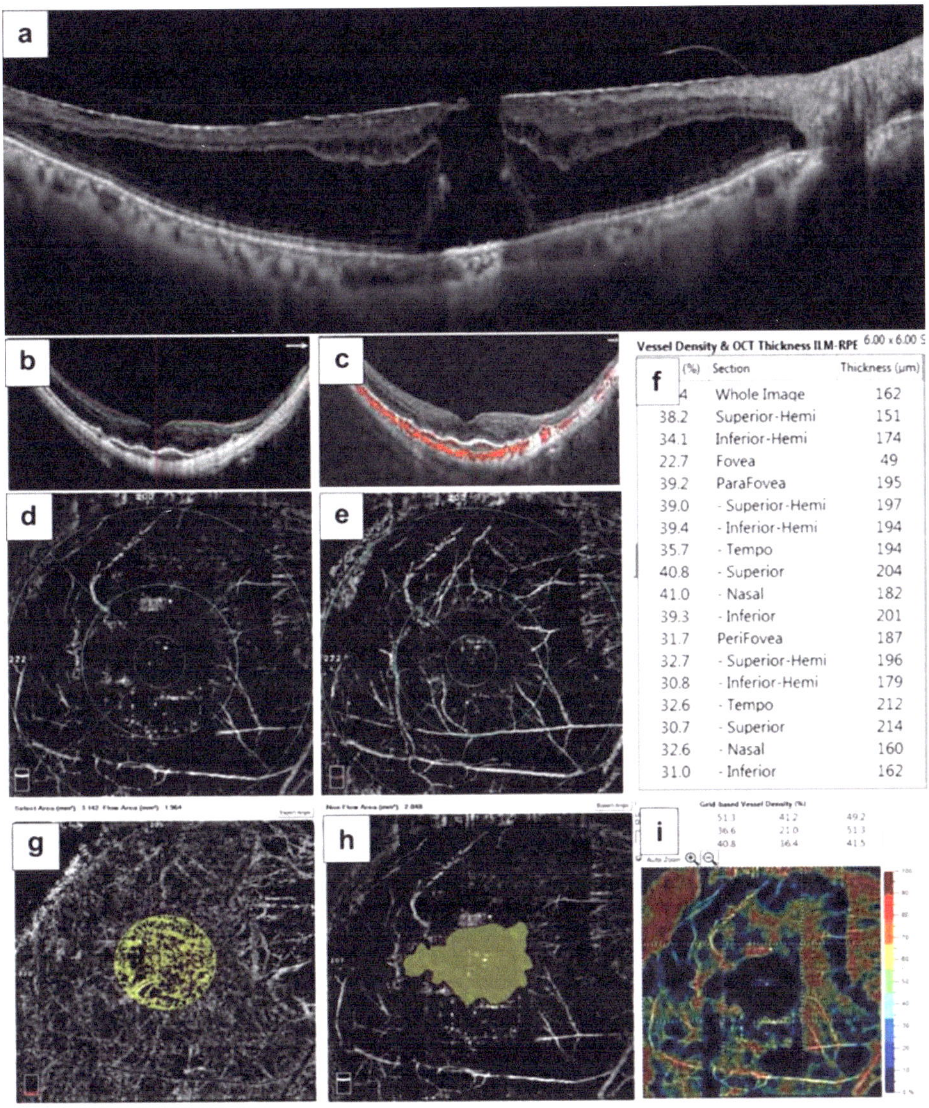

Fig. (7). ***Surgical case 4.*** A 41-year-old man with five months of disabling metamorphopsia, high myopia, and moderate PS. (**a**) Imaging depicts a high-definition enhanced grayscale 12 mm horizontal B scan of a preoperative SD-OCT of the affected eye having a severe full-thickness macular hole with persistent traction, epiretinal membrane proliferation and inner and outer retinal layer schisis-like thickening and severe tractional elongation of the Henle nerve fiber layer. This eye underwent vitreous and macular surgery consisting of a modified BBG dye-assisted ILM-peeling technique (inverted flap) and a 15% C_3F_8 long-acting nonexpandable gas tamponade. The preoperative BCVA was 20/400 (logMAR 1.30), and the axial length was 29.90 mm. After a 25-month follow-up, the final postoperative BCVA was 20/60 (logMAR 0.48). (**b**) and (**c**) Image shows long-term postoperative B scans with normal macular profiles and the presence of identifiable SD-OCT biomarkers, such as internal and external retina OCT layers, subfoveal IS/OS, ELM, and a well-preserved RPE layer. (**d**) and (**e**) Images depict comparisons between superficial and deep vascular plexuses. (**f**) Image shows the perfusion index deficiencies in both plexuses, which were considered lower than normal. (**g**) Image depicts the choriocapillaris flow of 1.964 mm^2, which was considered in the normal range. (**h**) Image depicts an irregular and enlarged foveal avascular zone of 2.848 mm^2, considered outside the mean; the pericapillary capillary net was not defined. (**i**) Image depicts the grid quadrants on angio-OCT with lower-than-normal vessel density perfusion index values expressed as percentages at the SVP that were considered lower than the mean. Modified figure adapted from [64] and is used under the Creative Commons Attribution 4.0 International License (https://creativecommons.org/licenses/by/4.0/).

Surgical Case 5

A 56-year-old woman with two months of slowly progressive decreased vision with metamorphopsia, high myopia, and severe PS underwent 25-G three-port pars plana vitrectomy and macular surgery on the phakic right eye for macular hole-related rhegmatogenous retinal detachment in three quadrants (Fig. **8a** and **b**). Preoperative SS-OCT confirmed MHRD (Fig. **8c** and **d**). This eye underwent vitreous and macular surgery consisting of the BBG dye-assisted ILM peeling technique (inverted-flap ILM-peeling technique) after reapplication of the detached retina and a 15% C_3F_8 long-acting non-expandable gas tamponade. The preoperative BCVA was 20/800 (logMAR 01.60), with a PS and an axial length of 31.40 mm. After a 14-month follow-up, the final postoperative BCVA was 20/100 (logMAR 0.70) and showed an SD-OCT pattern consistent with an abnormal macular profile and the presence of SD-OCT biomarkers, such as internal and external retina SD-OCT layers, subfoveal IS/OS (EZ), ELM line, and a well-preserved RPE layer (Fig. **8e** to **h**). The en face aspect depicted multiple deep defects at the level of the RPE (Fig. **8i**) with a very abnormal perfusion evaluation of the SVP (Fig. **8j**) and better perfusion evaluation on the DVP (Fig. **8k**). The choriocapillaris flow was very low (Fig. **8l**). The perfusion indices at the SVP (Fig. **8m**) were lower than the mean. The FAZ appeared irregular and larger (Fig. **8n**). The quantified perfusional indices in the DVP were lower than the mean (Fig. **8o**).

LITERATURE REVIEW AND DISCUSSION

Despite the reports of many retrospective observational studies and a handful of interventional studies on MTM, our understanding of this condition, its clinical course, and optimal management is still limited. Surgical treatments for MTM and its complications are limited by a lack of prospective trials and the small number of reported case series. We believe that vitreomacular traction is perhaps the primary mechanism for the development of MTM, but little has been reported in relation to potential perfusional mechanisms. Thus, vitrectomy and its variant techniques, with or without ILM removal and the use of different types of tamponade, are the most appropriate approaches [17]. Therefore, the present chapter aimed to report a long-term quantitative evaluation of perfusion indices (VD and flow index) at the macular level at different stages of successfully surgically operated MTM compared with normal controls. Our OCT angiography findings in perfusion indices (VD and flow index at different well-defined macular subregions) provided the mean and median with range perfusion data by macular subregion to build up the perfusion indices from surgically resolved eyes at different stages of MTM. In this study, we used different saved ILM and removal techniques without observing distinct and statistically significant differences in the quantitative evaluation of postoperative perfusion indices attributed to the technique. We detected decreased choroidal perfusion in myopic eyes in accordance with the report by Al-Sheikh *et al.* [39], and HD imaging OCT revealed choroidal thinning in the macular region as an age-related degenerative change described in high myopia and it has been documented that the decreased subfoveal choroidal thickness observed in the early stages of MTM may precede the development of retinoschisis [12, 26, 40].

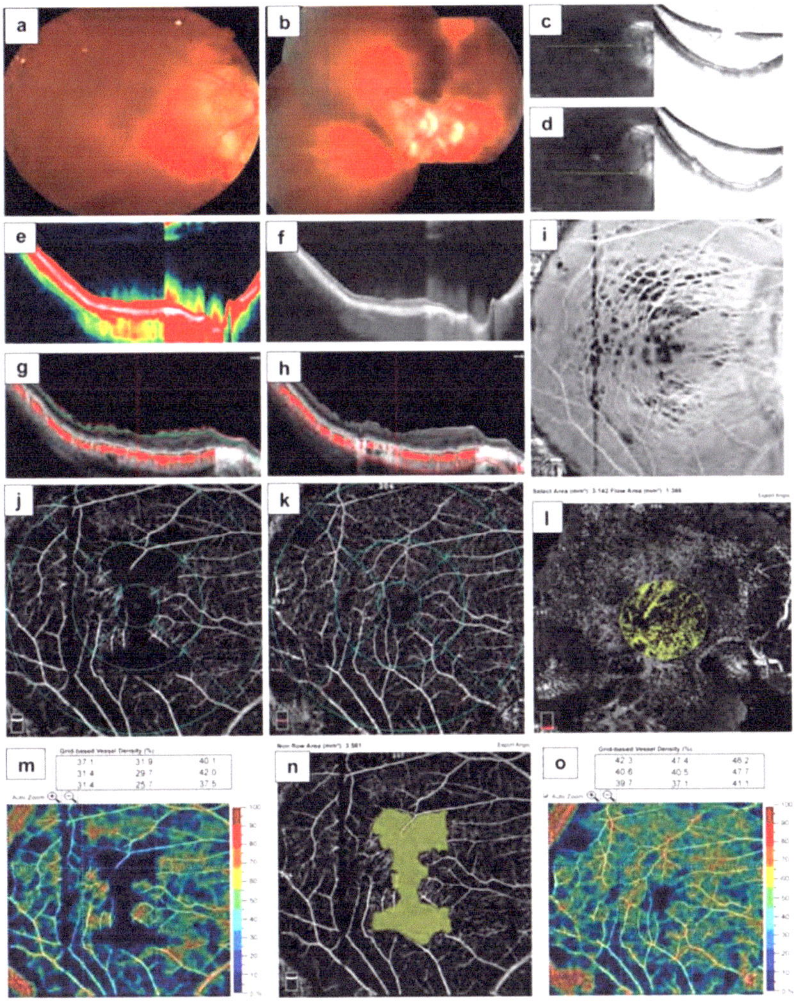

Fig. (8). ***Surgical case 5***. (**a**) and (**b**) Images depict color fundus photos of a 56-year-old woman with two months of slowly progressive decreased vision with metamorphopsia, high myopia, and an extensive rhegmatogenous retinal detachment in three quadrants associated with a macular hole. (**c**) and (**d**) Images of a Spectralis B scan examination consistent with retinal detachment and the confirmed presence of a full-thickness macular hole. This patient underwent 25-G three-port pars plana vitrectomy and macular surgery consisting of the BBG dye-assisted ILM-peeling technique (inverted-flap ILM-peeling technique) after reapplication of the detached retina and a 15% C_3F_8 long-acting nonexpandable gas tamponade. The preoperative BCVA was 20/800 (logMAR 01.60), with PS and an axial length of 31.40 mm. (**e**) and (**f**) Fourteen-month postoperative images depict high-definition 12 mm horizontal scans in brighter color and grayscale with the retina totally reattached and the macular hole closed, abnormal macular profile, presence of SD-OCT biomarkers such as inner and outer retina SD-OCT layers, disrupted subfoveal IS/OS (ellipsoid zone), irregular external limiting membrane line and a well-preserved RPE layer. (**g**) and (**h**) Images depict automated red and green segmentation lines with dissociated optic nerve fiber defects and irregular thinning of the inner layer of the retina. The red dots represent choroidal flow. (**i**) Image depicts the en face aspect of multiple deep defects at the level of the RPE and choroid. After a 14-month follow-up, the final postoperative BCVA was 20/100 (logMAR 0.70). (**j**) and (**k**) Images depict superficial and deep vascular plexuses considered lower than normal at the deferent macular subfield in the ETDRS grid over the OCT angio slabs. (**l**) Image depicts a deficient choriocapillaris flow index of 1.366 mm^2 considered under the mean value. (**m**) Image showing an irregular and enlarged superficial foveal avascular zone of 3.561 mm2. (**n**) and (**o**) Images show the vessel density expressed as the percentage at the 9 different macular quadrants denoted as lower than the mean perfusion indices. Modified figure adapted from [60] and is used under the Creative Commons Attribution 4.0 International License (https://creativecommons.org/licenses/by/4.0/).

Some studies have described the role of Müller cell integrity in traction maculopathies, since MTM is a pathology of Müller cell cones involving both inner traction from the ILM and outer stretch forces from the PS, as described by Wang *et al.* [20]. Structural changes in Müller cells are assumed to occur in eyes with retinoschisis [41]. As retinoschisis cavities enlarge, mechanical stretch forces may damage Müller cells and affect their function [42]. Therefore, we agree with the hypothesis that Müller cell dysfunction leads to visual impairment in eyes with retinoschisis-type MTM, as stated by Wang *et al.* [20].

Shimada *et al.* [19] performed a prospective and observational study of eight eyes with macular retinoschisis over an average follow-up period of 44 months and detected MH in two eyes. In one study, retinal detachment was associated with MH. While both eyes started with only foveomacular retinoschisis, both eyes developed partial detachment of the posterior hyaloid with persistent traction at the foveal level, whereas the rest of the patients in this study showed only progressive thickening of the macula, with data indicating foveomacular retinoschisis. Although the natural evolution of MH formation has recently been well described, its multiple pathogenic mechanisms have not been satisfactorily explained. In the report contained in this chapter, although this was not a target of our study, we were able to detect that the mean time to surgery on the fellow eye was 44.2±26.77 months, which coincides with the follow-up time at which surgery was required in the report by Benhamou *et al.* [34].

It is worthwhile to analyze the disease at its different stages. Although stages 1 and 2 have already been analyzed and discussed in Chapter 7, we will reiterate that most patients with stage 1 disease or MF presenting to a retina or macula specialist may be relatively asymptomatic, and the condition may persist at this stage for many years before significantly affecting vision [32, 43]. Therefore, we agree with Takano and Kishi [23], Shimada *et al.* [19], and Ichibe *et al.* [43], who proposed that MF is the earliest stage or direct precursor lesion of FRD or stage 2 disease. Uchida *et al.* [22] showed that at this stage, 80% of cases were resolved with only vitrectomy and gas tamponade, and in 20% of cases, it was necessary to add ILM-peeling techniques. We report a total resolution of foveoschisis in 87.1% of these eyes, although a modified ILM peeling technique was implemented in our cases with good anatomical and functional outcomes. 12.9% of these eyes showed progression to FRD or partial- or full-thickness MH during the follow-up. Hayashi *et al.* [44] observed a gradual progression of foveomacular retinoschisis to FRD in 41% of patients over a twelve-month follow-up period, which confirmed its importance as a significant clinical fact.

It has been reported that in patients diagnosed with MTM, 34.5% [16] to 41% of cases progress to FRD from an earlier stage [44], and the rate of progression to partial-thickness MH is 20.7% [16]. Focal irregularities and the thickness of the external retina have been described as initial findings, followed by the formation of an outer lamellar defect associated with small focal retinal detachment. As column-like structures exert traction, the lamellar defect is enlarged, elevating the upper edge of the retina and leading to FRD enlargement [44, 45]. Baba *et al.* [46] reported a 9% incidence of FRD in patients with posterior staphylomas.

Previous reports have shown that MF can be treated by only vitrectomy, posterior vitreous cortical remnant removal and gas tamponade with or without ILM-peeling [16, 24, 34, 47 - 50]. In a large case series [7], Panozzo and Mercanti concluded that the surgical resolution of vitreoretinal traction during the early stage of myopic FRD would allow reflattening of the macular center, thus preventing the development of full-thickness MH and emphasizing the high prevalence of ERM in highly myopic eyes with MF and FRD. However, this large case series lacked both perfusional and qualitative evaluations using fluorescein angiography and quantitative VD evaluation using AngioVue with OCT angiography, similar to the study by Wang *et al.* [20] and our study. Therefore, only mechanical tractional alteration was hypothesized without addressing the role of possible macular and choroidal perfusion abnormalities with lower-tha--normal quantified perfusion indices. Choroidal perfusion support, indicated by an increased VD in the choroid capillary layer, may help maintain a stable MF with a low rate of MTM progression and prevent FRD formation [50]. Al-Sheikh *et al.* [39] proposed that decreased choroidal perfusion and a lower VD pattern quality in myopic eyes with a reduced whole-macula VD, and consequently with lower macular perfusion, may result from mechanical stretch forces induced by eyeball elongation. As the foveal ILM is a part of the foveal Müller cell fibril, its surgical preservation may prevent further progression to more advanced stages of MTM [27, 51, 52].

Quantitatively, perfusion index evaluation to assess macular microcirculation is of paramount clinical importance, as even mild microcirculatory changes may lead to pathological changes with quality vision repercussions [53]. Small-vessel changes with lower VD value indices have been demonstrated in multiple retinal vascular diseases, including diabetic retinopathy, macular telangiectasia, and radiation retinopathy [54 - 56] and the MTM spectrum should be considered in this group.

In this chapter, owing to the reliability of the reproducibility of OCT angiography quantitative perfusion indices, we report a reliable statistical analysis evaluation. Our analysis showed that BCVA was positively correlated with the CFA, also known as the choriocapillaris subfoveal plexus (CSP), and tended to negatively correlate with CSFT (analysis performed with BCVA logMAR units showed a negative correlation with the CFA and a positive correlation with CSFT, although not statistically significant). The analysis of the results also revealed that structural defects in the EZ tended to correlate positively with the superficial FAZ area and ELM line defects. Similarly, structural defects in the ELM line tended to positively correlate with EZ defects and negatively correlate with the mean deep whole macular VD index. Thus, we report new information regarding the statistical analysis of normal-range vessel changes in normal emmetropic eyes, healthy highly myopic eyes, and different stages of surgically resolved cases of the MTM spectrum. However, this perfusional information and data need to be validated in further research. Our results indicated statistically non-significant changes in macular perfusion indices between the control groups and significant differences in the quantitative perfusion index evaluation between the different stages in the MTM study group. However, the data were highly significant when the microcirculation of the macula through the quantitative VD evaluation value was compared across groups; the difference between healthy eyes and eyes surgically resolved at different stages of MTM was highly significant ($p < 0.001$). These findings allowed us to speculate on the interrelation between tractional and perfusional mechanisms without concluding the physiopathogenic order.

Similar to You *et al.* [57], we found that the measurements of paracentral subfields were not affected by the FAZ area, and that the FAZ area had a lesser effect on the complete macular area evaluation. This result allowed us to conclude that the quantitative evaluation of macular VD in the paracentral macular area is as reliable as the measurement of the entire vascular macular area. Peng *et al.* [58, 59] also speculated that upregulated local cytokine production drove the resolution of myopic FRD after fovea-sparing ILM removal, thus implicating the vascular microenvironment together with alterations in microcirculation permeability in patients with MTM. Our study provides insights into the different stages of MTM, indicating that there are factors at the microcirculatory level involved in its tractional pathogenesis.

Several studies have correlated choroidal perfusion with VD. In this manner, choroidal perfusion (as reflected in the flow index) in eyes with advanced-stage MTM (such as MH and MHRD) should not be further temporarily diminished by transoperative perfusional alterations or permanently diminished by compression of the choroid secondary to macular buckling surgery, which may compress the choroid and further reduce choroidal perfusion [31]. FAZ distortion and enlargement of the juxtafoveal capillary net contribute to decreased VD perifoveal perfusion indices in MF. Subsequent impairment of visual acuity due to myopic FRD should be corrected by removing the mechanical stretching forces by peeling off the posterior hyaloid, ERM proliferation, and parafoveolar ILM. In our study and the study by Hwang *et al.* [31], there was a positive correlation between BCVA and mean macular perfusion indices in the SVP and the 1 mm selected foveal area of the choroid capillary layer across the different stages of MTM in the long-term postoperative perfusion evaluation compared with controls at the end of follow-up. However, no correlation was found in healthy highly myopic eyes in the control group in our study, suggesting that choroidal capillary vascular density flow abnormalities or deficiencies detected by quantifying the CFA and reflected in a low value of choroidal thickness itself may not directly affect vision, but this important hypothetical concept needs further perfusional research.

Our report shows that as the disease progresses, additional more complex techniques for macular surgery need to be employed, especially those related to manipulation or free flap transplantation of the ILM. The evaluation of perfusion as the disease progressed, as observed in our study, showed more altered and consequently lower perfusion indices. We speculate that this is due to progressive deterioration at the structural level, perhaps induced by factors at the level of microcirculation.

Several surgical techniques have been described for treating stage 2 (FRD) MTM. Most of these patients are symptomatic of metamorphopsia and show progressive vision loss. Reported techniques range from vitrectomy and tamponade (with long-acting gases and no ILM removal in primary cases) to vitrectomy and classical ILM removal. However, better modified techniques such as fovea-sparing ILM peeling with long-term gas are recommended in both refractory and primary cases, resulting in foveal reattachment and significant visual improvement [25, 28, 29, 32]. These observations suggest that modified ILM removal may be beneficial despite the risks inherent to ILM removal. Shimada *et al.* [27] tried to avoid some of these risks by using a modified technique called the fovea-sparing ILM removal technique; no eyes developed an MH after treatment with this technique, and 16.7% of eyes developed a full-thickness MH after treatment with the total classical technique or non-sparing ILM removal. Gaucher *et al.* [24] reported FRD in 10 (34.5%) of 29 eyes. Several authors have considered that the presence of MF/FRD may be a factor indicative of poor prognosis, leading to MH formation [16, 23, 25, 34]; we would consider the development of an FRD, a case of impending MH formation [60]. In our series, the eyes showed FRD, and the best postoperative final logMAR vision was found after treatment with modified fovea-sparing ILM peeling and long-acting gas, after treatment with observed MH formation in one case (3.8%) compared with the MF/FRD eyes that underwent the classical ILM peeling technique (9.7%).

The development of full-thickness MH may be spontaneous as part of the natural course of the disease or secondary to ILM removal by classical macular surgery, as mentioned by some authors [10, 23, 25, 34] and observed in our surgical experience. Gaucher *et al.* [24] stated that the pathogenesis of myopic MH might be different from that of idiopathic MH. Highly myopic eyes with total posterior vitreous detachment are not protected from the traction exerted by cortical remnants adhering to the macula; hypothetical ILM and retinal vessel rigidity also contribute [5]. In addition, enhanced-depth OCT imaging has revealed choroidal thinning in the macular region to be the consequence of age-related degenerative changes [11, 12]; we believe this also contributes to reduced macular perfusion. The formation of an MH is always preceded by FRD, where the foveola becomes extremely thin, and the tangential traction exerted by a tense ILM or persistent posterior vitreous remnants might explain the occurrence of an MH. In our series, for eyes with full-thickness MH, a better success rate of MH closure and better vision was achieved with the ILM-modified inverted-flap technique, regardless of the tamponade used. However, there was no significant difference between the surgical techniques or tamponade types used, and no statistically significant correlation was observed in the long-term perfusion rates of these patients. Thus, the carefully modified inverted-flap ILM manipulation technique is of paramount importance for MH closure.

Rhegmatogenous retinal detachment associated with MH formation is a therapeutic challenge. Several surgical approaches are routinely used, including vitrectomy, retinal membrane peeling, and ILM peeling, with classical or modified peeling techniques and various tamponades [51, 52]. Several surgical approaches have also been described, including gas tamponade, silicone oil tamponade, additional laser treatment of the hole margin, and episcleral buckling of the macula area [59, 61, 62]. Autologous neurosensory retinal grafting techniques for the MHRD surgical approach are not analyzed in this chapter.

The reported success rate of vitrectomy with long-acting gas for eyes with MHRD varies between 45 and 68%, but higher success rates of up to 79% and 89% have been described with silicone oil as tamponade [63 - 68]. As mentioned by other authors [66], chorioretinal tissue loss and RPE atrophy contribute to both a deficit in reapplication of the retina and poor visual recovery, as shown in this group of eyes, where obvious trophic alterations were observed in the neurosensory macula and RPE. Hence, this could be a possible explanation for the poor visual recovery in these eyes in the stage 4 (MHRD) group, in addition to considering the severe alterations in the perfusion indices found in these patients, which definitely contributes to poor visual recovery once the macula has been reattached. Kadonosono *et al.* [47] revealed that myofibroblasts on the ILM surface contract around these MHs, resulting in ILM or ILM remnants playing a role in hole reopening, delayed hole closure, or even subsequent retinal detachment. Thus, the type of tamponade plays a secondary role in the incidence of MH closure and in depurative macular surgery, with the ILM peeling technique as the main factor of hole closure. It has also been reported that removing the ILM and overlaying the ERM may increase the flexibility of the detached retina, inverting the ILM flap, or inverting multi-layer ILM flap techniques, thereby contributing to MH sealing, even in the presence of PS [69 - 71]. Several reports have emphasized the importance of appropriate ILM manipulation using intraoperative microscope-integrated SD-OCT to improve anatomical and functional outcomes. This new technology has not yet been integrated into our regular surgical practice but appears promising for achieving better macular surgery with better control of membrane and ILM stripping [72, 73].

Finally, new surgical approaches [74], a new method of automated choroidal segmentation to quantitatively measure choroidal thickness [75], and calculation of the choroidal vascular index (CVI) in binary images will be published soon.

We acknowledge the inherent limitations of the retrospective series analysis, including the relatively small number of eyes. The information analyzed in this chapter was primarily related to the strict exclusion criteria we applied to limit our study to successfully surgically corrected eyes at different stages of MTM in a long-term assessment. We note that OCT-A currently lacks sufficient resolution for accurate assessment of the CVI and retinal mid-periphery, where perfusional deficits are also expected. An abundance of artifacts must be manually or digitally compensated.

The study also lacked a serial or longitudinal data analysis. However, it has the benefits of long-term correlations revealed by SD-OCT, SS-OCT, and OCT angiography, and includes an evaluation of quantitative perfusional changes in macular perfusion indices. We anticipate that the scientific retina community will appreciate our findings due to the sparsity of published material on perfused macular assessment at different stages of operated highly myopic eyes with MTM.

Several strengths were noted, such as the long follow-up of the analyzed data, the presence of data also allowing the approximate time of disease occurrence in the fellow eye to be inferred, and the inclusion of a significant group of fellow eyes. Additionally, due to a long longitudinal follow-up, this condition could be detected at earlier stages. In a previous report [60], it was clinically observed that a group of fellow eyes showed significantly better final postoperative BCVA values, and most of these eyes underwent surgery at early stages, leading to better functional and structural results. No fellow eyes underwent surgical intervention at stage IV (MHRD); 85.7% of fellow eyes were treated at an early stage of MTM.

To evaluate choroidal perfusion, in recent years, the choroidal vascularity index (CVI) has emerged as a new tool to fill this need due to its ease of use and the noninvasiveness of its calculation [76 - 78]. The CVI was calculated from the OCT images *via* a series of digital binarization and quantification steps. In principle, it is the ratio of the number of dark and light pixels, corresponding to luminal (luminal choroidal area; LCA) and stromal (stromal choroidal area; SCA) areas, as a percentage, with the luminal area representing the vascular structures within the choroid [79, 80]. As CVI captures both the vascular and stromal changes within the choroid, it provides a more informative characterization of the state of the choroidal structure than choroidal thickness.

Since the initial introduction of CVI, a series of studies have linked changes in CVI with the pathogenesis and progression of a variety of retinal diseases [78, 81, 82]. CVI has been shown to capture some of the microcirculatory changes in the retina [83 - 85] and has demonstrated correlations with visual function [83]. As retinal diseases typically involve multiple processes that affect the choroid (*e.g.*, inflammation, edema, and leakage), CVI has been suggested as a potentially useful biomarker for assessing the integrity of the vascular network within the choroid [84]. Furthermore, earlier studies found that CVI is not sensitive to various confounding factors, such as axial length, blood pressure, or intraocular pressure [85].

The MTM is a vision-threatening condition. MTM may evolve to form more severe retinal complications [86]. Frequently, eyes with FRD and macular foveoschisis develop MH [7, 87]. Furthermore, highly myopic eyes have been shown to develop macular foveoschisis in nearly 34% of patients [5 - 12, 87]. In this context, monitoring disease and treatment outcomes through noninvasive methods such as CVI could substantially improve the management of MTM [88].

CONCLUDING REMARKS

In summary, according to the perfusional, structural, and functional outcomes analyzed in this chapter, there was significant visual improvement when eyes were surgically treated in the early stages of MTM, as opposed to poor postoperative visual improvement ($p<0.05$) when eyes underwent surgery for advanced stages of MTM. Likewise, perfusion indices were significantly lower when the eyes were operated on at advanced stages ($p<0.005$) or when they underwent more than one surgical procedure. By analyzing the prevalence and need for surgery in the second eye, we can conclude that these highly myopic patients are at a high risk of developing profound and irreversible loss of vision when they undergo surgery in the late stages of this myopic condition, especially if abnormalities in the perfusion indices are detected in the postoperative period, meaning that the prognosis for visual recovery will be poor. Thus, careful prospective and longitudinal evaluations of highly myopic eyes are advised to detect the early stages of this condition and make an early surgical choice considering different macular surgical techniques to optimize visual outcomes. Further prospective randomized clinical trials are needed to better establish the pathogenesis of MTM and to determine the most appropriate surgical procedures to address this severe condition.

Further investigations, including randomized multicenter quantitative evaluation of perfusion indices and histopathological studies, are necessary to confirm the role of *live* perfusional macular mechanisms in the pathogenesis of MTM. These studies would help elucidate the role of microvascular perfusion mechanisms in maintaining Müller cell integrity in traction maculopathies, as MTM is a pathology of Müller cell cones involving the inner traction from the ILM and the outer stretch forces from the slow development of the PS. Thus, the perfusional mechanisms must be investigated in detail in the future.

Myopic Traction Maculopathy

Supplemental Statistical File

The data for this chapter study were collected from the Retina Specialists Unit at Oftalmologia Integral ABC. The institutional review board of the facility approved the study and provided access to the patients' medical records for analysis. Written informed consent was obtained from all patients in accordance with the institutional guidelines. Data are available from the Imagenology Laboratory in the retina department at oftalmologiaintegralabc.com.

The study groups and inclusion criteria are listed in Table **1**. The surgery group included consecutively enrolled patients who underwent vitrectomy with successful and uncomplicated macular surgery using different ILM surgical techniques for symptomatic MTM. The disease was staged according to the description of the previous stages.

Table 1. Summary of study groups and inclusion criteria.

Study group	Inclusion criteria
Control emmetropia (n = 25)	No previous disease history, BCVA ≥ 20/20, intraocular pressure ≥ 10 to ≤ 21 mmHg, no abnormalities on dilated fundus examination and OCT scan
Control high myopia (n = 20)	Spherical equivalent refractive error of > -6.0 diopters or axial length > 26.5 mm
Surgical treatment group (n = 46)	**Stage 1** - Eyes exhibiting MF **Stage 2** - Eyes with evidence of FRD **Stage 3** - Eyes with evidence of a partial- or full-thickness MH **Stage 4** - Eyes with posterior pole MHRD

BCVA; best-corrected visual acuity, FRD; foveoretinal detachment, MF; myopic foveoschisis, MH; macular hole, MHRD; macular hole retinal detachment.

None of the selected eyes included in the study received intravitreal injections or laser photocoagulation during the study period. The study participants were matched for age, sex, study period, and follow-up durations. Patients were evaluated based on the standardized protocol of every month for six months and then every six months until the last follow-up visit. The surgical procedures were performed by a single highly experienced retina surgeon (MAQR). The same inclusion and exclusion criteria were used for the referrals.

In the surgical group, the previously described surgical technique was performed in the included patients. All the selected eyes had an axial length of >26.5 mm with no evidence of patchy foveal-affected chorioretinal atrophy, diffuse macular chorioretinal atrophy, or quiescent or active myopic choroidal neovascularization according to the amyloid. Tau, neurodegeneration (ATN) classification [35]. In the surgical groups, a diagnosis of different stages of MTM was confirmed using spectral-domain OCT (SD-OCT) findings. Only eyes with posterior staphyloma determined by fundus examination and by B-scan ultrasonography were included. Eyes with patchy or diffuse chorioretinal atrophy affecting the center of the macula and active or involuted fibrous myopic choroidal pathological neovascularization and Fuchs spots affecting the fovea were not included. All eyes were followed up for more than six months and examined between four and twelve months until the last follow-up visit. Only patients who completed a postoperative follow-up period of at least six months and a long-term OCT-A postoperative perfusional evaluation in the last follow-up visit were included in the statistical analysis.

Postoperative Perfusional Findings in MTM

Postoperative perfusional and quantitative VD and choroidal flow evaluations (perfusion indices) were performed using an OCT angiography device (RTVue XR OCT Avanti with AngioVue Software; OptoVue, Inc., Fremont, CA, USA). The AngioVue OCT angiography system was used for imaging, which uses a split-spectrum amplitude-decorrelation angiography software algorithm and acquires 70,000 A-scans/s to compose OCT angiography volumes consisting of 304 × 304 A-scans, achieving high axial resolution at depths of up to 5 μm and minimizing motion artifacts. Each OCT angiography cube scan consisted of 304 × 304 A-scans within a 3 mm × 3 mm square centered on the fovea, which yielded 304 B-scans. Each B-scan output displayed an average of at least two individual scans. The AngioVue software includes a built-in projection artifact removal algorithm and has four default en face retinal imaging settings for automatic segmentation of the superficial vascular plexus (SVP), deep vascular plexus (DVP), outer retina layer, and choriocapillaris flow area (CFA). The autosegmentation errors were corrected by automated adjustment of the contour and location of each segmentation line. An independent reader interpreted the imaging data from each patient. The quality of the OCT angiography images was assessed using the signal strength index (SSI).

The foveal avascular zone (FAZ) area in the SVP slab was evaluated by analyzing en face images saved as PNG files in the AngioVue system. Each FAZ area was automatically outlined following AngioAnalytics with angiometrics in the AngioVue software system to facilitate the measurements. Only scans with > 46 SSI were included. Projection artifacts were automatically excluded with digital outlining of the FAZ in the SVP. The superficial FAZ area was quantitatively calculated. A built-in tool in the AngioVue system measured the VD [36, 37], automatically generating a quantitative evaluation of SVP and DVP. The in-built automated software processes the image-information generating sets of VD and flow index (perfusion indices) for four en face sections of the retina. We defined perfusion indices represented by VD as the proportion of the vessel area with blood flow over the total measured area, and whole-macula VD and CFA as density values within a 3 mm × 3 mm square and a 1-mm-diameter circle automatically selected in the foveal area, respectively.

Outcome Measures

Macula quantitative perfusion indices (superficial and deep vessel density at different subdivided sections of the macula), anatomical outcomes and functional improvements were compared in terms of logarithm of the minimum angle of resolution (logMAR) units. Anatomical success was defined by a significant reduction or disappearance of MF, clinical and tomographic resolution of the FRD, closure of the myopic MH or reattachment of the macula and retina before the final visit regardless of the number of surgical procedures. The SD-OCT and OCT-A findings obtained preoperatively and at the last follow-up evaluation, respectively, were used to perform statistical analysis. At the least, a long-term high-quality OCT-A evaluation was performed, and the results were analyzed; data were collected by two other macula and retina specialists masked to other information, and a third observer evaluated the SD-OCT readings in case of disagreements.

STATISTICAL ANALYSIS

Data were collected in Microsoft Excel and transferred to GraphPad Prism version 8.2.1 and SPSS version 28. The data were assessed for normal distribution, and statistical tests were chosen based on the data normality: one-way analysis of variance (ANOVA) for parametric analysis and the Kruskal–Wallis test for nonparametric analysis. Dunnett's test was used for post hoc analysis. The Spearman correlation test was used to compare perfusion indices with the final visual outcome. The Wilcoxon matched signed-rank test was used to compare preoperative and postoperative BCVA (logMAR). For functional evaluations among stages, types of tamponade and surgical variants, only the final postoperative BCVA was included in the statistical analysis. P values of <0.05 were considered statistically significant.

General Outcome

In Stage 1 (MF) group, macular hole was evident in 1/5 eyes post-surgery (20%). The mean postoperative BCVA was significantly better when compared with the preoperative BCVA (Fig. **3**). In Stage 2 (FRD) group, the median preoperative and postoperative BCVAs in this group were 1.00 (0.60 to 1.30) logMAR and 0.30 (0.09 to 1.00) logMAR, respectively, which differed significantly ($P < 0.001$). In Stage 3 (MH) group, the median preoperative and postoperative BCVAs in this group were 1.15 (0.54 to 1.30) logMAR, and 0.49 (0.09 to 1.00) logMAR, respectively, which differed significantly ($P < 0.001$). In the Stage 4 (MHRD) group, the median preoperative and postoperative BCVAs in this group were 1.15 (0.54 to 1.30) logMAR, and 0.60 (0.30 to 1.00) logMAR, respectively, which differed significantly ($P < 0.001$).

The postoperative BCVA improved significantly in all stages of the disease ($p < 0.001$). The graphs show the median with range for each individual stage of the disease. The postoperative BCVA in the surgically treated groups remained poorer than that in the emmetropic control groups (p <0.0001). Stage two disease resulted in a better BCVA than the other three stages (p <0.0001).

The postoperative follow-up period was longest in stage 4 disease (40 months, 6–67; median, range). Across all surgical eyes, the mean (SD) preoperative evolution of MTM was 11.34 (7.12) months, the postoperative time for myopic FRD resolution was 5.48 (2.22) weeks, and the postoperative follow-up time was 23.96 (15.04) months (Table **2**).

Table 2. Patients' demographic dataand preoperative clinical characteristics.

Study groups	Female (%)	Median age (min to max, years)	Preoperative median BCVA (min to max, logMAR)	Axial length (mean ± SD, mm)	Postoperative follow-up months (median, range)
Control emmetropic group (n = 25)	76	52 (22 to 66)	0.00 (-0.12 to 0.09)	20.53 ± 0.09	-
Control myopic group (n = 20)	70	60 (48 to 70)	0.00 (0.00 to 0.09)	29.45 ± 1.49	-
Surgical Group (n = 46)					
Stage 1 (n = 5)	84.60	59 (44 to 70)	0.69 (0.60 to 1.00)	30.54 ± 1.51	13 (6-58)
Stage 2 (n = 26)	75.40	59 (43 to 76)	1.00 (0.60 To 1.30)	29.38 ± 1.64	27 (6–67)
Stage 3 (n = 4)	90.00	61 (46 to 70)	1.15 (0.54 to 1.30)	30.10 ± 1.33	15.50 (6–62)
Stage 4 (n = 11)	71.4	58 (43 to 82)	1.30 (0.60 to 1.30)	29.94 ± 1.71	40 (6-67)
p value	0.009	0.012	<0.0001	<0.0001	>0.05

BCVA; best-corrected visual acuity; SD, standard deviation.

Diffuse chorioretinal atrophy (DCRA) with secondary macular atrophy was the most common complication across all stages of the disease. Full-thickness MH development was the most common complication observed in the MF/FRD stages (12.9%) followed by rhegmatogenous retinal detachment (5%), three eyes (6.5%) showed refractory FRD after surgery, and six eyes (13.1%) showed an open but sealed MH at the end of follow-up (Table **3**).

Table 3. List of complications.

Stage	Normal	DCRA	Macular atrophy	ERM	FRD	Closed hole	Foveoschisis	Macular hole development	Open but sealed hole
Stage 1	2	-	-	-	-	-	-	1	1
Stage 2	23	2	1	-	-	-	1	3	-
Stage 3	1	1	1	-	-	3	-	-	1
Stage 4	-	2	2	2	1	7	2	-	4
Total (%)	26 (50)	4 (8.7)	4 (8.7)	2 (4.3)	1(2.8)	10 (21.7)	3 (6.5)	(12.9%) *	6 (13.1)

DCRA; diffuse chorioretinal atrophy, ERM; epiretinal membrane, FRD; foveal retinal detachment; * denotes consideration only from stage 1 and 2.

Perfusion Analysis Among Groups

A microstructural analysis of the SD-OCT findings was conducted based on the International Nomenclature for Optical Coherence Tomography (IN•OCT) Panel [38]. The results of the functional, structural and perfusional outcomes across treatment groups and different stages of the diseases are summarized in Table **4**. The quantitative evaluation of macular perfusion and central subfoveal thickness across study groups is depicted in Table **4**. The postoperative BCVA in the surgically treated groups remained poorer than that in the emmetropic control groups ($p < 0.0001$) (Table **4**). Stage 2 disease resulted in a better BCVA than the other three stages ($p < 0.0001$). Briefly, the perfusion analysis showed that the superficial FAZ area in the control emmetropic groups was significantly smaller than that in all other groups ($p < 0.0001$). The superficial foveal VD in the emmetropic group differed only from stage 3 to stage 4 of the disease ($p < 0.0001$). Deep foveal VD differed only between emmetropic and stage 3 disease ($p = 0.0058$). Similarly, the CFA was significantly larger in the emmetropic group ($p < 0.0001$).

Decreased superficial foveal VD correlated with poor visual outcome in stage 4 disease ($p = 0.014$). Similarly, a smaller CFA was associated with poorer visual outcome ($p = 0.048$) in stage 3 disease. Additionally, CSFT tended to correlate negatively with the final BCVA (Table **4**). The correlation of final visual outcomes with the perfusion indices are depicted in Table **5**. Preoperative and final BCVAs by stage, group and surgical procedures are compared in Table **6**, which shows that final visual acuities were significantly better across all the study variables.

Table 4. Quantitative evaluation of macular perfusion and central subfoveal thickness across study groups.

Study groups	Superficial FAZ area (mm^2, mean ± SD)	Superficial foveal VD (%, mean ± SD)	Deep foveal VD (%, mean ± SD)	Superficial parafoveal VD (%, mean ± SD)	Deep parafoveal VD (%, mean ± SD)	Superficial whole-macula VD (%, mean ± SD)	Deep whole-macula VD (%, mean ± SD)	CFA (mm^2, mean ± SD)	CSFT (μm, mean ± SD)	Postoperative median BCVA (Min to max, logMAR)
Control emmetropic group (n = 25)	0.33 ± 0.04	27.17 ± 3.40	31.39 ± 3.06	58.76 ± 3.03	59.17 ± 2.60	56.93 ± 4.27	58.50 ± 3.66	2.51 ± 0.24	246.40 ± 21.12	0.00 (-0.12 to 0.09)
Control high-myopia group (n = 20)	0.64 ± 0.12*	27.57 ± 3.91	32.11 ± 4.27	55.24 ± 2.56*	54.98 ±2.051*	46.35 ± 3.36*	48.55 ± 2.65*	2.25 ± 0.22	264.9 ± 37.91	0.00 (0.00 to 0.09)
Surgically Treated Group (n = 105)										
Stage 1 (n = 5)	0.74 ± 0.29*	28.53 ± 5.47	31.13 ± 4.56	49.66 ± 6.79*	51.53 ± 6.28*	48.81 ± 4.84*	50.13 ± 5.47*	1.90 ± 0.12*	228.60 ± 48.54	0.47 (0.09 to 0.60)*
Stage 2 (n = 26)	0.77 ± 0.25*	28.95 ± 5.72	31.45 ± 5.12	49.71 ± 4.58*	50.83 ± 4.72*	50.26 ± 3.97*	50.37 ± 4.02*	1.85 ± 0.28*	208.70 ± 29.97*	0.30 (0.09 to 1.00)*
Stage 3 (n = 4)	1.28 ± 0.35*	21.27 ± 4.35*	25.51 ± 4.17*	37.14 ± 4.61*	39.58 ± 4.30*	40.29 ± 4.21*	41.46 ± 3.92*	1.35 ± 0.18*	194.70 ± 10.86*	0.49 (0.09 to 1.00)*
Stage 4 (n = 11)	1.66 ± 0.40*	22.64 ± 4.13*	23.71 ± 3.50	27.91 ± 4.39*	29.81 ± 4.79*	31.41 ± 4.09*	33.69 ± 3.43*	1.35 ± 0.22*	214.80 ± 22.01*	0.60 (0.30 to 1.00)*
Comparison with the control emmetropic group (p values)	0.0001	0.0001	0.0058	0.0001	0.0001	0.0001	0.0001	0.0001	0.0001	0.0001

*Indicates the groups in which the data differed significantly ($p<0.05$) from those of the control emmetropic group. The BCVA in the control emmetropic and control high-myopia groups was compared with the postoperative BCVA in the surgical groups. Abbreviations – CSFT; central subfield foveal thickness, CFA; choriocapillaris flow area, FAZ; foveal avascular zone, VD; vessel density, SD; standard deviation.

Table 5. The correlation of final visual outcome with the perfusion indices (vessel density and flow index). Data indicate p values and Spearman correlation coefficients.

Study groups	Superficial FAZ area, p value (r coefficient)	Superficial foveal VD, p value (r coefficient)	Deep foveal VD, p value (r coefficient)	Superficial parafoveal VD, p value (r coefficient)	Deep parafoveal VD, p value (r coefficient)	Superficial whole-macula VD, p value (r coefficient)	Deep whole-macula VD, p value (r coefficient)	CFA, p value (r coefficient)	CSFT, p value (r coefficient)
Stage 1 (n = 5)	0.12 (-0.55)	0.55 (0.24)	0.96 (0.03)	0.89 (0.06)	0.75 (0.13)	0.96 (-0.03)	0.50 (-0.25)	0.47 (0.29)	0.68 (0.17)
Stage 2 (n = 26)	0.77 (0.03)	0.78 (-0.03)	0.76 (-0.04)	0.65 (0.06)	0.58 (0.07)	0.74 (-0.04)	0.96 (0.007)	0.91 (0.01)	0.29 (-0.14)

(Table 5) cont.....

Stage 3 (n = 4)	0.39 (-0.32)	0.59 (0.20)	0.73 (0.13)	0.76 (-0.11)	0.73 (-0.13)	0.73 (-0.13)	0.64 (-0.17)	**0.04* (0.69)**	0.71 (-0.14)
Stage 4 (n = 11)	0.50 (0.16)	**0.01* (0.56)**	0.07 (0.42)	0.75 (-0.07)	0.92 (0.02)	0.85 (-0.04)	0.63 (0.11)	0.85 (-0.04)	0.48 (-0.17)

*Indicates the groups in which a positive correlation to the final BCVA was observed ($p<0.05$). Abbreviations – CSFT; central subfoveal thickness, CFA; choriocapillaris flow area, FAZ; foveal avascular zone, VD; vessel density, SD; standard deviation.

Table 6. Comparison between the preoperative and the final BCVA by stage, group and surgical procedures (logMAR, median, interquartile range).

Variable	Preoperative	Final	P*
First eye	1.00 (0.95-1.45)	0.48 (0.30-0.70)	< 0.001
Fellow eye	1.00 (0.90-1.30)	0.18 (0.12-0.53)	< 0.001
Single eye	1.60 (1.00-2.30)	0.65 (0.30-1.00)	< 0.001
Tamponade	-	-	-
Gas	1.00 (0.90-1.30)	0.30 (0.16-0.54)	< 0.001
Silicon	1.60 (1.00-2.30)	0.70 (0.48-0.70)	< 0.001
Single surgery	-	-	-
Yes	1.00 (0.90-1.30)	0.30 (0.18-0.62)	< 0.001
No	1.60 (1.00-2.30)	0.70 (0.53-1.08)	< 0.001

BCVA; best corrected visual acuity.

Correlation Between BCVA, EZ Defects, ELM Line Defects, and Biomarkers

Statistical analysis may reveal biomarkers for functional BCVA, anatomical CSFT, and structural defects in the EZ and ELM layers. The analysis results showed that BCVA was positively correlated with CFA (analysis was performed with BCVA converted to the logMAR scale, which showed a negative correlation with the CFA) (Table 7). In the surgical group, the superficial FAZ area was found to positively correlate with postoperative changes in BCVA (Table **8**). Analysis also revealed that anatomical CSFT was positively correlated with superficial foveal VD (Table **9**). The presence of EZ defects was found to be positively correlated with superficial whole-macula VD and negatively correlated with deep whole-macula VD (Table **10**). Last, the presence of ELM line defects was found to be negatively correlated with deep parafoveal VD (Table **11**). It is worth noting that none of the p values were very small, with the smallest being $p = 0.006$ in the analysis of ELM defects.

Table 7. Correlation analysis with BCVA.

-	Coefficient estimate	Std. Error	P value[a]
Superficial FAZ area	0.029432	0.0823	0.721231
Superficial foveal VD	0.01164	0.007505	0.123457
Deep foveal VD	-0.0123	0.008353	0.143257
Superficial parafoveal VD	-0.01839	0.013467	0.174563
Deep parafoveal VD	0.003908	0.014757	0.791562
Superficial whole-macula VD	0.001586	0.01407	0.91045
Deep whole-macula VD	-0.00627	0.015801	0.692299
CFA	-0.14168	0.069464	0.043495

[a] adjusted p values < 0.05 are highlighted in gray. BCVA; best corrected visual acuity, CFA; choriocapillaris flow area, FAZ; foveal avascular zone, VD; vessel density

Table 8. Correlation analysis with change in BCVA.

-	Coefficient estimate	Std. Error	P value[a]
Superficial FAZ area	-0.23678	0.108903	0.032641
Superficial foveal VD	0.021504	0.014501	0.142019
Deep foveal VD	-0.00727	0.015772	0.646134
Superficial parafoveal VD	-0.00526	0.019355	0.786597
Deep parafoveal VD	0.045014	0.023161	0.055467
Superficial whole-macula VD	-0.03708	0.022449	0.102498
Deep whole-macula VD	-0.01217	0.022497	0.589995
CFA	0.029959	0.119834	0.803228

[a] adjusted p values < 0.05 are highlighted in gray. BCVA; best corrected visual acuity, CFA; choriocapillaris flow area, FAZ; foveal avascular zone, VD; vessel density

Table 9. Correlation analysis with CSFT.

-	Coefficient estimate	Std. Error	P value[a]
Superficial FAZ area	12.12241	9.745091	0.217106
Superficial foveal VD	3.1662	1.296561	0.016784
Deep foveal VD	-1.82231	1.409868	0.199845
Superficial parafoveal VD	-1.50448	1.732746	0.387816
Deep parafoveal VD	-1.44119	2.072449	0.488792
Superficial whole-macula VD	2.317136	2.001291	0.25034
Deep whole-macula VD	1.369357	2.000286	0.495563
CFA	5.582436	10.71017	0.60363

[a] adjusted p values < 0.05 are highlighted in gray. CSFT; central subfoveal thickness, CFA; choriocapillaris flow area, FAZ; foveal avascular zone, VD; vessel density

Table 10. Correlation analysis with ellipsoid zone defects.

-	Coefficient estimate	Std. Error	P value[a]
Superficial FAZ area	0.303649	0.156077	0.055183
Superficial foveal VD	0.03115	0.020766	0.137478
Deep foveal VD	-0.03391	0.02258	0.137023
Superficial parafoveal VD	0.015817	0.027752	0.57028
Deep parafoveal VD	-0.02563	0.033192	0.442278
Superficial whole-macula VD	0.082885	0.032053	0.011503
Deep whole-macula VD	-0.083	0.032037	0.011352
CFA	-0.15003	0.171534	0.384352

[a] adjusted p values < 0.05 are highlighted in gray. CFA; choriocapillaris flow area, FAZ; foveal avascular zone, VD; vessel density.

Table 11. Correlation analysis with external limiting membrane line defects.

-	Coefficient estimate	Std. Error	P value[a]
Superficial FAZ area	-0.12694	0.135478	0.351542
Superficial foveal VD	0.01827	0.018025	0.31379
Deep foveal VD	0.000158	0.0196	0.993581
Superficial parafoveal VD	0.041901	0.024089	0.085757
Deep parafoveal VD	-0.08165	0.028812	0.005803
Superficial whole-macula VD	-0.0044	0.027822	0.874688
Deep whole-macula VD	0.014054	0.027808	0.614671
CFA	-0.27117	0.148895	0.072267

[a] adjusted p values < 0.05 are highlighted in gray. CFA; choriocapillaris flow area, FAZ; foveal avascular zone, VD; vessel density

PATIENT CONSENT

Written informed consent in accordance with the institutional guidelines was obtained from all the patients.

LIST OF ABBREVIATIONS

BBG	Brilliant Blue G
BCVA	Best-corrected visual acuity
CFA	Choriocapillaris flow area
CSP	Choriocapillaris subfoveal plexus
CVI	Choroidal vascularity index

DCRA	Diffuse chorioretinal atrophy
DRT	Diffuse retinal thinning
DVP	Deep vascular plexus
ELM	External limiting membrane
ERM	Epiretinal membranes
EZ	Ellipsoid zone
FAZ	Foveal avascular zone
FRD	Foveoretinal detachment
ILM	Internal limiting membrane
IS/OS	Internal segment/outer segment
LCA	Luminal choroidal area
logMAR	Logarithm of minimum angle of resolution
MF	Myopic foveoschisis
MH	Macular hole
MHRD	Macular hole retinal detachment
MTM	Myopic traction maculopathy
OCT angiography	Optical coherence tomography angiography
PPV	Pars plana vitrectomy
PS	Posterior staphyloma
RPE	Retinal pigment epithelium
RRD	Rhegmatogenous retinal detachment
SCA	Stromal choroidal area
SD-OCT	Spectral-domain optical coherence tomography
SRF	Subretinal fluid
SVP	Superficial vascular plexus
VD	Vessel density
VMT	Vitreomacular traction

DISCLAIMER

All scientific comments issued in this chapter are solely the responsibility of the authors and not of the institutions with which they are affiliated.

ACKNOWLEDGMENTS

We express our deep appreciation to the technical staff of the Retina Specialists Unit at the Oftalmologia Integral ABC Medical Center (Nonprofit Medical and

Surgical Organization) affiliated with the Postgraduate Division Studies at the National Autonomous University of Mexico.

REFERENCES

[1] Morgan IG, French AN, Ashby RS, *et al.* The epidemics of myopia: Aetiology and prevention. Prog Retin Eye Res 2018; 62: 134-49. [http://dx.doi.org/10.1016/j.preteyeres.2017.09.004] [PMID: 28951126]

[2] Iwase A, Araie M, Tomidokoro A, Yamamoto T, Shimizu H, Kitazawa Y. Prevalence and causes of low vision and blindness in a Japanese adult population: The Tajimi Study. Ophthalmology 2006; 113(8): 1354-1362.e1. [http://dx.doi.org/10.1016/j.ophtha.2006.04.022] [PMID: 16877074]

[3] Xu L, Wang Y, Li Y, *et al.* Causes of blindness and visual impairment in urban and rural areas in Beijing: The Beijing Eye Study. Ophthalmology 2006; 113(7): 1134.e1-1134.e11. [http://dx.doi.org/10.1016/j.ophtha.2006.01.035] [PMID: 16647133]

[4] Vitale S, Sperduto RD, Ferris FL III. Increased prevalence of myopia in the United States between 1971-1972 and 1999-2004. Arch Ophthalmol 2009; 127(12): 1632-9. [http://dx.doi.org/10.1001/archophthalmol.2009.303] [PMID: 20008719]

[5] Ikuno Y, Tano Y. Early macular holes with retinoschisis in highly myopic eyes. Am J Ophthalmol 2003; 136(4): 741-4. [http://dx.doi.org/10.1016/S0002-9394(03)00319-2] [PMID: 14516820]

[6] Sayanagi K, Ikuno Y, Gomi F, Tano Y. Retinal vascular microfolds in highly myopic eyes. Am J Ophthalmol 2005; 139(4): 658-63. [http://dx.doi.org/10.1016/j.ajo.2004.11.025] [PMID: 15808161]

[7] Panozzo G, Mercanti A. Optical coherence tomography findings in myopic traction maculopathy. Arch Ophthalmol 2004; 122(10): 1455-60. [http://dx.doi.org/10.1001/archopht.122.10.1455] [PMID: 15477456]

[8] Panozzo G, Mercanti A. Vitrectomy for myopic traction maculopathy. Arch Ophthalmol 2007; 125(6): 767-72. [http://dx.doi.org/10.1001/archopht.125.6.767] [PMID: 17562987]

[9] Curtin BJ. The myopias. Basic Sci Clin Manag 1985; 6: 132.

[10] Summers Rada JA, Shelton S, Norton TT. The sclera and myopia. Exp Eye Res 2006; 82(2): 185-200. [http://dx.doi.org/10.1016/j.exer.2005.08.009] [PMID: 16202407]

[11] Imamura Y, Fujiwara T, Margolis R, Spaide RF. Enhanced depth imaging optical coherence tomography of the choroid in central serous chorioretinopathy. Retina 2009; 29(10): 1469-73. [http://dx.doi.org/10.1097/IAE.0b013e3181be0a83] [PMID: 19898183]

[12] Margolis R, Spaide RF. A pilot study of enhanced depth imaging optical coherence tomography of the choroid in normal eyes. Am J Ophthalmol 2009; 147(5): 811-5. [http://dx.doi.org/10.1016/j.ajo.2008.12.008] [PMID: 19232559]

[13] Parolini B, Palmieri M, Finzi A, Besozzi G, Frisina R. Myopic traction maculopathy: A new perspective on classification and management. Asia Pac J Ophthalmol 2021; 10(1): 49-59. [http://dx.doi.org/10.1097/APO.0000000000000347] [PMID: 33481391]

[14] Parolini B, Palmieri M, Finzi A, *et al.* The new myopic traction maculopathy staging system. Eur J Ophthalmol 2021; 31(3): 1299-312. [http://dx.doi.org/10.1177/1120672120930590] [PMID: 32506945]

[15] Quiroz-Reyes MA, Moreno-Andrade B, Quiroz-Gonzalez EA. Long-term postoperative structural and functional evaluation in myopic foveoretinal detachment. Int J Ophthalmol Clin Res 2021; 8: 132.

[16] Ikuno Y, Gomi F, Tano Y. Potent retinal arteriolar traction as a possible cause of myopic foveoschisis. Am J Ophthalmol 2005; 139(3): 462-7.
[http://dx.doi.org/10.1016/j.ajo.2004.09.078] [PMID: 15767054]

[17] Todorich B, Scott IU, Flynn HW Jr, Chang S. Macular retinoschisis associated with pathologic myopia. Retina 2013; 33(4): 678-83.
[http://dx.doi.org/10.1097/IAE.0b013e318285d0a3] [PMID: 23492947]

[18] Sun CB, Liu Z, Xue AQ, Yao K. Natural evolution from macular retinoschisis to full-thickness macular hole in highly myopic eyes. Eye (Lond) 2010; 24(12): 1787-91.
[http://dx.doi.org/10.1038/eye.2010.123] [PMID: 20829889]

[19] Shimada N, Tanaka Y, Tokoro T, Ohno-Matsui K. Natural course of myopic traction maculopathy and factors associated with progression or resolution. Am J Ophthalmol 2013; 156(5): 948-957.e1.
[http://dx.doi.org/10.1016/j.ajo.2013.06.031] [PMID: 23972301]

[20] Wang SW, Hsia Y, Huang CJ, Hung KC, Chen MS, Ho TC. Biomarkers in the pathogenesis of epiretinal membrane and myopic traction maculopathy: Effects of internal limiting membrane incompliance and posterior staphyloma. Photodiagn Photodyn Ther 2021; 33: 102208.
[http://dx.doi.org/10.1016/j.pdpdt.2021.102208] [PMID: 33561575]

[21] Oie Y, Ikuno Y, Fujikado T, Tano Y. Relation of posterior staphyloma in highly myopic eyes with macular hole and retinal detachment. Jpn J Ophthalmol 2005; 49(6): 530-2.
[http://dx.doi.org/10.1007/s10384-005-0249-1] [PMID: 16365803]

[22] Uchida A, Shinoda H, Koto T, *et al.* Vitrectomy for myopic foveoschisis with internal limiting membrane peeling and no gas tamponade. Retina 2014; 34(3): 455-60.
[http://dx.doi.org/10.1097/IAE.0b013e3182a0e477] [PMID: 23917541]

[23] Takano M, Kishi S. Foveal retinoschisis and retinal detachment in severely myopic eyes with posterior staphyloma. Am J Ophthalmol 1999; 128(4): 472-6.
[http://dx.doi.org/10.1016/S0002-9394(99)00186-5] [PMID: 10577588]

[24] Gaucher D, Haouchine B, Tadayoni R, *et al.* Long-term follow-up of high myopic foveoschisis: Natural course and surgical outcome. Am J Ophthalmol 2007; 143(3): 455-462.e1.
[http://dx.doi.org/10.1016/j.ajo.2006.10.053] [PMID: 17222382]

[25] Kobayashi H, Kishi S. Vitreous surgery for highly myopic eyes with foveal detachment and retinoschisis11The authors have no proprietary interest in any aspect of this study. Ophthalmology 2003; 110(9): 1702-7.
[http://dx.doi.org/10.1016/S0161-6420(03)00714-0] [PMID: 13129865]

[26] Alkabes M, Mateo C. Macular buckle technique in myopic traction maculopathy: A 16-year review of the literature and a comparison with vitreous surgery. Graefes Arch Clin Exp Ophthalmol 2018; 256(5): 863-77.
[http://dx.doi.org/10.1007/s00417-018-3947-3] [PMID: 29589106]

[27] Shimada N, Sugamoto Y, Ogawa M, Takase H, Ohno-Matsui K. Fovea-sparing internal limiting membrane peeling for myopic traction maculopathy. Am J Ophthalmol 2012; 154(4): 693-701.
[http://dx.doi.org/10.1016/j.ajo.2012.04.013] [PMID: 22835515]

[28] Kwok AKH, Lai TY, Yip WW. Vitrectomy and gas tamponade without internal limiting membrane peeling for myopic foveoschisis. Br J Ophthalmol 2005; 89(9): 1180-3.
[http://dx.doi.org/10.1136/bjo.2005.069427] [PMID: 16113377]

[29] Sayanagi K, Ikuno Y, Tano Y. Reoperation for persistent myopic foveoschisis after primary vitrectomy. Am J Ophthalmol 2006; 141(2): 414-7.
[http://dx.doi.org/10.1016/j.ajo.2005.09.009] [PMID: 16458717]

[30] Ho AC, Yannuzzi LA, Guyer DR, Slakter JS, Sorenson JA, Orlock DA. Intraretinal leakage of indocyanine green dye. Ophthalmology 1994; 101(3): 534-41.
[http://dx.doi.org/10.1016/S0161-6420(94)31323-6] [PMID: 7510380]

[31] Hwang TS, Zhang M, Bhavsar K, *et al.* Visualization of 3 distinct retinal plexuses by projection-resolved optical coherence tomography angiography in diabetic retinopathy. JAMA Ophthalmol 2016; 134(12): 1411-9.
[http://dx.doi.org/10.1001/jamaophthalmol.2016.4272] [PMID: 27812696]

[32] Angel Quiroz-Reyes M, Andres Quiroz-Gonzalez E, Esparza-Correa F, *et al.* Structural and perfusional study of successfully repaired diabetic tractional retinal detachment involving the macula. Int J Ophthal Vis Sci 2021; 6(4): 187-98.
[http://dx.doi.org/10.11648/j.ijovs.20210604.12]

[33] Quiroz-Reyes M, Quiroz-Gonzalez E, Esparza-Correa F, Kim-Lee J, Morales-Navarro J. Outcomes for successfully repaired macula-off diabetic tractional retinal detachment. Int J Ophthalmol Clin Res 2021; 8: 131.

[34] Benhamou N, Massin P, Haouchine B, Erginay A, Gaudric A. Macular retinoschisis in highly myopic eyes. Am J Ophthalmol 2002; 133(6): 794-800.
[http://dx.doi.org/10.1016/S0002-9394(02)01394-6] [PMID: 12036671]

[35] Ruiz-Medrano J, Flores-Moreno I, Ohno-Matsui K, Cheung CMG, Silva R, Ruiz-Moreno JM. Validation of the recently developed atn classification and grading system for myopic maculopathy. Retina 2020; 40(11): 2113-8.
[http://dx.doi.org/10.1097/IAE.0000000000002725] [PMID: 32073545]

[36] Klufas MA, Phasukkijwatana N, Iafe NA, *et al.* Optical coherence tomography angiography reveals choriocapillaris flow reduction in placoid chorioretinitis. Ophthalmol Retina 2017; 1(1): 77-91.
[http://dx.doi.org/10.1016/j.oret.2016.08.008] [PMID: 31047399]

[37] Kuehlewein L, Bansal M, Lenis TL, *et al.* Optical coherence tomography angiography of type 1 neovascularization in age-related macular degeneration. Am J Ophthalmol 2015; 160(4): 739-748.e2.
[http://dx.doi.org/10.1016/j.ajo.2015.06.030] [PMID: 26164826]

[38] Staurenghi G, Sadda S, Chakravarthy U, Spaide RF. Proposed lexicon for anatomic landmarks in normal posterior segment spectral-domain optical coherence tomography: the IN•OCT consensus. Ophthalmology 2014; 121(8): 1572-8.
[http://dx.doi.org/10.1016/j.ophtha.2014.02.023] [PMID: 24755005]

[39] Al-Sheikh M, Phasukkijwatana N, Dolz-Marco R, *et al.* Quantitative OCT angiography of the retinal microvasculature and the choriocapillaris in myopic eyes. Invest Ophthalmol Vis Sci 2017; 58(4): 2063-9.
[http://dx.doi.org/10.1167/iovs.16-21289] [PMID: 28388703]

[40] Sebag J. Anomalous posterior vitreous detachment: a unifying concept in vitreo-retinal disease. Graefes Arch Clin Exp Ophthalmol 2004; 242(8): 690-8.
[http://dx.doi.org/10.1007/s00417-004-0980-1] [PMID: 15309558]

[41] Tang J, Rivers MB, Moshfeghi AA, Flynn HW, Chan CC. Pathology of macular foveoschisis associated with degenerative myopia. J Ophthalmol 2010; 2010: 1-4.
[http://dx.doi.org/10.1155/2010/175613] [PMID: 20814547]

[42] Park S, Lee YJ. Nano-mechanical compliance of Müller cells investigated by atomic force microscopy. Int J Biol Sci 2013; 9(7): 702-6.
[http://dx.doi.org/10.7150/ijbs.6473] [PMID: 23904794]

[43] Ichibe M, Baba E, Funaki S, Yoshizawa T, Abe H. Retinoschisis in a highly myopic eye without vision impairment. Retina 2004; 24(2): 331-3.
[http://dx.doi.org/10.1097/00006982-200404000-00033] [PMID: 15097909]

[44] Hayashi K, Ohno-Matsui K, Shimada N, *et al.* Long-term pattern of progression of myopic maculopathy: A natural history study. Ophthalmology 2010; 117(8): 1595-611.
[http://dx.doi.org/10.1016/j.ophtha.2009.11.003] [PMID: 20207005]

[45] Shimada N, Ohno-Matsui K, Yoshida T, Sugamoto Y, Tokoro T, Mochizuki M. Progression from

macular retinoschisis to retinal detachment in highly myopic eyes is associated with outer lamellar hole formation. Br J Ophthalmol 2008; 92(6): 762-4. [http://dx.doi.org/10.1136/bjo.2007.131359] [PMID: 18523081]

[46] Baba T, Ohno-Matsui K, Futagami S, *et al.* Prevalence and characteristics of foveal retinal detachment without macular hole in high myopia. Am J Ophthalmol 2003; 135(3): 338-42. [http://dx.doi.org/10.1016/S0002-9394(02)01937-2] [PMID: 12614751]

[47] Kadonosono K, Yazama F, Itoh N, *et al.* Treatment of retinal detachment resulting from myopic macular hole with internal limiting membrane removal. Am J Ophthalmol 2001; 131(2): 203-7. [http://dx.doi.org/10.1016/S0002-9394(00)00728-5] [PMID: 11228296]

[48] Spaide RF, Fisher Y. Removal of adherent cortical vitreous plaques without removing the internal limiting membrane in the repair of macular detachments in highly myopic eyes. Retina 2005; 25(3): 290-5. [http://dx.doi.org/10.1097/00006982-200504000-00007] [PMID: 15805905]

[49] Hirakata A, Hida T. Vitrectomy for myopic posterior retinoschisis or foveal detachment. Jpn J Ophthalmol 2006; 50(1): 53-61. [http://dx.doi.org/10.1007/s10384-005-0270-4] [PMID: 16453188]

[50] Kumagai K, Furukawa M, Ogino N, Larson E. Factors correlated with postoperative visual acuity after vitrectomy and internal limiting membrane peeling for myopic foveoschisis. Retina 2010; 30(6): 874-80. [http://dx.doi.org/10.1097/IAE.0b013e3181c703fc] [PMID: 20094010]

[51] Shiraki N, Wakabayashi T, Ikuno Y, *et al.* Fovea-sparing versus standard internal limiting membrane peeling for myopic traction maculopathy: A study of 102 consecutive cases. Ophthalmol Retina 2020; 4(12): 1170-80. [http://dx.doi.org/10.1016/j.oret.2020.05.016] [PMID: 32470651]

[52] Ho TC, Yang CM, Huang JS, *et al.* Long-term outcome of foveolar internal limiting membrane nonpeeling for myopic traction maculopathy. Retina 2014; 34(9): 1833-40. [http://dx.doi.org/10.1097/IAE.0000000000000149] [PMID: 24787384]

[53] Yu DY, Cringle SJ. Oxygen distribution and consumption within the retina in vascularised and avascular retinas and in animal models of retinal disease. Prog Retin Eye Res 2001; 20(2): 175-208. [http://dx.doi.org/10.1016/S1350-9462(00)00027-6] [PMID: 11173251]

[54] Sakata K, Funatsu H, Harino S, Noma H, Hori S. Relationship between macular microcirculation and progression of diabetic macular edema. Ophthalmology 2006; 113(8): 1385-91. [http://dx.doi.org/10.1016/j.ophtha.2006.04.023] [PMID: 16877077]

[55] Chin EK, Kim DY, Hunter AA III, *et al.* Staging of macular telangiectasia: Power-Doppler optical coherence tomography and macular pigment optical density. Invest Ophthalmol Vis Sci 2013; 54(7): 4459-70. [http://dx.doi.org/10.1167/iovs.12-11116] [PMID: 23716628]

[56] Veverka KK, AbouChehade JE, Iezzi R Jr, Pulido JS. Noninvasive grading of radiation retinopathy: The use of optical coherence tomography angiography. Retina 2015; 35(11): 2400-10. [http://dx.doi.org/10.1097/IAE.0000000000000844] [PMID: 26502009]

[57] You Q, Freeman WR, Weinreb RN, *et al.* Reproducibility of vessel density measurement with optical coherence tomography angiography in eyes with and without retinopathy. Retina 2017; 37(8): 1475-82. [http://dx.doi.org/10.1097/IAE.0000000000001407] [PMID: 27930458]

[58] Peng M, Wei Y, Zhang Z, *et al.* Increased levels of DKK1 in vitreous fluid of patients with pathological myopia and the correlation between DKK1 levels and axial length. Curr Eye Res 2020; 45(1): 104-10. [http://dx.doi.org/10.1080/02713683.2019.1646772] [PMID: 31335221]

[59] Mitamura Y, Takeuchi S, Tsuruoka M. Macular buckling combined with pars plana vitrectomy for complicated retinal detachment due to macular hole. Retina 2000; 20(6): 669-72. [http://dx.doi.org/10.1097/00006982-200006000-00016] [PMID: 11131424]

[60] Quiroz-Reyes MA, Nieto-Jordan A, Quiroz-Gonzalez EA, *et al.* Timing of vitrectomy in myopic traction maculopathy: A long term follow up report of a hispanic population. Am J Med Surg 2020; 1: 7-14.

[61] Gonvers M, Machemer R. A new approach to treating retinal detachment with macular hole. Am J Ophthalmol 1982; 94(4): 468-72. [http://dx.doi.org/10.1016/0002-9394(82)90240-9] [PMID: 7137271]

[62] Ripandelli G, Parisi V, Friberg TR, Coppé AM, Scassa C, Stirpe M. Retinal detachment associated with macular hole in high myopia*1Using the vitreous anatomy to optimize the surgical approach. Ophthalmology 2004; 111(4): 726-31. [http://dx.doi.org/10.1016/j.ophtha.2003.08.026] [PMID: 15051205]

[63] Seike C, Kusaka S, Sakagami K, Ohashi Y. Reopening of macular holes in highly myopic eyes with retinal detachments. Retina 1997; 17(1): 2-6. [http://dx.doi.org/10.1097/00006982-199701000-00001] [PMID: 9051834]

[64] Quiroz-Reyes MA, Quiroz-Gonzalez EA, Morales-Navarro J, Nieto-Jordan A. Postoperative perfusion findings in highly myopic eyes: case series report. J Ophthalmol Vis Sci 2022; 7: 1062.

[65] Rouhette H, Cauchi O, Zur C, Gastaud P. Retinal detachment due to macular holes in highly myopic eyes. prognostic factors. J Fr Ophtalmol 2001; 24(1): 49-53. [PMID: 11240471]

[66] Haut J, Faure JF, Larricart P, Monin C, Le Mer Y. Treatment by internal tamponade of retinal detachment with a macular hole. J Fr Ophtalmol 1987; 10(11): 707-15. [PMID: 3448126]

[67] Meng L, Wei W, Li Y, Han X, Shi X, Yang M. Treatment of retinal detachment secondary to macular hole in highly myopic eyes: Pars plana vitrectomy with internal limiting membrane peel and silicone oil tamponade. Retina 2014; 34(3): 470-6. [http://dx.doi.org/10.1097/IAE.0b013e31829d004b] [PMID: 23881229]

[68] Nishimura A, Kimura M, Saito Y, Sugiyama K. Efficacy of primary silicone oil tamponade for the treatment of retinal detachment caused by macular hole in high myopia. Am J Ophthalmol 2011; 151(1): 148-55. [http://dx.doi.org/10.1016/j.ajo.2010.07.023] [PMID: 21130979]

[69] Matsumura N, Ikuno Y, Tano Y. Posterior vitreous detachment and macular hole formation in myopic foveoschisis. Am J Ophthalmol 2004; 138(6): 1071-3. [http://dx.doi.org/10.1016/j.ajo.2004.06.064] [PMID: 15629315]

[70] Abdelkader E, Lois N. Internal limiting membrane peeling in vitreo-retinal surgery. Surv Ophthalmol 2008; 53(4): 368-96. [http://dx.doi.org/10.1016/j.survophthal.2008.04.006] [PMID: 18572054]

[71] Christensen UC, Krøyer K, Sander B, *et al.* Value of internal limiting membrane peeling in surgery for idiopathic macular hole stage 2 and 3: A randomised clinical trial. Br J Ophthalmol 2009; 93(8): 1005-15. [http://dx.doi.org/10.1136/bjo.2008.151266] [PMID: 19028741]

[72] Pichi F, Alkabes M, Nucci P, Ciardella AP. Intraoperative SD-OCT in macular surgery. Ophthalmic Surg Lasers Imaging Retina 2012; 43(6) (Suppl.): S54-60. [http://dx.doi.org/10.3928/15428877-20121001-08] [PMID: 23357325]

[73] Lytvynchuk LM, Falkner-Radler CI, Krepler K, *et al.* Dynamic intraoperative optical coherence tomography for inverted internal limiting membrane flap technique in large macular hole surgery. Graefes Arch Clin Exp Ophthalmol 2019; 257(8): 1649-59.

[http://dx.doi.org/10.1007/s00417-019-04364-5] [PMID: 31139918]

[74] Wang X, Zhu Y, Xu H. Inverted multi-layer internal limiting membrane flap for macular hole retinal detachment in high myopia. Sci Rep 2022; 12(1): 10593. [http://dx.doi.org/10.1038/s41598-022-14716-7] [PMID: 35732799]

[75] Li M, Zhou J, Chen Q, *et al.* Automatic segmentation and thickness quantification on swept-source optical coherence tomography images of highly myopic patients. Ann Transl Med 2022; 10(11): 620. [http://dx.doi.org/10.21037/atm-21-6736]

[76] Agarwal A, Agrawal R, Khandelwal N, *et al.* Choroidal structural changes in tubercular multifocal serpiginoid choroiditis. Ocul Immunol Inflamm 2018; 26(6): 838-44. [http://dx.doi.org/10.1080/09273948.2017.1370650] [PMID: 29020533]

[77] Agrawal R, Gupta P, Tan KA, Cheung CMG, Wong TY, Cheng CY. Choroidal vascularity index as a measure of vascular status of the choroid: Measurements in healthy eyes from a population-based study. Sci Rep 2016; 6(1): 21090. [http://dx.doi.org/10.1038/srep21090] [PMID: 26868048]

[78] Agrawal R, Li LKH, Nakhate V, Khandelwal N, Mahendradas P. Choroidal vascularity index in vogt-koyanagi-harada disease: An EDI-OCT derived tool for monitoring disease progression. Transl Vis Sci Technol 2016; 5(4): 7. [http://dx.doi.org/10.1167/tvst.5.4.7] [PMID: 27525196]

[79] Yazdani N, Ehsaei A, Hoseini-Yazdi H, Shoeibi N, Alonso-Caneiro D, Collins MJ. Wide□field choroidal thickness and vascularity index in myopes and emmetropes. Ophthalmic Physiol Opt 2021; 41(6): 1308-19. [http://dx.doi.org/10.1111/opo.12875] [PMID: 34487376]

[80] Iovino C, Au A, Hilely A, *et al.* Evaluation of the choroid in eyes with retinitis pigmentosa and cystoid macular edema. Invest Ophthalmol Vis Sci 2019; 60(15): 5000-6. [http://dx.doi.org/10.1167/iovs.19-27300] [PMID: 31794599]

[81] Agrawal R, Salman M, Tan KA, *et al.* Choroidal vascularity index (CVI)--a novel optical coherence tomography parameter for monitoring patients with panuveitis? PLoS One 2016; 11(1): e0146344. [http://dx.doi.org/10.1371/journal.pone.0146344] [PMID: 26751702]

[82] Aribas YK, Hondur AM, Tezel TH. Choroidal vascularity index and choriocapillary changes in retinal vein occlusions. Graefes Arch Clin Exp Ophthalmol 2020; 258(11): 2389-97. [http://dx.doi.org/10.1007/s00417-020-04886-3] [PMID: 32860575]

[83] Marques JH, Marta A, Castro C, *et al.* Choroidal changes and associations with visual acuity in diabetic patients. Int J Retina Vitreous 2022; 8(1): 6. [http://dx.doi.org/10.1186/s40942-021-00355-z] [PMID: 34998439]

[84] Kim M, Kim RY, Park YH. Choroidal vascularity index and choroidal thickness in human leukocyte antigen-B27-associated uveitis. Ocul Immunol Inflamm 2019; 27(8): 1280-7. [http://dx.doi.org/10.1080/09273948.2018.1530364] [PMID: 30285514]

[85] Singh SR, Invernizzi A, Rasheed MA, *et al.* Wide-field choroidal vascularity in healthy eyes. Am J Ophthalmol 2018; 193: 100-5. [http://dx.doi.org/10.1016/j.ajo.2018.06.016] [PMID: 29958821]

[86] Ohno-Matsui K, Kawasaki R, Jonas JB, *et al.* International photographic classification and grading system for myopic maculopathy. Am J Ophthalmol 2015; 159(5): 877-883.e7. [http://dx.doi.org/10.1016/j.ajo.2015.01.022] [PMID: 25634530]

[87] Shimada N, Ohno-Matsui K, Baba T, Futagami S, Tokoro T, Mochizuki M. Natural course of macular retinoschisis in highly myopic eyes without macular hole or retinal detachment. Am J Ophthalmol 2006; 142(3): 497-500. [http://dx.doi.org/10.1016/j.ajo.2006.03.048] [PMID: 16935601]

[88] Fan H, Chen HY, Ma HJ, *et al.* Reduced macular vascular density in myopic eyes. Chin Med J 2017; 130(4): 445-51.
[http://dx.doi.org/10.4103/0366-6999.199844] [PMID: 28218219]

CHAPTER 4

Postoperative Ocular Perfusional Findings in Successfully Reattached Severe Proliferative Vitreoretinopathy, An OCT-A Evaluation

Juan Pablo Dávila-Gonzalez[1,*] and **José Dalma-Weiszhausz**[2]

[1] *Dalma y Asociados SC. Mexico City, Mexico*

[2] *Asociacion para prevenir la Ceguera en Mexico, Mexico City, Mexico*

Abstract: Rhegmatogenous retinal detachment (RRD) is the separation of the neurosensory retina from the underlying retinal pigment epithelium (RPE) and is one of the leading causes of severe vision loss when it involves the macula or proliferative vitreoretinopathy (PVR) in different stages. Optical coherence tomography (OCT) and Optical coherence tomography - angiography (OCT-A) have opened a new scenario in the investigation of macular microstructural abnormalities in RRD.

Findings in the preoperative retinal detachment structural B-scans in OCT such as ellipsoid zone (EZ)/external limiting membrane (ELM) integrity, cavities along the inner nuclear layer (INL) or outer nuclear layer (ONL), retinal height of detachment at the fovea, presence of retinal folds and subfoveal choroidal thickness may predict the functional and structural outcomes.

Structural and en-face analysis with OCT-A in RRD with PVR has demonstrated an enlarged foveal avascular zone, and changes in the flow at the superficial, intermediate and deep capillary plexus during 6 months postoperative follow up. High resolution and deep enhancing imaging OCT-A technology will provide an important role regarding the choriocapillaris and choroid and their potential correlation with visual acuity recovery.

OCT and OCT-A will provide preoperative prognostic biomarkers and adequate vascular retinochoroidal layers may influence a postoperative outcome.

Keywords: Angiography, Outer nuclear layer (ONL), Rhegmatogenous retinal detachment (RRD), Retinal morphology, Retinal pigment epithelium (RPE).

INTRODUCTION

Rhegmatogenous retinal detachment (RRD) is the separation of the neurosensory retina from the underlying retinal pigment epithelium (RPE). In normal eyes, the rate of RRD is approximately 5 per 100,000 people per year [1]. It often causes severe vision loss when it involves the macula or proliferative vitreoretinopathy

* **Corresponding author Juan Pablo Dávila-Gonzalez:** Dalma y Asociados SC. Mexico City, Mexico; Tel: +52 55 5540-3428; E-mail: juan_pablo_davila@doctor.com

Miguel A. Quiroz-Reyes and Virgilio Lima-Gomez (Eds.)

(PVR) in different stages. The incidence of PVR ranges from 5.1 to 11.7%, and remains the most common cause of failed repair rhegmatogenous retinal detachment. The risk factors for PVR are well known pre, intra and postoperative clinical findings [1]. Retinal pigment epithelium (RPE) cells are the key factor triggering PVR development in addition to multiple inflammatory and proliferative factors that induce non-vascular fibrocellular epiretinal membrane, intraretinal membranes and subretinal bands proliferation and contraction. Histologically, PVR membranes may appear gliotic, fibrovascular or fibroglial. PVR is believed to form from inward migration and proliferation of glial cells normally present in the nerve fiber and ganglion cell layers. Aside from glial cells, PVR membranes may also contain fibroblast and RPE cells [1, 2].

Various treatments can be performed to reattach the retina, including vitrectomy, scleral buckling, a combination of the two, pneumatic retinopexy, laser or cryocoagulation or newer techniques like tissue adhesive or retinal autografts in addition to multiples tamponades like SF_6 or C_3F_8 gas or silicon oil tamponade extensively used in the presence of advanced PVR [1, 2].

However, even after successful anatomic reattachment, the functional results show a wide range of visual outcomes. Poor visual acuity, permanent functional damage, persistent metamorphopsia or color vision defects can remain after surgery. Factors that affect the visual outcomes include the macula-off RRD, preoperative visual acuity, age of the patient, duration of the detachment, extension of the detachment, concomitant choroidal detachment, any degree of PVR, vitreous hemorrhage along with other ophthalmic conditions such as preretinal membrane formation, macular cysts or holes, senile cataracts or glaucoma [1, 2].

Optical coherence tomography (OCT) is the most accurate method to image the macular structure. The utilization of OCT in clinical practice has dramatically increased the ability to diagnose vitreomacular abnormalities, providing subclinical information and allowing physicians to visualize, classify and monitor the vitreomacular interface, retina and choroid with better accuracy. Findings in the preoperative retinal detachment structural B-scans in OCT such as ellipsoid zone (EZ) / external limiting membrane (ELM) integrity, cavities along the inner nuclear layer (INL) or outer nuclear layer (ONL), retinal height of detachment at the fovea, presence of retinal folds and subfoveal choroidal thickness may predict the functional and structural outcomes [3, 4].

In the last decades, the use of fluorescein angiography has revealed abnormalities in the retinal perfusion of patients with RRD. Some findings include vascular dilation and hyperpermeability because of tissue hypoxia [5].

Emerging evidence using OCT-Angiography (OCT-A), a new imaging technology represents one of the latest revolutions in retinal imaging.

OCT-A has opened a new scenario in the investigation of macular microstructural abnormalities in RRD. OCT-A has revealed the existence of microscopic macular changes, even in cases where retinal morphology appears normal on the fundus biomicroscopy. Despite the increased rate of successful anatomical retinal reattachment after surgery in non-complicated or complicated RDD, a substantial proportion of patients have unexpected limited visual outcomes, indicating that the functional status of the macula may not be entirely restored. It is possible that circulatory changes at the macular capillary level may explain this low visual recovery. The microcirculation system of the macula consists of retinal and choroidal capillary networks. The superficial capillary plexus (SCP) and the deep capillary plexus (DCP) are located within the ganglion cell layer and the inner nuclear layer, respectively. They are responsible for providing nourishment to the inner retinal layer and removing metabolic products. The intermediate capillary plexus (ICP), located in between the SCP and DCP, is a distinct vascular network whose formation seems to depend more on hypoxia-induced factors than the other capillary plexus [5 - 8].

Macular microvascular disturbance has been previously shown to be present in RRD eyes even without macular involvement. Scanning-laser doppler flowmetry has shown macular flow velocity decrease, probably due to an autoregulation phenomenon secondary to tissue hypoxia [7].

There is little quantitative analysis information considering the association between OCT-A characteristics and the final visual acuity in RRD and PVR after successful surgery. Changes in the macular capillary plexus after RRD may indicate the presence of ischemic damage in the fovea leading to poor visual outcomes. The first analysis of OCT-A characteristics after RRD surgery was published by Sato and colleagues in 2017, who demonstrated, in 22 eyes, no association of FAZ area changes with the SCP and DCP with visual acuity (VA) at 1, 3 and 6 months after vitrectomy. In 2018, Woo and co-authors published 34 cases with and without macular involvement and found that both superficial and especially deep FAZ were markedly larger in the macula-off after 2 months. In addition, DCP flow deficit was affected probably due to the watershed zone and lower oxygen saturation, making this deep plexus more vulnerable to hypoxia compared to the SCP directly related to large retinal arterioles, which have higher perfusion pressure. Patients with macula-on postoperative FAZ were not significantly different from the control group, so changes in FAZ observed may indicate ischemic changes leading to suboptimal visual recovery. Observations by Yui and co-authors in some patients with RDD and PVR suggest that preoperative visual function is related to reduced superficial vascular density even after successful surgery. According to Wang and collaborators' reports in 2019, the flow density in SCP and DCP, and choriocapillaris flow density (CCP FD) were decreased after 2 weeks postoperatively, with a gradual recovery over time from two to twelve months in all retinal layers but not reaching the values of the unaffected normal eye [9 - 12].

Other findings from Bonfiglio or Agarwal and co-authors described that vascular density in the parafovea was decreased, an explanation to their findings according to experimental model findings showed Müller cell activation due to inflammation (highly increased in PVR) even in the non-detached retina. Activation seemed to be connected with local blood flow changes in the inner retina secondary, leading to a decrease in capillary flow density [8].

There are also reports by Nam SH or Sato T which found no negative correlation between the vascular findings and the final visual acuity. Discrepancies in between results might be affected due to the unique baseline characteristics of the subjects, duration of the follow-up period, macula region analyzed, or different OCT-A technology employed [9]. In all studies, only a few patients presented with advanced stages of PVR. Mostly all studies published on pars plana vitrectomy (PPV) refer to cases treated exclusively with gas tamponade. Silicon oil is preferably used in PPV in complicated macula-off RRD and advanced PVR poor vision, which make the OCT-A scanning acquisition difficult, typically with low intensity signals and artifacts. OCT findings in postoperative RRD and PVR showremnants of proliferative tissue even months after the surgery. If epiretinal or subretinal macular contraction is present in patients with RRD and PVR, standardized FAZ quantification, vascular flow and vascular density analysis algorithms in the different retinal plexus are prone to appear more affected because of a wrong segmentation. Prospective comparative studies are required to investigate whether the use of silicon oil implicates a higher vascular alteration. Another aspect that needs consideration is the fact that most reported series have a small number of cases with PVR and shorter ranges of follow up [8 - 13].

REFERENCES

[1] Donald J D'Amico. Clinical practice. primary retinal detachment. N Engl J Med 2008; 359(22): 2346-54.
[http://dx.doi.org/10.1056/NEJMcp0804591] [PMID: 19038880]

[2] Kwon OW, Song JH, Roh MI. Retinal detachment and proliferative vitreoretinopathy. Dev Ophthalmol 2016; 55: 154-62.
[http://dx.doi.org/10.1159/000438972] [PMID: 26501375]

[3] Hostovsky A, Trussart R, AlAli A, Kertes PJ, Eng KT. Pre-operative optical coherence tomography findings in macula-off retinal detachments and visual outcome. Eye 2021; 35(12): 3285-91.
[http://dx.doi.org/10.1038/s41433-021-01399-z] [PMID: 33514905]

[4] Baba T, Hirose A, Moriyama M, Mochizuki M. Tomographic image and visual recovery of acute macula-off rhegmatogenous retinal detachment. Graefes Arch Clin Exp Ophthalmol 2004; 242(7): 576-81.
[http://dx.doi.org/10.1007/s00417-004-0884-0] [PMID: 14997321]

[5] Spaide RF, Klancnik JM Jr, Cooney MJ. Retinal vascular layers imaged by fluorescein angiography and optical coherence tomography angiography. JAMA Ophthalmol 2015; 133(1): 45-50.
[http://dx.doi.org/10.1001/jamaophthalmol.2014.3616] [PMID: 25317632]

[6] Woo JM, Yoon YS, Woo JE, Min JK. Foveal avascular zone area changes analyzed using oct angiography after successful rhegmatogenous retinal detachment repair. Curr Eye Res 2018; 43(5): 674-8.
[http://dx.doi.org/10.1080/02713683.2018.1437922] [PMID: 29451996]

[7] Hong EH, Cho H, Kim DR, Kang MH, Shin YU, Seong M. Changes in retinal vessel and retinal layer thickness after vitrectomy in retinal detachment *via* swept-source oct angiography. Invest Ophthalmol Vis Sci 2020; 61(2): 35.
[http://dx.doi.org/10.1167/iovs.61.2.35] [PMID: 32084264]

[8] Bonfiglio V, Ortisi E, Scollo D, *et al.* Vascular changes after vitrectomy for rhegmatogenous retinal detachment: Optical coherence tomography angiography study. Acta Ophthalmol 2020; 98(5): e563-9.
[http://dx.doi.org/10.1111/aos.14315] [PMID: 31773840]

[9] Christou EE, Stavrakas P, Batsos G, Christodoulou E, Stefaniotou M. Association of OCT-A characteristics with postoperative visual acuity after rhegmatogenous retinal detachment surgery: A review of the literature. Int Ophthalmol 2021; 41(6): 2283-92.
[http://dx.doi.org/10.1007/s10792-021-01777-2] [PMID: 33745033]

[10] Adhi MI, Siyal N, Aziz S. Anatomical and functional outcomes of retinectomies in retinal detachments complicated by proliferative vitreoretinopathy. Saudi J Ophthalmol 2017; 31(4): 216-23.
[http://dx.doi.org/10.1016/j.sjopt.2017.09.005] [PMID: 29234222]

[11] Barca F, Bacherini D, Dragotto F, *et al.* OCT angiography findings in macula-on and macula-off rhegmatogenous retinal detachment: A prospective study. J Clin Med 2020; 9(12): 3982.
[http://dx.doi.org/10.3390/jcm9123982] [PMID: 33316923]

[12] Takahashi H, Uramoto K, Ohno-Matsui K. Ultra-widefield optical coherence tomography for retinal detachment with proliferative vitreoretinopathy. Retin Cases Brief Rep 2022; 16(3): 355-9.
[http://dx.doi.org/10.1097/ICB.0000000000000980] [PMID: 32032288]

[13] Bacherini D, Mastropasqua R, Borrelli E, *et al.* OCT-A in the management of vitreoretinal diseases and surgery. Asia Pac J Ophthalmol 2021; 10(1): 12-9.
[http://dx.doi.org/10.1097/APO.0000000000000373] [PMID: 33512825]

CHAPTER 5

Polypoidal Choroidal Vasculopathy and Pachychoroid Neovasculopathy Represent Different Manifestations of the Same Disease

Erick A. Quiroz-Gonzalez[1,2,*], **Miguel A. Quiroz-Reyes, MD**[1] and **Zixuan Shao**[3]

[1] *Oftalmologia Integral ABC, Retina Department, Medical and Surgical Assistance Institution (Nonprofit Organization), Affiliated with the Postgraduate Studies Division, National Autonomous University of Mexico, Mexico City, Mexico*

[2] *Institute of Ophthalmology, Fundacion Conde de Valenciana, Private Assistance Institution (Nonprofit Organization), Mexico City, Mexico*

[3] *Division of Chemistry and Chemical Engineering, California Institute of Technology, Pasadena, CA, USA*

Abstract: The pachychoroid spectrum has various clinical manifestations. There are three major characteristics, all of which have an unknown etiology and controversial pathogenesis: pachychoroid, presence of pachyvessels at the external choroid, and inner choroidal attenuation. This study describes a patient with clinical and multimodal manifestations in the pachychoroid spectrum, in which different clinical variants are presented in both eyes simultaneously. Specifically, the patient had an acute visual loss and massive hemorrhagic maculopathy in the right eye, and a chronic decrease in visual acuity and metamorphopsia in the left eye accompanied by pigmentary changes and subretinal fluid at the geometric center of the fovea. The patient underwent a complete ophthalmological examination and multimodal imaging and was diagnosed with polypoidal choroidal vasculopathy (PCV) and pachychoroid neovasculopathy (PNV); two different manifestations of the same disease spectrum occur simultaneously.

Owing to the active nature of the disease, the patient received three doses of intravitreal antiangiogenic agents in each eye. Many different degenerative etiologies have been considered, such as pathological choroidal neovascularization due to age-related macular degeneration (AMD) and pachychoroid spectrum. Evaluation of the choroid vasculature using swept-source optical coherent tomography (SS-OCT) and OCT angiography (OCT-A) revealed the origin of the disease to be idiopathic. PCV and PNV are considered to represent a single end-stage of the pachychoroid spectrum with

* **Corresponding author Erick A. Quiroz-Gonzalez:** Oftalmologia Integral ABC, Retina Department, Medical and Surgical Assistance Institution (Nonprofit Organization), Affiliated with the Postgraduate Studies Division, National Autonomous University of Mexico, Mexico City, Mexico; E-mail: erwick-andrew@hotmail.com

Miguel A. Quiroz-Reyes and Virgilio Lima-Gomez (Eds.)

different manifestations; the former presents with aneurysmatic characteristics, whereas the latter lacks this anomaly.

Keywords: Central serous chorioretinopathy, Choroidal neovascularization, Hemorrhagic maculopathy, Pachychoroid neovasculopathy, Pachychoroid spectrum, Peripapillary pachychoroid syndrome, Pachychoroid neovasculopathy polypoidal choroidal vasculopathy, Polypoidal choroidal neovascularization, Retinal angiomatous proliferation.

INTRODUCTION

The pachychoroid spectrum comprises several manifestations of a single disease [1]. The word pachychoroid is derived from Greek, meaning "thick" choroid. Three major characteristics are associated with the pachychoroid spectrum. First, although there is no precise cutoff point of choroidal thickness for diagnosis (probably due to physiological fluctuations influenced by the circadian cycle, blood pressure, hydration status, sex, axial length, and other factors [2]), recent studies have reported that a thickness of >270-300 microns indicates the presence of pachychoroid [3, 4]. Second, pachyvessels or a dilated Haller's plexus cause compression of the Sattler's plexus and choriocapillaris, decreasing the oxygen concentration at the Ruysch's complex (retinal pigment epithelium (RPE), Bruch's membrane, and choriocapillaris). Third, inner choroidal attenuation has also been observed in this disease [5].

The etiology of pachychoroid disease is not well understood; however, both exogenous and endogenous factors (including genetic background) are likely involved. Some reports point to choroidal congestion as a possible contributor to disease progression [6], yet the exact pathogenesis remains controversial. Additionally, mineralocorticoid and corticosteroid receptors are abundantly expressed in the choroidal vasculature, contributing to the increase in choroidal thickness [4, 7] and functional anomalies secondary to hydrostatic pressure alteration [8]. Altogether, these three main characteristics, in particular, the attenuation of choriocapillaris, lead to retinal pigment epithelium (RPE) dysfunction, photoreceptor atrophy, and subsequent development of choroidal neovascularization (CNV) in response to significant choroidal ischemia [5, 9] and sub-RPE endothelial cell proliferation due to pigmentary epithelium detachments (PEDs) [10].

The pachychoroid spectrum comprises central serous chorioretinopathy (CSC), pachychoroid pigment epitheliopathy (PPE), polypoidal choroidal vasculopathy (PCV), pachychoroid neovasculopathy (PNV), focal choroidal excavation (FCE), and peripapillary pachychoroid syndrome (PPS) [2, 7]. PCV has been described as an area of choroidal vasculature proliferation immediately beneath the RPE, forming a branching vascular network (BVN) with edges exhibiting vascular dilatations or aneurysms, controversially named polyps, because this word refers to dilatation of a mucous membrane, and it is more accurate to use the term aneurysm instead of polyp, as proposed by the CONAN group [11]. The presence of this aneurysmatic lesion develops serous or hemorrhagic PEDs and evolves into massive hemorrhagic maculopathy with areas of lipid exudation [7] (Fig. **1**).

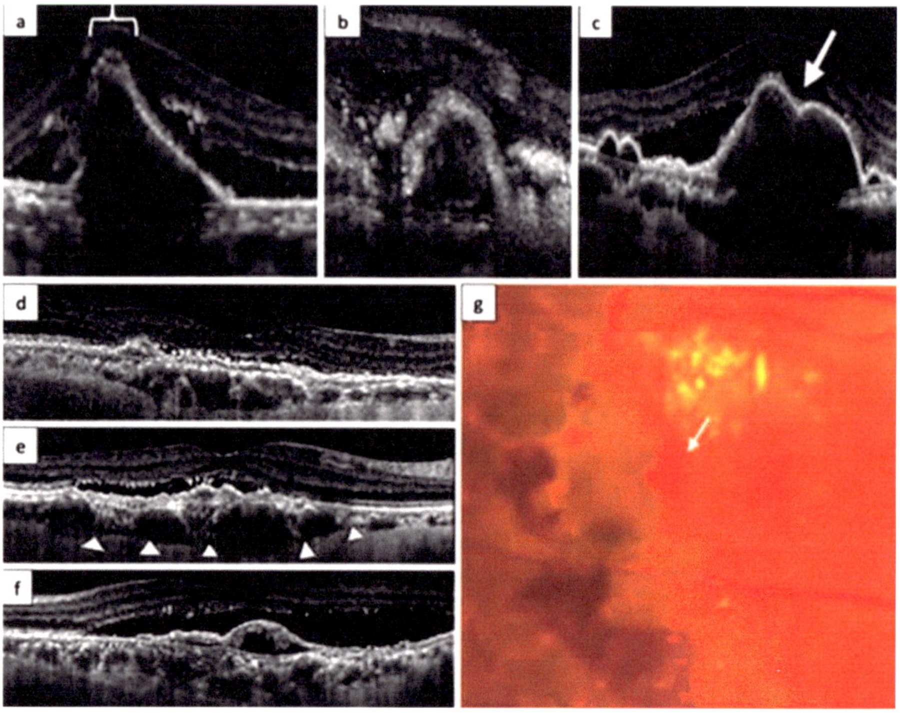

Fig. (1). Reference images for 7 selected features evaluated for inclusion into the final set of polypoid choroidal vasculopathy diagnostic criteria. (**a**) Sharp-peaked pigment epithelial detachment (PED). (**b**) Subretinal pigment detachment ring-like lesion. (**c**) Complex or multilobular PED (arrow highlighting the notch within the outline of the PED). (**d**), Double-layer sign or shallow, irregular retinal pigment epithelium (RPE) elevation. (**e**), Thick choroid with dilated Haller's layer vessels (scleral choroidal interface shown by arrowheads). (**f**), Predominance of subretinal fluid and Complex RPE elevation observed with in OCT. (**g**) Orange nodule (white arrow). This modified multipanel figure was originally published by the Asia-Pacific Ocular Imaging Society PCV Workgroup. Ophthalmology 2021; 128:443-452 by the American Academy of Ophthalmology. This is an open access article under the CC BY-NC-ND license (http://creativecommons.org/licenses/by-nc-nd/4.0/).

This disease is classified as a variant of age-related macular degeneration (AMD), and many authors believe that 1 in 10 pachychoroid patients is misdiagnosed with neovascular AMD [2, 12], particularly when choroidal imaging is not performed [13]. PNV can be considered the final stage of CSC or PPE due to type 1 CNV formation, leading to chronic disease and subsequent photoreceptor destruction. In contrast to AMD patients, CSC patients are typically diagnosed at a young age with idiopathic neovascular membranes, without pigmentary alterations or drusen [10]. The diagnosis of PCV was based on the gold standard indocyanine green angiography evaluation, which demonstrates early nodular hyperfluorescence signifying the polyp with additional features, such as an abnormal vascular network (AVN). Due to the lack of access to this study in some centers, there has been a tendency to use optical coherence tomography (OCT) and optical coherence tomography angiography (OCT-A) as the main tools to achieve diagnosis. Recalling that OCT works as a reflectance detector of the different retinal tissues, depending on their composition, and the OCT-A functions comparing OCT reflectance at the same point in consecutive scans, analyzing the correlation between scans. This means that a zone of decorrelation corresponds to an area of movement, which in turn correlates with blood cells passing through a vessel [14]. Making these technologies are excellent tools for diagnosing PCV, monitoring disease activity, and decision-making regarding the type of therapy treatment (Figs. **2** and **3**).

It is important to highlight the necessity of using swept-source (SS) OCT or Enhanced Depth Imaging (EDI-OCT) to characterize the choroidal features due to the penetration of light through thick tissues and blood, deriving a more reliable image. In addition, this technology brings a new approach, the possibility of binarizing a retinal image and making precise measurements of different parameters, such as the luminal and stromal area deriving into the choroidal vascularity index (CVI), leading to a functional measurement instead of only an anatomical measure from a single OCT [8].

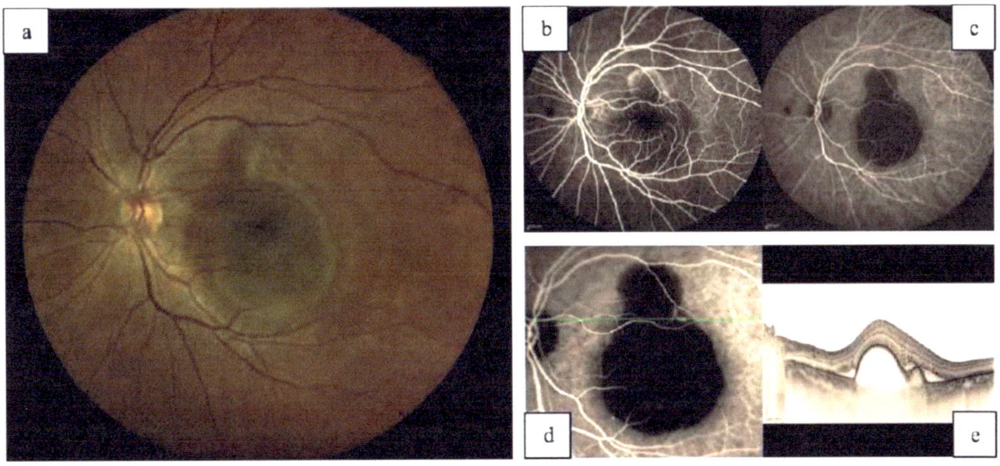

Fig. (2). Fundus image **(a)**, fluorescein angiography **(b)**, indocyanine green angiography **(c, d)** and SD- OCT **(e)** images of a 54-year-old woman with polypoidal choroidal vasculopathy on her left eye, showing the polyp visible in the ICGA corresponding with the PED notch. (courtesy of EQG).

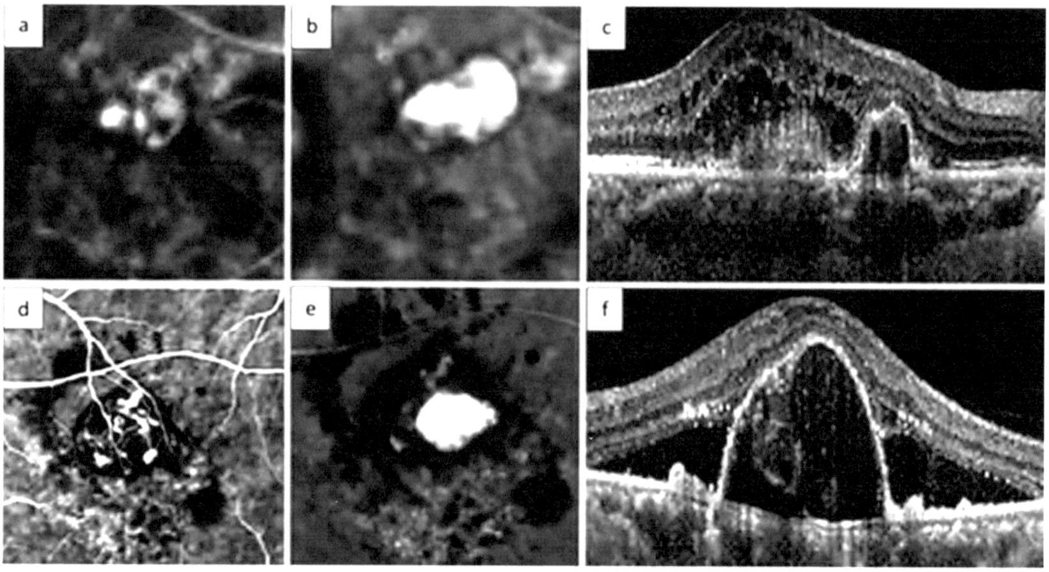

Fig. (3). Images depicting analysis of indocyanine green angiography (ICGA) in 2 patients. (**a**) to (**c**), Patient 1: (**a**) early phase ICGA (25 seconds) image shows that a combination of saccular and fusiform vascular dilatation was visible, but these cannot be discerned individually in (**b**) the mid-phase image (5 minutes). (**c**) corresponding cross-sectional SD-OCT image depicts a sharp-peaked pigment epithelial detachment (PED) with subretinal pigment epithelium ring-like lesion and thick choroid with dilated Haller's layer. (**d**)-(**f**), Patient 2: (**d**) early phase ICGA image shows a complex vascular network with dilatation at the terminal and (**e**) mid-phase ICGA image depicts no perceivable individual characteristic and the lesion appearing as a single structure filled with dye. (**f**), Cross-sectional SD-OCT image in which the internal structure appears to be present within the large PED. This modified multipanel figure was originally published by the Asia-Pacific Ocular Imaging Society PCV Workgroup. Ophthalmology 2021; 128:443-452 by the American Academy of Ophthalmology. This is an open access article under the CC BY-NC-ND license (http://creativecommons.org/licenses/by-nc-nd/4.0/).

Current treatment options include photodynamic therapy, which modifies choroidal perfusion, and antiangiogenic agents that inhibit vascular endothelial growth factor (VEGF) levels [15]. However, anti-VEGF treatment does not resolve pachychoroid characteristics, and the response is typically weaker than that of non-pachychoroid neovascularization [4]. This chapter provides detailed OCT observations complemented by OCT-A imaging evaluation from one clinical case that developed different manifestations of pachychoroid disease in both eyes simultaneously.

CASE PRESENTATION

A 54-year-old Latin man presented to the *Institute of Ophthalmology, Conde de Valenciana Foundation* in Mexico City, Mexico, with a 1-month history of erythropsia and low vision in the right eye. In addition, he had a 1-year history of metamorphopsia and painless vision loss in the left eye. The patient had no relevant medical history. Ophthalmic examination revealed a best-corrected visual acuity (BCVA) of 20/400 in the right eye and 20/50 in the left eye. Intraocular pressure and anterior segment biomicroscopy findings were unremarkable in both eyes.

Fundus examination of the right eye revealed a clear vitreous cavity and orange optic nerve without abnormalities. The macula presented foveolar elevation due to subretinal fluid and a large red spot beneath the vessels, corresponding to a subretinal hemorrhage with hard exudates (Fig. **4**a). The hemorrhages extended out of the vascular network to the inferior nasal and temporal retina in the mid-peripheral region following an irregular pattern (Fig. **4**b). The contralateral eye showed normal vitreous and optic nerves, with pigmentary changes inferior to the fovea and slight elevation (Fig. **4**c). The periphery was unremarkable (Fig. **4d**).

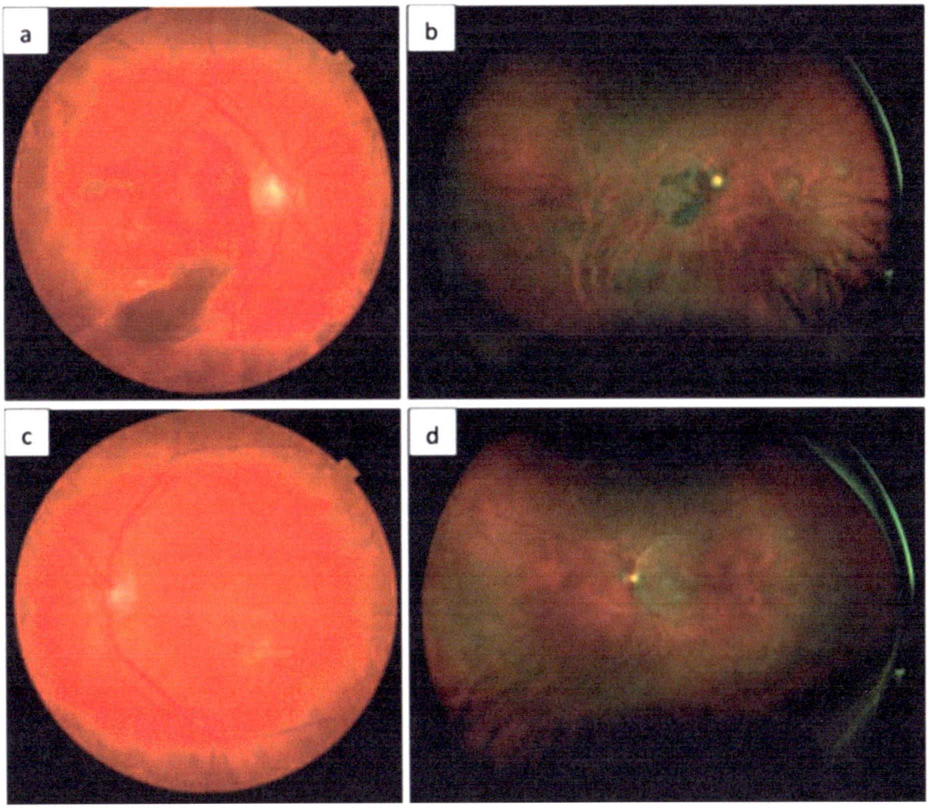

Fig. (4). (**a**) The fundus of the right eye shows a clear vitreous, normal optic nerve, and vasculature without anomalies. A large red spot associated with subretinal fluid and hard exudates can be observed at the macular level. (**b**) Ultrawide field photo shows subretinal blood at the inferior nasal and temporal retina in the mid-peripheral region that does not follow the distribution of the vasculature. (**c**) Left eye fundus shows pigmentary alterations only at the center of the fovea and slight foveal elevation, indicating the presence of subretinal fluid. (**d**) Ultrawide field photo showing an unremarkable periphery.

CNV was suspected because of the characteristics of the subretinal fluid. Therefore, autofluorescence imaging and fundus fluorescein angiography (FFA) of the retina were performed to define the pattern, area of extension, and morphology of the disease in both eyes. A hypoautofluorescence pattern was observed in the right eye, corresponding to areas of hemorrhage, with a slight hyperautofluorescent ring around the fovea. In the early arterial–venous phase, adequate filling of the arteries and veins was observed, as well as multiple areas of hypofluorescence secondary to blockage due to subretinal hemorrhages. Subsequently, multiple points of superior and nasal perifoveal hypofluorescence were observed in the late phases, which increased over time in both extension and intensity, corresponding to a filtration pattern consistent with CNV (Fig. **5**). In the left eye, autofluorescence images showed a well-defined hyperautofluorescent ring around the fovea, with gravitational extension. FFA in this area showed hyperfluorescence that increased in intensity throughout the study, consistent with the pattern of accumulation (Fig. **6**).

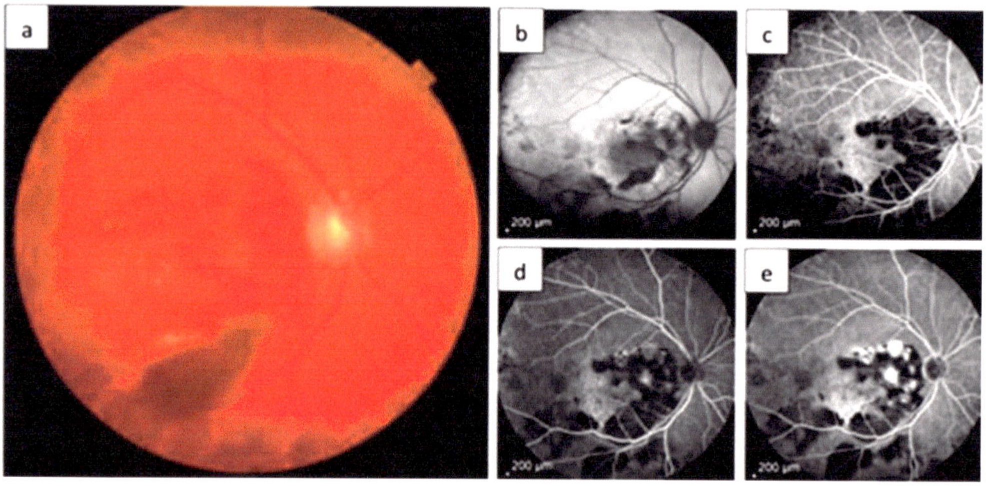

Fig. (5). (**a**) Right eye with hemorrhagic maculopathy. (**b** and **c**) Autofluorescence and fluorangiography images show a hypoautofluorescent area corresponding to blood and a hyperautofluorescent ring around the geometric center of the fovea. (**d**) In the early stages of fluorangiography, there is a block pattern due to hypofluorescence secondary to the presence of blood. (**e**) In the advanced stages, multiple hyperfluorescent areas can be observed with increased extension and intensity.

SS-OCT was performed to analyze the characteristics of the choriocapillaris and the integrity of the RPE and Bruch's membrane. SS-OCT revealed loss of the foveomacular profile in the right eye, disruption and disorganization of the outer layers of the retina, presence of subretinal fluid with multiple hyperreflective points in the region temporal to the fovea, and multiple high PEDs containing heterogeneous hyporeflective material, consistent with hemorrhagic PEDs. These detachments had notches and the double-layer sign showed disruption within the

RPE and Bruch's membrane. The subfoveal choroidal thickness was measured to be 366 µm, with attenuation of the choriocapillaris and dilated vessels in Haller's layer, indicating pachyvessels (Fig. **7**). In the left eye, the inner layers of the neurosensory retina were intact, whereas disorganization of the outer layers and loss of the ellipsoid zone (EZ) were observed at the subfoveal level. Subretinal fluid with hyperreflective material was also noted in the foveal area, corresponding to shaggy photoreceptors and atrophy of the outer segments of the rest of the retina. A mottled pattern was observed at the RPE, along with multiple small extrafoveal-plane PEDs. The choroid was 290 µm thick, where pachyvessels and choriocapillaris attenuation were detected (Fig. **8**), as well as a disproportionate luminal area and CVI seen in the binarized image of the left eye (Fig. **9**).

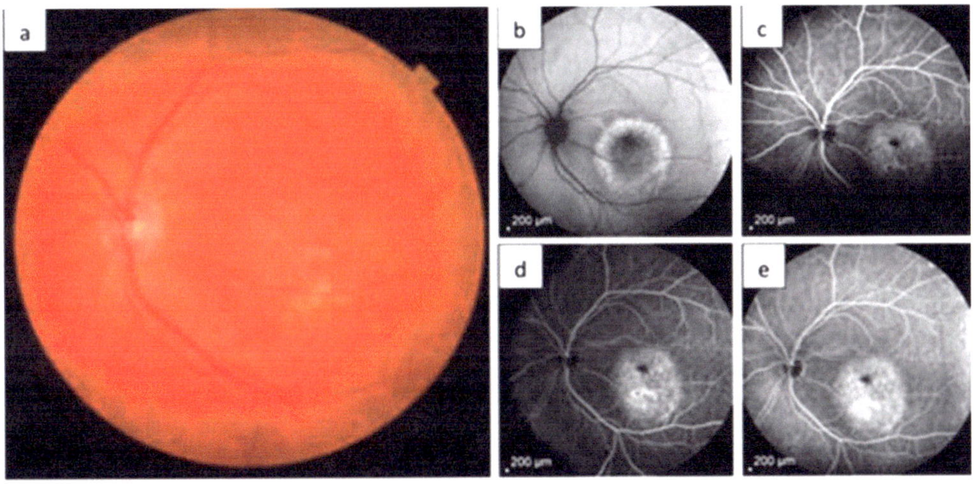

Fig. (6). (**a**) Fundus color photo of the left macula shows irregular central whitish mottling. (**b**) Left eye macula autofluorescence at the center of the macula. (**c** and **d**) Fluorangiography images show a hypoautofluorescent area surrounded by a hyperautofluorescent ring forming in a gravitational fashion, indicating the chronic presence of subretinal fluid. (**e**) At the mid-stages, fluorangiography shows a hyperfluorescent area around the fovea that increased in intensity throughout the study period.

Because FFA did not demonstrate any changes in the left eye, OCT angiography was performed to explore the presence of CNV. OCT angiography evaluation of the right eye showed blood flow in the upper portion of the nasal PED on the b-scan. The en face scan highlighted the presence of a hyperreflective spot in the outer layers, probably corresponding to an aneurysm, as marked by the red arrow (Fig. **10**). In the left eye, a reduction in flow was seen in the choriocapillaris with inferior foveal predominance, and an extrafoveal area of blood flow was observed below the RPE in the horizontal b-scan, indicating type 1 CNV (Fig. **11**).

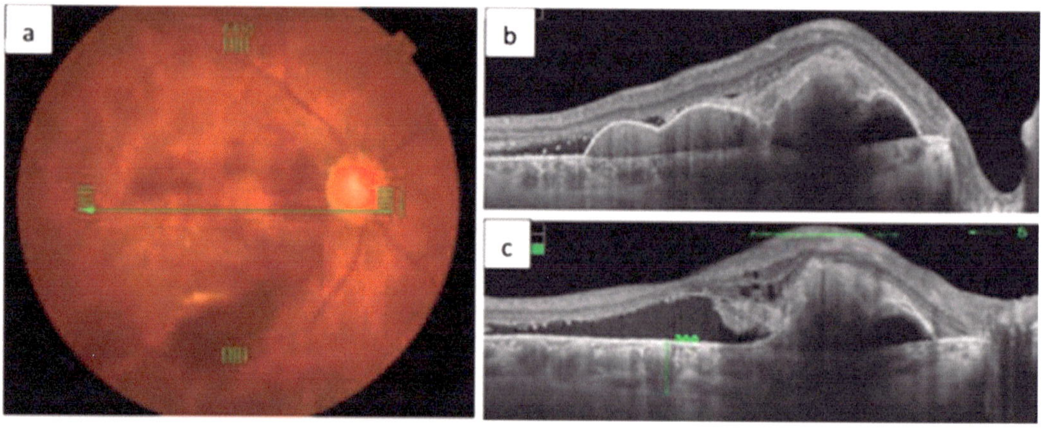

Fig. (7). (**a**) Right eye fundus color photo of the hemorrhagic macula with the corresponding green horizontal tracking line. (**b**) Right eye SS-OCT image shows disruption of the normal foveomacular profile with internal layer integrity associated with marked disruption of outer retina layers and the presence of subretinal fluid. Multiple large and notched serohemorrhagic PEDs with a double layer sign are present. (**c**) In addition to a pachychoroid 366 microns in thickness, signs of pachyvessels and internal choroidal vasculature attenuation are present.

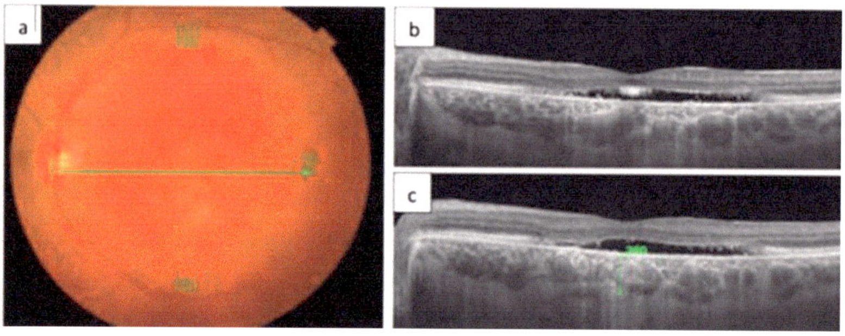

Fig. (8). (**a**) Fundus color photo of the left eye with irregular whitish central mottling. (**b**) Left eye SS-OCT image shows a normal foveo-macular profile with internal layer integrity and disruption of the external layer, particularly at the ellipsoid zone and external limiting membrane layer. Subretinal fluid with hyperreflective material resembling shaggy photoreceptors is also present. (**c**) Presence of a mottled RPE with flat PEDs. Pachychoroid 290 microns in thickness and extremely large pachyvessels can be observed.

The four-month evaluation after a series of three-monthly intravitreal injections of aflibercept showed that the right eye had shallow detachment of the central macula and thickening of the macula without loss of inner and outer biomarkers, while the pachychoroid persisted (Fig. **12**). Structural evaluation inferior to the center of the macula revealed persistent macular thickening. The inner and outer layers of the neurosensory macula were structurally preserved, with evidence of large choroid vessels and diffuse thickening of the choroid (Fig. **12**b and **c**). The eye had a final BCVA of 20/200 at the last follow-up visit.

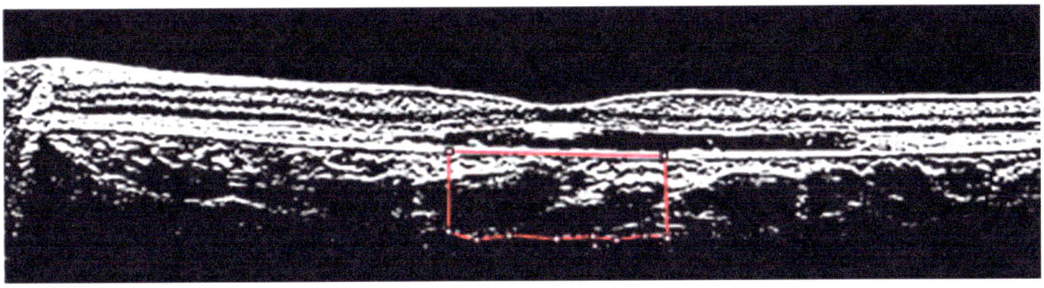

Fig. (9). Left eye, central OCT scan, binarized using the ImageJ program (version 1.53; NIH, Rasband and contributors, USA, public domain). First of all, the original OCT image was changed to an 8-bit format. Then, the brightness was lowered until the pachyvessels were fully visible. Subsequently, the image was binarized using the Otsu threshold. After that, the choroid was measured manually using the center of the fovea as a reference point, then the boundaries were limit between 750 µm nasal and 750 µm temporal in a horizontal fashion and vertically from Bruch's membrane to the uveoscleral junction. Finally, the luminal area was identified as the dark pixels and the stromal area as the white ones. The luminal area (0.61mm^2) was divided by the total choroidal area (0.82mm^2) to produce the choroidal vascular index (75.87%). Being this result totally out of normal proportion, resulting in a huge luminal area and choroidal vascular index as a result of the presence of pachyvessels.

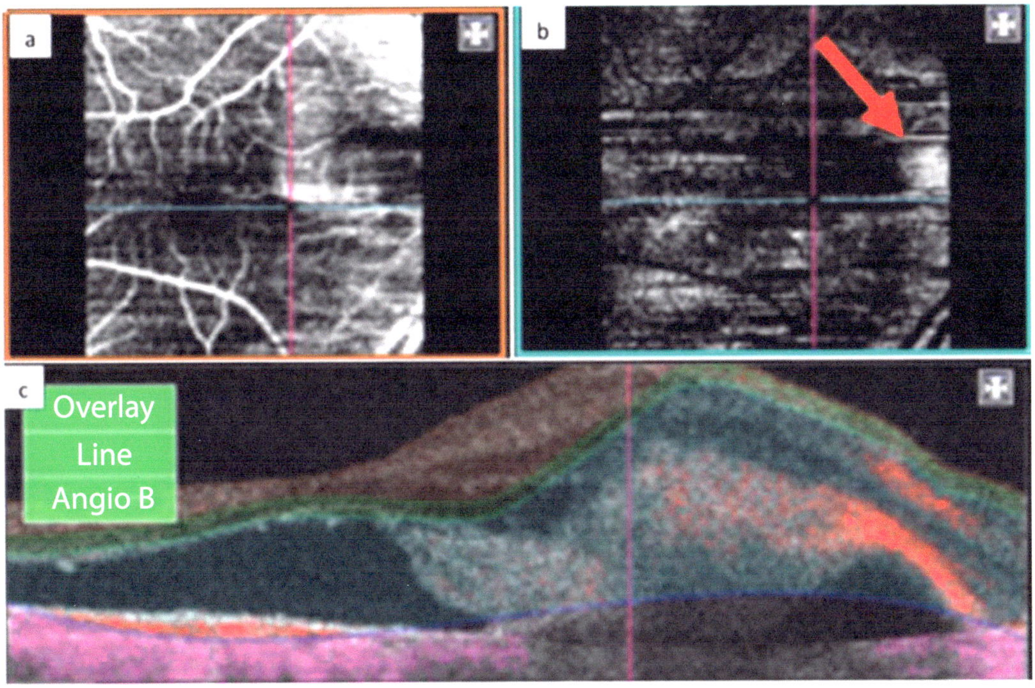

Fig. (10). (**a**) Right eye SS-OCT angiography image of the superficial vascular plexus. (**b**) The deep vascular plexus slab shows a hyperreflective zone (red arrow) corresponding to the polyp. (**c**) SS-OCT horizontal B-scan with evidence of hemorrhagic multilobulated PEDs and the presence of hemorrhagic material. The red dots represent blood flow visible nasally at the top of the PED, correlating with flow inside the aneurysm and an area of non-flow due hemorrhagic component beneath the RPE. Inner and outer retinal layer biomarkers are difficult to identify.

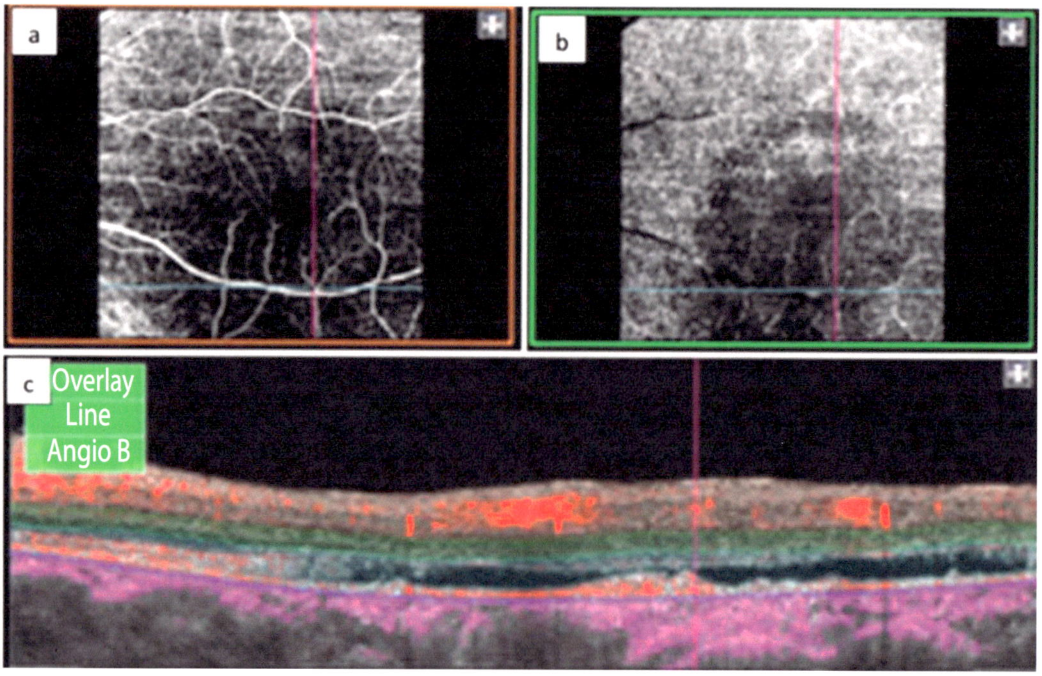

Fig. (11). (**a**) and (**b**) Images of the left eye show pretreatment superficial and deep vascular plexus slabs, with the latter showing multiple vascular deficiencies. (**c**) SS-OCT horizontal B-scan shows irregular RPE in the presence of an extrafoveal type 1 CNV. Segmentation lines reveal thin outer retinal layers in the presence of blood within the PEDs inferior to the fovea. The red dots represent hemorrhagic superficial components and qualitatively diminished vascular choriocapillaris flow.

The last structural evaluation of the left eye identified important changes in the RPE with an irregular well-defined central area of hypoautofluorescence, along with central persistent shallow submacular fluid, and the presence of persistent hyperreflective material still resembling shaggy photoreceptors (Fig. **13**a). Pachychoroids and extremely large pachyvessels were also observed. Dots of hyperreflective material were present in the inner layer of the macula (Fig. **13**b). Parafoveal SS-OCT examination showed a thin RPE with a very shallow presence of subretinal fluid and pachychoroid-like appearance of the choroidal layer (Fig. **13**c). The left eye exhibited low-grade activity, and a final BCVA of 20/30. After four months of careful monitoring and a series of three-monthly injections of aflibercept, this was considered a refractive case of PCV in the right eye and PNV in the left eye. The patient refused further treatment with half doses of photodynamic verteporfin therapy.

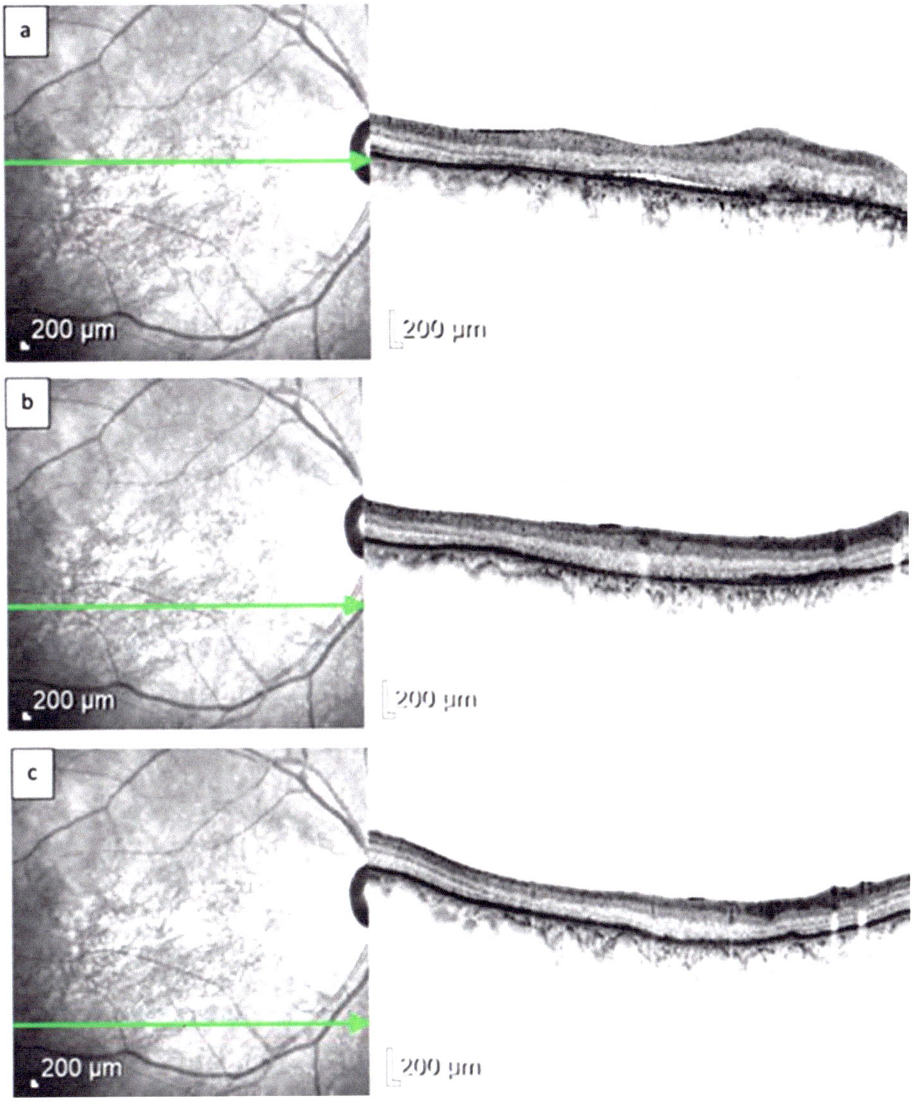

Fig. (12). (**a**) En face red-free image with a foveal green tracking line. Fine pigment mottling at the RPE is seen. The structural analysis depicts retinal thickening of the nasal fovea with a mild presence of central submacular fluid. Choroidal thickening is evident. (**b** and **c**) Images of the juxtafoveal and parafoveal macular regions, respectively, depict mild neurosensorial thickening with preservation of the inner and outer retina layer biomarkers.

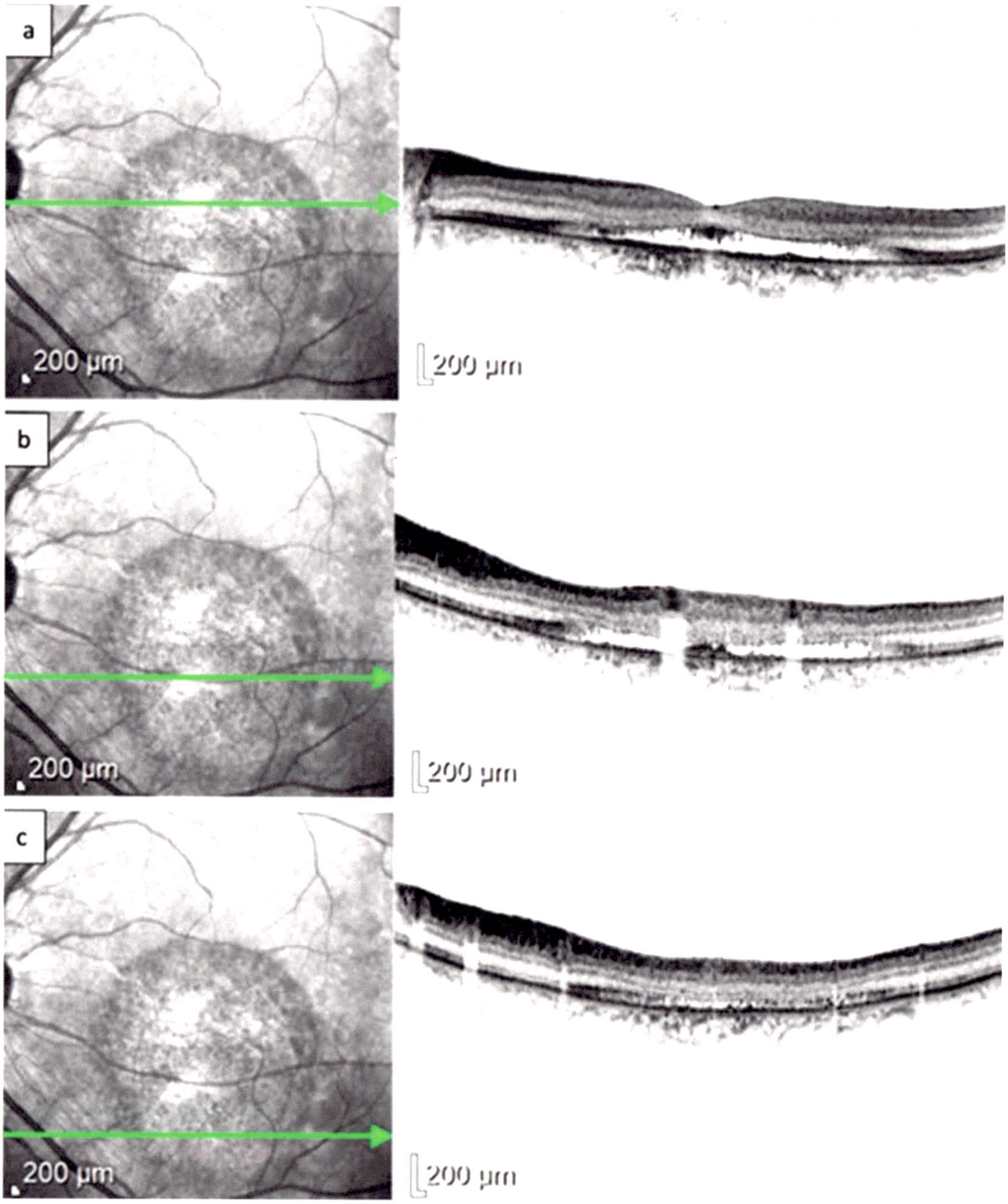

Fig. (13). (**a**) SS-OCT structural evaluation of the left eye showed changes in the RPE with a well-defined central area of hypoautofluorescence. (**b**) Central persistent shallow submacular fluid and the presence of persistent hyperreflective material resembling shaggy photoreceptors. The RPE appears mottled with pachychoroid and extremely large pachyvessels. Dots of hyperreflective material are seen in the inner layer of the macula. (**c**) Parafoveal SD-OCT shows a thin RPE with a very shallow presence of subretinal fluid and a pachychoroid-like appearance of the choroidal layer.

Considering the clinical, fluorescein angiographic, and tomographic findings, we concluded that CNV was present in both eyes at different stages with different manifestations. Large serohemorrhagic PEDs with notches and a double-layer sign indicated PCV in the right eye without indocyanine green angiography (ICGA) confirmation, as per recent reports [16, 17] that defined FFA imaging and SD-OCT criteria to diagnose PCV without ICGA. Additionally, Eraydin *et al.* [18] concluded that OCT has a sensitivity of 75.3% and a specificity of 75% for PCV diagnosis. The OCT angiography findings correlated with the polyp findings reported by others, in which the aneurysmatic lesion tended to be located just below the top of the serohemorrhagic PED and was more visible in the en face slabs [14]. OCT angiography findings in the left eye indicated PNV due to chronic subretinal and subfoveal fluid accumulation associated with blood flow, consistent with observations by Demirel *et al.* [19] and others.

The results of the Everest II and Planet studies [4] indicate that anti-angiogenic treatment is a sound option for patients with PCV. While no large randomized clinical trials have been conducted on PNV, a meta-analysis of retrospective series has demonstrated the efficacy of antiangiogenic applications [9]. Therefore, we decided to inject three monthly doses of aflibercept (Wetlia, Bayer) in both eyes.

DISCUSSION

CNVs can be classified according to their location with respect to the RPE. Etiology is another way to classify these conditions, with degeneration (specifically AMD) being the most common. Other causes, usually rare in nature, include inflammatory diseases, dystrophies, neoplasms, pachychoroid spectrum diseases, and idiopathic CNVs. The two forms of PCV can occur simultaneously without a shared origin, as shown in Fig. (**14**).

There is no universally accepted definition of PCV, but it shares characteristics with two other diseases: 1) type 1 neovascular membrane resembles AMD, and 2) choroidal vascular hyperpermeability and choroidal abnormalities resemble CSC [20]. Unlike the thin vasculature and drusen observed in AMD, the choroid in PCV is typically thick without drusen; thus, many authors believe that PCV is a different disease and is often misdiagnosed before the advent of SS-OCT and enhanced depth imaging OCT (EDI-OCT) [3]. Nevertheless, PCV has been described by Chang and Cheng [3] and other authors as having a biphasic pattern; one form tends to exhibit a larger number of polyps without increased subfoveal choroidal thickness (polypoidal choroidal neovascularization; PCN), and the other has pachychoroid characteristics (typical PCV). The first subtype has more features of AMD than CSC; in contrast, the pachychoroid subtype is more similar to CSC than AMD. The second subtype is more common in younger patients and shows a decreased response to anti-VEGF therapy. Although the exact reason for this is unknown, it has been proposed that increased subfoveal choroidal thickness leads to hydrostatic alterations, disrupts RPE tight junctions, and causes secondary ischemia with a low VEGF concentration [18]. In contrast, PCN is characterized by high VEGF levels, which respond better to anti-VEGF therapy (Fig. **15**), although the pathogenic implications are likely worse in later stages [3, 9, 21].

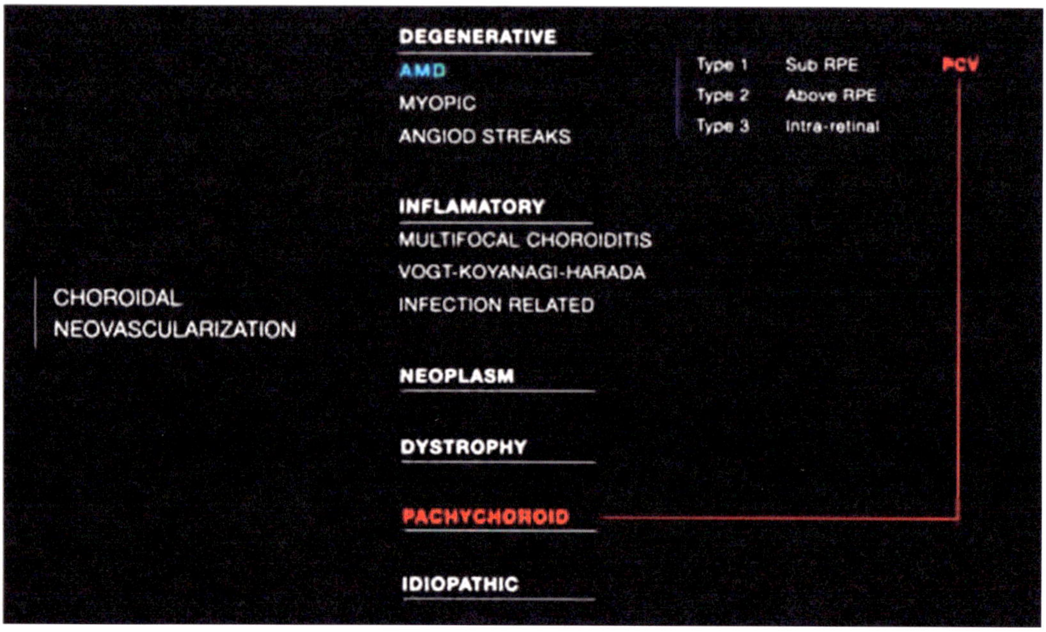

Fig. (14). Choroidal neovascularization has multiple etiologies. There are multiple causes of pachychoroid spectrum diseases, where polypoidal choroidal vasculopathy (PCV) can be classified as a subtype of age-related macular degeneration (AMD) or as part of the pachychoroid spectrum. RPE, retinal pigment epithelium.

As previously described, PNV has pachychoroid characteristics that are different from those of AMD and are similar to those of PCV. Although there are also features that differ from PCV, including the presence of flat PEDs and the lack of subretinal hemorrhages and polyps, the ultimate development of CNV in the presence of the pachychoroid spectrum is similar to PCV [10]. We believe that CSC, PPE, PCV, and PNV are the same diseases at different stages, but they do not necessarily evolve from one stage to another. Additionally, the genetic background likely plays an important role in the pathogenesis of this disease. PCV and PNV represent the end stages of the disease, indicating that the pachychoroid spectrum can follow two paths if CSC or PPE becomes chronic. As seen in the case presented above, these two paths could occur in the same patient, but with different clinical manifestations and complications, such as time of evolution, initial BCVA, and prognosis. Specifically, the progression of the condition in the patient's right eye was rapid and severe, whereas the left eye presented a more latent and benign condition. The patient initially developed CSC in the left eye, which evolved into a neovascular membrane. This condition subsequently occurred in the right eye, rapidly progressing to the final stage but with a CNV that had aneurysmal characteristics.

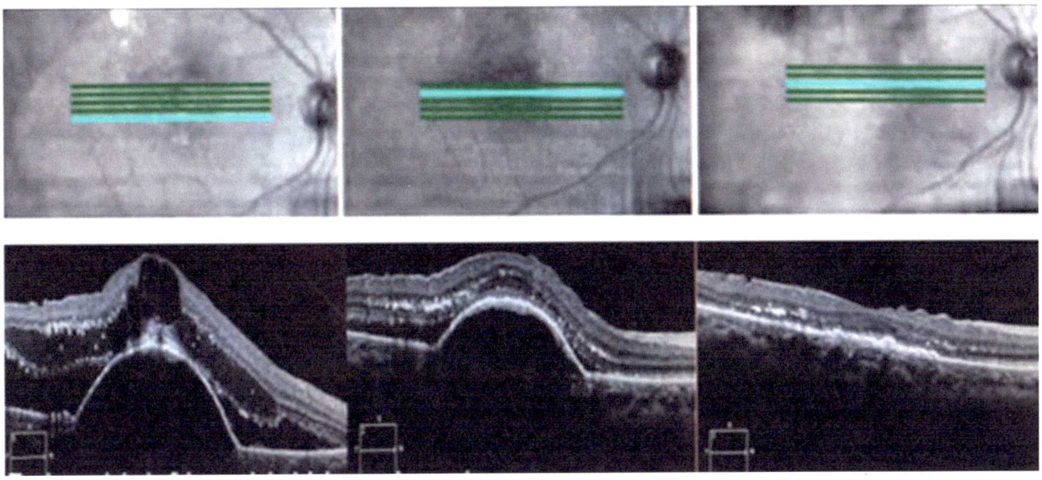

Fig. (15). SD-OCT of polypoidal choroidal vasculopathy before and after treatment. This image was originally published on the Retina Image Bank® website. Author –Aristofanes Canamary Jr, M.D. Photographer –Fábio Canamary. Retina Image Bank. Jan 31, 2019; 28843. © the American Society of Retina Specialists.

In addition, in making a differential diagnosis between retinal angiomatous proliferation (RAP) in AMD and the pachychoroid spectrum (Fig. **16**), genetic factors constitute an important characteristic of these diseases [22, 23]. Hwang, D.DJ. *et al.* [24]. have published recent advances in deep learning technology, such as convolutional neural networks (CNNs), providing a new technological retinal image acquisition with a high accuracy level in detecting retinal diseases such as PCV. (Fig. **16**) illustrates the main PCV characteristics that differentiate them from RAP characteristics using a deep CNN model that uses OCT scans. Additionally, using gradient-weighted class activation mapping (Grad-CAM) heat maps, specific features determined by the proposed model were visualized to facilitate the understanding of structural differences between RAP and PCV [25].

As proposed by Yamashiro *et al.* [26], complement factor H (CFH) appears to be a key gene; the CFH rs800292 G allele acts as a risk gene for AMD development and is protective against pachychoroid spectrum diseases, whereas the CFH rs800292 A allele has the opposite effect [9]. The reason why an allele can be protective in one disease and a risk factor for another is unknown. ARMS2/HTRA1 is the second susceptibility gene related to drusen formation and is a risk factor for AMD while being protective against CSC [27]. Additionally, this gene is associated only with severe PCV and not with mild PCV. These novel genetic concepts support that the pachychoroid spectrum is a different entity from AMD and is not genetically exclusive. Other components contribute to the multifactorial nature of these diseases by combining the genetic basis with environmental factors.

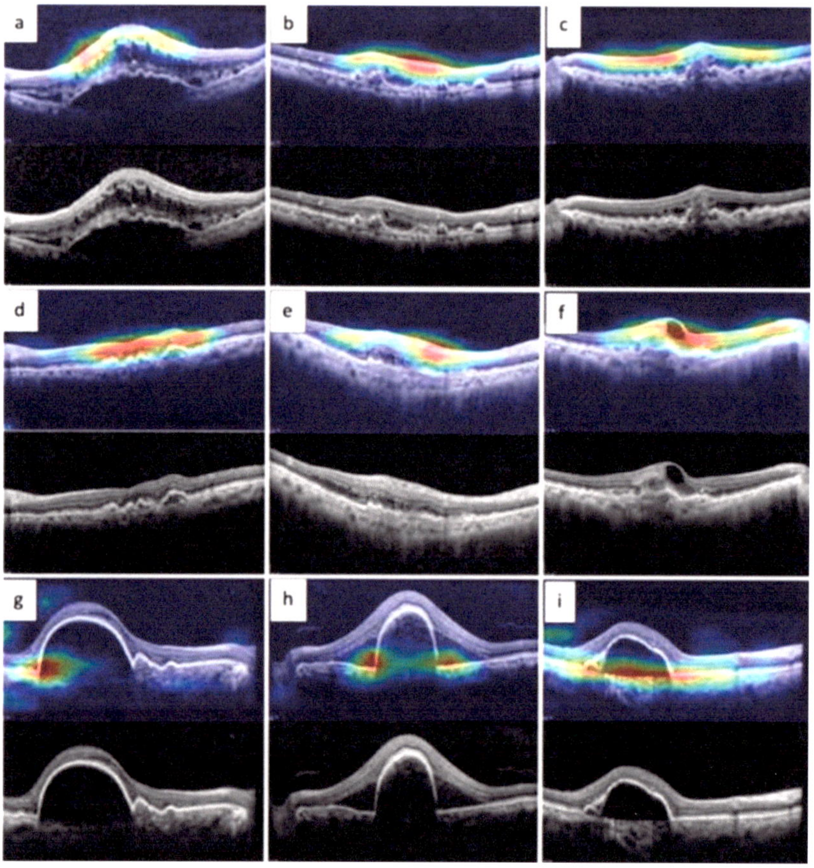

Fig. (16). Gradient-weighted class activation mapping (Grad-CAM) of the model for six RAP images (a) to (f) and three PCV images (g) to (i). The Grad-CAM images display the heat maps of regions used by the model for classifying polypoidal choroidal vasculopathy (PCV) and retinal angiomatous proliferation (RAP) images. Grad-CAM was able to identify pathologic regions on the spectral-domain optical coherence tomography images. In PCV cases, Grad-CAM emphasized the sharp edge of the steeper retinal pigment epithelial detachment (RPED). In one of these PCV cases, the Bruch membrane directly under the RPED was also emphasized. Grad-CAM, gradient-weighted class activation mapping. This multipanel unchanged figure was taken from Hwang. D:DJ *et al.* [21], and is used under the Creative Commons Attribution 4.0 International License (https://creativecommons.org/licenses/by/4.0/).

There is no well-established difference between the management of neovascular AMD and pachychoroid spectrum diseases, as anti-VEGF injection is effective for both. However, an inferior response is typically observed when an increase in choroidal thickness is present. Anti-VEGF drugs are effective as monotherapy for PCV by improving patients' visual acuity, but they have minimal impact on reducing polyps compared with photodynamic therapy (PDT) alone or combined [4]. The treat-and-extend anti-VEGF regimen is the first-line treatment for PNV, with PDT reserved for treating chronic or recurrent fluid accumulation that induces choroidal hypoperfusion [9]. Anti-VEGF therapy has also been shown to reduce choroidal thickness without significantly improving visual acuity [28]. Additionally, multiple studies have found VEGF levels to be much lower in pachychoroid disease than in wet AMD [29, 30], suggesting that VEGF may play a less significant role in the pathology.

More recently, subthreshold micropulse laser (SML) therapy has gained recognition as an alternative to PDT and anti-VEGF for CSCs with the advantage of inflicting less damage to the RPE [31, 32]. SML is thought to improve RPE metabolism and function while decreasing subretinal fluid accumulation and VEGF levels. Although studies thus far suggest that SML is effective and safe, outcomes may be limited in eyes with more advanced RPE defects [33]. Moreover, SML may also be therapeutic in the management of PNV; however, to date, no studies have been conducted to evaluate this application.

CONCLUDING REMARKS

In summary, the differential diagnoses of CNV are extensive, ranging from degenerative etiologies to less common and specific causes. Currently, multimodal imaging is the best tool to differentiate between these diseases and determine an idiopathic etiology. Evaluation of the thickness and characteristics of the choroid must be performed to exclude pachychoroid spectrum diseases. Keeping this spectrum in mind can avoid the misdiagnosis of AMD and provide a more accurate prediction of treatment response and prognosis.

PATIENT CONSENT

Written informed consent in accordance with the institutional guidelines was obtained from all the patients.

LIST OF ABBREVIATIONS

AMD Age-related macular degeneration

BVN Branching vascular network

BCVA Best-corrected visual acuity

CNV	Choroidal neovascularization
CSC	Central serous chorioretinopathy
CFH	Complement factor H
CNNs	Convolutional neural networks
EDI-OCT	Enhanced depth imaging OCT
EZ	Ellipsoid zone
FCE	Focal choroidal excavation
FFA	Fundus fluorescein angiography
Grad-CAM	Gradient-weighted class activation mapping
ICGA	Indocyanine green angiography
OCT-A	OCT angiography
PNV	Pachychoroid neovasculopathy
PED	Pigmentary epithelium detachments
PCV	Polypoidal choroidal vasculopathy
PDT	Photodynamic therapy
PNV	Pachychoroid neovasculopathy
PPE	Pachychoroid pigment epitheliopathy
PPS	Peripapillary pachychoroid syndrome
RAP	Retinal angiomatous proliferation
RPED	Retinal pigment epithelial detachment
SML	Subthreshold micropulse laser
SS-OCT	Swept-source optical coherent tomography
VEGF	Vascular endothelial growth factor

DISCLAIMER

All scientific comments issued in this chapter are solely the responsibility of the authors and not of the institutions with which they are affiliated.

ACKNOWLEDGMENTS

We express our deep appreciation to the technical staff of the Retina Specialists Unit at Oftalmologia Integral ABC (Nonprofit Medical and Surgical Organization) and Instituto de Oftalmologia, Fundacion Conde de Valenciana, Mexico City, Mexico, which are affiliated with The Postgraduate Division Studies at the National Autonomous University of Mexico.

REFERENCES

[1] Akkaya S. Spectrum of pachychoroid diseases. Int Ophthalmol 2018; 38(5): 2239-46. [http://dx.doi.org/10.1007/s10792-017-0666-4] [PMID: 28766279]

[2] Borooah S, Sim PY, Phatak S, *et al.* Pachychoroid spectrum disease. Acta Ophthalmol 2021; 99(6): e806-22. [http://dx.doi.org/10.1111/aos.14683] [PMID: 33258304]

[3] Chang YC, Cheng CK. Difference between pachychoroid and nonpachychoroid polypoidal choroidal vasculopathy and their response to anti–vascular endothelial growth factor therapy. Retina 2020; 40(7): 1403-11. [http://dx.doi.org/10.1097/IAE.0000000000002583] [PMID: 31181038]

[4] Cheung CMG, Lai TYY, Ruamviboonsuk P, *et al.* Polypoidal choroidal vasculopathy. Ophthalmology 2018; 125(5): 708-24. [http://dx.doi.org/10.1016/j.ophtha.2017.11.019] [PMID: 29331556]

[5] Moraru A, Costin D, Moraru R, Costuleanu M, Brănișteanu D. Current diagnosis and management strategies in pachychoroid spectrum of diseases (Review). Exp Ther Med 2020; 20(4): 3528-35. [http://dx.doi.org/10.3892/etm.2020.9094] [PMID: 32905090]

[6] Yanagi Y. Pachychoroid disease: A new perspective on exudative maculopathy. Jpn J Ophthalmol 2020; 64(4): 323-37. [http://dx.doi.org/10.1007/s10384-020-00740-5] [PMID: 32318919]

[7] Cheung CMG, Lee WK, Koizumi H, Dansingani K, Lai TYY, Freund KB. Pachychoroid disease. Eye 2019; 33(1): 14-33. [http://dx.doi.org/10.1038/s41433-018-0158-4] [PMID: 29995841]

[8] Demirel S, Değirmenci MFK, Batıoğlu F, Özmert E. Evaluation of the choroidal features in pachychoroid spectrum diseases by optical coherence tomography and optical coherence tomography angiography. Eur J Ophthalmol 2021; 31(1): 184-93. [http://dx.doi.org/10.1177/1120672119887095] [PMID: 31684767]

[9] Sartini F, Figus M, Casini G, Nardi M, Posarelli C. Pachychoroid neovasculopathy: A type-1 choroidal neovascularization belonging to the pachychoroid spectrum—pathogenesis, imaging and available treatment options. Int Ophthalmol 2020; 40(12): 3577-89. [http://dx.doi.org/10.1007/s10792-020-01522-1] [PMID: 32729062]

[10] Pang CE, Freund KB. Pachychoroid neovasculopathy. Retina 2015; 35(1): 1-9. [http://dx.doi.org/10.1097/IAE.0000000000000331] [PMID: 25158945]

[11] Spaide RF, Jaffe GJ, Sarraf D, *et al.* Consensus nomenclature for reporting neovascular age-related macular degeneration data. Ophthalmology 2020; 127(5): 616-36. [http://dx.doi.org/10.1016/j.ophtha.2019.11.004] [PMID: 31864668]

[12] Keidel LF, Schworm B, Priglinger SG, Siedlecki J. Pachychoroid neovasculopathy disguising as age-related macular degeneration treated by spironolactone and anti-vegf combination therapy. Case Rep Ophthalmol 2021; 12(1): 116-23. [http://dx.doi.org/10.1159/000510828] [PMID: 33976667]

[13] Gallego-Pinazo R, Dolz-Marco R, Gómez-Ulla F, Mrejen S, Freund KB. Pachychoroid diseases of the macula. Med Hypothesis Discov Innov Ophthalmol 2014; 3(4): 111-5. [PMID: 25756060]

[14] Wang M, Zhou Y, Gao SS, *et al.* Evaluating polypoidal choroidal vasculopathy with optical coherence tomography angiography. Invest Ophthalmol Vis Sci 2016; 57(9): OCT526-32. [http://dx.doi.org/10.1167/iovs.15-18955] [PMID: 27472276]

[15] Iu LPL, Chan HY, Ho M, *et al.* The contemporary role of photodynamic therapy in the treatment of pachychoroid diseases. J Ophthalmol 2021; 2021: 1-9. [http://dx.doi.org/10.1155/2021/6590230] [PMID: 34725570]

[16] Bautista-Barba A, Andres Quiroz-Gonzalez E, Angel Quiroz-Reyes M, *et al.* Optical coherence tomography as an alternative for diagnosing polypoidal choroidal vasculopathy in developing countries. Int J Ophthalm Vis Sci 2021; 6(4): 219.
[http://dx.doi.org/10.11648/j.ijovs.20210604.17]

[17] Cheung CMG, Lai TYY, Teo K, *et al.* Polypoidal choroidal vasculopathy. Ophthalmology 2021; 128(3): 443-52.
[http://dx.doi.org/10.1016/j.ophtha.2020.08.006] [PMID: 32795496]

[18] Eraydin B, Koçak N, Birinci H. The comparison of spectral domain optical coherence tomography and indocyanine green angiography in the diagnosis of polypoidal choroidal vasculopathy. Int Ophthalmol 2021; 41(2): 659-65.
[http://dx.doi.org/10.1007/s10792-020-01622-y] [PMID: 33057916]

[19] Demirel S, Yanık Ö, Nalcı H, Batıoğlu F, Özmert E. The use of optical coherence tomography angiography in pachychoroid spectrum diseases: A concurrent comparison with dye angiography. Graefes Arch Clin Exp Ophthalmol 2017; 255(12): 2317-24.
[http://dx.doi.org/10.1007/s00417-017-3793-8] [PMID: 28891028]

[20] Liu ZY, Li B, Xia S, Chen YX. Analysis of choroidal morphology and comparison of imaging findings of subtypes of polypoidal choroidal vasculopathy: A new classification system. Int J Ophthalmol 2020; 13(5): 731-6.
[http://dx.doi.org/10.18240/ijo.2020.05.06] [PMID: 32420219]

[21] Jang JW, Kim JM, Kang SW, Kim SJ, Bae K, Kim KT. Typical polypoidal choroidal vasculopathy and polypoidal choroidal neovascularization. Retina 2019; 39(10): 1995-2003.
[http://dx.doi.org/10.1097/IAE.0000000000002259] [PMID: 30024574]

[22] Lehmann M, Bousquet E, Beydoun T, Behar-Cohen F. PACHYCHOROID: An inherited condition? Retina 2015; 35(1): 10-6.
[http://dx.doi.org/10.1097/IAE.0000000000000287] [PMID: 25046398]

[23] DeAngelis MM, Owen LA, Morrison MA, *et al.* Genetics of age-related macular degeneration (AMD). Hum Mol Genet 2017; 26(R1): R45-50.
[http://dx.doi.org/10.1093/hmg/ddx228] [PMID: 28854576]

[24] Hwang DDJ, Choi S, Ko J, *et al.* Distinguishing retinal angiomatous proliferation from polypoidal choroidal vasculopathy with a deep neural network based on optical coherence tomography. Sci Rep 2021; 11(1): 9275.
[http://dx.doi.org/10.1038/s41598-021-88543-7] [PMID: 33927240]

[25] Selvaraju RR, Cogswell M, Das A, Vedantam R, Parikh D, Batra D. Grad-CAM: Visual Explanations from Deep Networks *via* Gradient-Based Localization, 2017 IEEE International Conference on Computer Vision (ICCV), Venice, Italy 2017; 618-26.
[http://dx.doi.org/10.1109/ICCV.2017.74.1]

[26] Yamashiro K, Hosoda Y, Miyake M, Ooto S, Tsujikawa A. Characteristics of pachychoroid diseases and age-related macular degeneration: Multimodal imaging and genetic backgrounds. J Clin Med 2020; 9(7): 2034.
[http://dx.doi.org/10.3390/jcm9072034] [PMID: 32610483]

[27] Miyake M, Ooto S, Yamashiro K, *et al.* Pachychoroid neovasculopathy and age-related macular degeneration. Sci Rep 2015; 5(1): 16204.
[http://dx.doi.org/10.1038/srep16204] [PMID: 26542071]

[28] Shimizu Y, Miyata M, Ooto S, *et al.* Pachychoroid-phenotype effects on 5-year visual outcomes of anti-VEGF monotherapy in polypoidal choroidal vasculopathy. Acta Ophthalmol 2022; 100(4): e943-9.
[http://dx.doi.org/10.1111/aos.15015] [PMID: 34533280]

[29] Hata M, Yamashiro K, Ooto S, *et al.* Intraocular vascular endothelial growth factor levels in

pachychoroid neovasculopathy and neovascular age-related macular degeneration. Invest Ophthalmol Vis Sci 2017; 58(1): 292-8.
[http://dx.doi.org/10.1167/iovs.16-20967] [PMID: 28114590]

[30] Terao N, Koizumi H, Kojima K, *et al.* Distinct aqueous humour cytokine profiles of patients with pachychoroid neovasculopathy and neovascular age-related macular degeneration. Sci Rep 2018; 8(1): 10520.
[http://dx.doi.org/10.1038/s41598-018-28484-w] [PMID: 30002400]

[31] Long H, Liu M, Hu Q, Li X. 577 nm subthreshold micropulse laser treatment for acute central serous chorioretinopathy: A comparative study. BMC Ophthalmol 2022; 22(1): 105.
[http://dx.doi.org/10.1186/s12886-022-02330-0] [PMID: 35248003]

[32] Zhou L, Lai K, Jin L, *et al.* Subthreshold micropulse laser vs. conventional laser for central serous chorioretinopathy: A randomized controlled clinical trial. Front Med 2021; 8: 682264.
[http://dx.doi.org/10.3389/fmed.2021.682264] [PMID: 34336888]

[33] Kaymak H, Funk S, Fricke A, *et al.* Efficacy of nanosecond laser treatment in central serous chorioretinopathy with and without atrophy of retinal pigment epithelium. Int J Retina Vitreous 2020; 6(1): 11.
[http://dx.doi.org/10.1186/s40942-020-00214-3] [PMID: 32518690]

CHAPTER 6

The Current Role of OCTA in the Management of Pathological Choroidal Neovascularization with Anti-VEGF Therapy

Miguel A. Quiroz-Reyes, MD[1,*], **Zixuan Shao**[2] and **Erick A. Quiroz-Gonzalez**[1,3]

[1] *Oftalmologia Integral ABC, Retina Department, Medical and Surgical Assistance Institution (Nonprofit Organization), Affiliated with the Postgraduate Studies Division, National Autonomous University of Mexico, Mexico City, Mexico*

[2] *Division of Chemistry and Chemical Engineering, California Institute of Technology, Pasadena, CA, USA*

[3] *Institute of Ophthalmology, Fundacion Conde de Valenciana, Private Assistance Institution (Nonprofit organization), Mexico City, Mexico*

Abstract: Optical coherence tomography angiography (OCT-A) is an emerging technology that captures flow motion within the retinal vasculature to produce angiograms. Compared to dye-based angiography techniques, OCTA is a noninvasive and fast method that enables detailed visualization of the vasculature, which is not easily observable using previously available techniques. Over the past decade, OCT-A has been used to characterize the pathological features of choroidal neovascularization (CNV) associated with several retinal diseases, including neovascular age-related macular degeneration (AMD). In eyes at risk of developing CNV, OCT-A has demonstrated the capability to detect subclinical signs of neovascularization (NV) that may enable early treatment and better visual outcomes. Various CNV conditions are now routinely treated with intravitreal injections of anti-vascular endothelial growth factor (anti-VEGF). OCT-A was used to identify the characteristics of CNV at various stages, before and after anti-VEGF therapy. Although preliminary, OCT-A has demonstrated the potential to help guide treatment decisions in CNV cases that respond differently to anti-VEGF therapy.

Despite its multiple advantages and applications, the clinical use of OCT-A remains limited. OCT-A has several limitations, including visualization of a small area, the presence of artifacts, and results that are challenging to interpret. However, OCTA technology continues to advance as some of the early limitations have been resolved. Overall, OCT-A promises to be a significant step forward in our current ability to

* **Corresponding author Miguel A. Quiroz-Reyes, MD:** Oftalmologia Integral ABC, Retina Department, Medical and Surgical Assistance Institution (Nonprofit Organization), Affiliated with the Postgraduate Studies Division, National Autonomous University of Mexico, Mexico City, Mexico; Tel.: +52 55 5217 2732; Fax: +52 55 1664 7180; E-mails: drquiroz@prodigy.net.mx and drquirozreyes7@gmail.com

visualize pathological CNV, and has the potential to improve both the diagnosis and management of a variety of retinal diseases.

Keywords: Age-related macular degeneration, Anti–vascular endothelial growth factor, Myopic choroidal neovascularization, Central serous chorioretinopathy, Choroidal neovascularization, Geographic atrophy, Ischemic macula, Optical coherence tomography angiography, Pathological choroidal neovascularization, Type I and Type II choroidal neovascularization, Vascular endothelial growth factor.

INTRODUCTION

Choroidal neovascularization (CNV) is characterized by abnormal blood vessel growth from the choroidal vasculature through Brunch's membrane into the retina. The majority of CNV cases are observed in neovascular age-related macular degeneration (AMD); however, CNV can also be found in numerous other conditions, including myopic degeneration, chronic central serous chorioretinopathy, and choroidal tumors. CNV consists of clusters of ill-developed immature vessels that are prone to fluid leakage, leading to retinal edema and hemorrhage that subsequently cause a rapid decline in visual function. Among the biological factors involved in this process, the vascular endothelial growth factor (VEGF) plays a central role in stimulating and sustaining pathological angiogenesis in the retina [1]. Thus, targeting VEGF has become a central strategy in the treatment of multiple retinal conditions characterized by abnormal angiogenesis and fluid exudation.

CNV is currently routinely managed by anti-VEGF drugs that have largely replaced earlier treatment options such as laser photocoagulation and photodynamic therapy [2]. Anti-VEGF drugs are typically administered via intravitreal injection into the vitreous, whereas the more recent approval of Susvimo provides a refillable, implantable delivery option with slow drug release for up to six months [3]. Mechanistically, anti-VEGF blocks the activity of VEGF protein to reduce fluid leakage and rescue vision loss. However, continued treatment is needed to optimize visual outcomes, and cases with persistent fluid despite intervention are frequently observed [1].

Optical coherence tomography (OCT) was first developed in the early 1990s and is currently widely used for the diagnosis and management of retinal diseases [4]. OCT's popularity of OCT can be attributed to its non-invasive characteristics while simultaneously capturing high-resolution, cross-sectional images of the retina and surrounding tissues. These characteristics make OCT particularly valuable in diagnosing retinal diseases where microscopic observation of the tissue through biopsy is not available [5].

In principle, OCT images are obtained by casting light that is divided into reference and sample beams to obtain a reflectivity versus depth profile for the retina. Specifically, the retina backscatters light waves, which interfere with the reference beam and create interference patterns that can be used to derive the light echoes versus the depth profile of the retina *in vivo* [4].

OCT technology has evolved substantially over the past three decades since its introduction. The initial instruments available used time-domain OCT technology (TD-OCT) technology, which has a very slow imaging speed and poor image quality [5]. It was not until the introduction of the first commercially available spectral domain OCT (SD-OCT) in 2006 that the adaptation of OCT truly took off [6]. SD-OCT uses a Fourier domain detection technique and improves TD-OCT with substantial upgrades in both imaging speed and image quality, reaching a level of detail that parallels histopathology [7].

Swept-source OCT (SS-OCT) is another modern OCT technology that uses a Fourier domain detection technique [5]. Unlike SD-OCT, which utilizes a near-infrared broadband light source and a combination of a spectrometer and a high-speed line-scan camera as the detector system, SS-OCT uses a rapidly sweeping tunable laser and a point photodetector as the detector [5, 8]. Compared to SD-OCT, SS-OCT is much faster in scan acquisition, reaching speeds of up to 400 thousand A-scans/second, which enables longer B-scans for widefield imaging [9, 10]. Additionally, SS-OCT platforms use a light source centered at a longer wavelength than SD-OCT (1050 nm *vs.* 840 nm in SD-OCT), allowing better tissue penetration and clearer visualization of the choroid and lamina cribrosa. However, longer wavelengths also reduce the image resolution, which becomes more severe in certain cases, such as in the presence of a thickened choroid or drusen. Additionally, SD-OCT's ability to image the outer retina can be improved with enhanced depth imaging (EDI) technologies that are available in all modern machines. Overall, the current rate of adoption of SS-OCT remains limited, mainly because of its high cost and lack of clear advantages over SD-OCT [11].

First commercialized in 2014, OCT angiography (OCT-A) is a relatively new technology that captures flow motion within the retinal and choroidal vasculature without using conventional contrast agents [12]. Unlike standard structural OCT, OCTA analyzes temporal changes in the OCT signal in addition to reflected light [13]. Through repeated B-scans at the same retinal location, OCT-A can isolate the temporal scattering changes caused by erythrocytes moving through vessels, and use the resultant fluctuation in the OCT signal to generate angiographic images [14]. This process can be repeated over consecutive locations to create volumetric visualization of the retinal vasculature [15]. It is worth emphasizing that blood vessels with slow or obstructed flow may be missed on OCT-A due to a lack of erythrocyte migration, which is a requirement for detection [16]. Vessels at greater retinal depths or aligned with the optical beam are also more difficult to visualize [17], but various processing approaches have been proposed to improve visualization [14].

There are four main OCT-A devices currently available: two based on SD-OCT technology (Optovue Avanti with Angiovue by Visionix and Spectralis OCT-A by Heidelberg Engineering) and two based on SS-OCT technology (Plex Elite by Carl Zeiss Meditec and Triton by Topcon). Among these, SS-OCT machines have higher scanning speeds (100,000-200,000 A-scans/sec *vs.* 70,000-85,000 A-scans/sec in SD-OCT) and field of view (45-56° *vs.* 30-40° in SD-OCT) but lack in axial resolution (6.3-8μm *vs.* 3.9-5μm in SD-OCT) [10]. Other companies that provide products with OCT-A capabilities include Canon, Optopol, and Nidek [14].

Before the advent of OCT-A, visualization of the retinal microvasculature typically relied on fluorescein angiography and indocyanine green angiography (Fig. **1**) [12]. These techniques are invasive procedures that require intravenous injection of the dye that subsequently travels to the eye to enable detection [18]. Additionally, these imaging techniques generate a 2-dimensional view of the retinal vasculature and are not compatible with more segmented visualization of the individual retinal capillary plexuses (deep retinal capillaries and choriocapillaris are not clearly visualized). Furthermore, the dye-based angiography approach is relatively expensive and time-consuming, limiting its repeatability in the longitudinal management of diseases. Although rare, the dyes used are also associated with side effects, such as allergic reactions, nausea, and even life-threatening anaphylaxis [18].

In comparison, OCT-A is a noninvasive technique that produces en face images that can be easily scrolled to visualize various retinal layers, including the choriocapillaris, to visualize the structure of CNV (Fig. **2**). In a study of 80 eyes that presented with a variety of CNV in neovascular AMD eyes, a high 90-95% concordance was identified between treatment diagnoses using OCT-A and traditional multimodal imaging techniques (fluorescein angiography, indocyanine green angiography, and OCT) [19]. Another study found a lower agreement (80%) among 30 eyes imaged using both OCT-A and fluorescein angiography [20]. These findings were corroborated by a study by Soomro and Talks, which also concluded that OCT-A was useful in diagnosing cases where evidence of CNV was inconclusive following conventional dye-based angiography [21]. A meta-analysis conducted in 2022 consisting of seven primary studies found both high sensitivity and specificity for the diagnostic accuracy of OCT-A in identifying CNV in AMD [22]. Notably, OCT-A has been reported to be slightly less consistent in the diagnosis of CNV in central serous chorioretinopathy [23]. Overall, OCT-A's ability of OCT-A to generate a substantial volume of data on the retinal vasculature in vivo without invasive dye injection has propelled its wide use in both academic research and clinical management of retinal diseases.

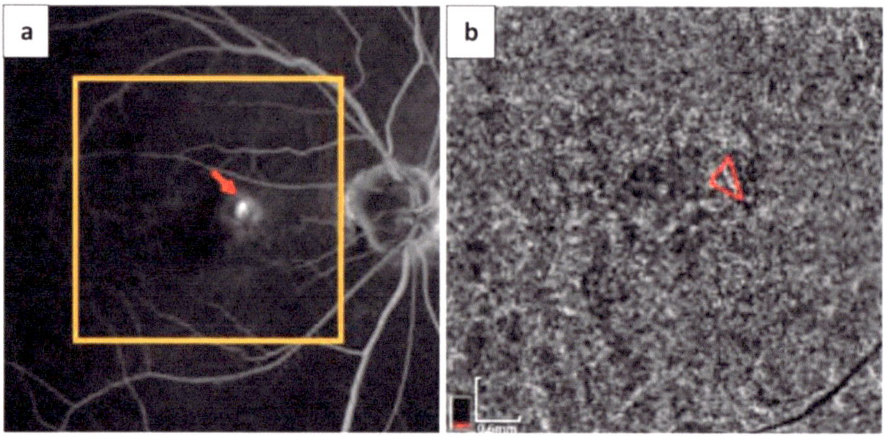

Fig. (1). Comparison of (**a**) fluorescein angiography and (**b**) optical coherence tomography angiography (OCTA) images. (**a**) Dye leakage on fluorescein angiography (red arrow) reveals the location of choroidal neovascularization. The orange square represents the smaller 3x3 mm area that is typically imaged by OCTA. (**b**) The CNV is detected after choroidal segmentation. This modified copyright-free figure was obtained from Cheng, Lin, Hsiao, and Chang. Detection of Choroidal Neovascularization by Optical Coherence Tomography Angiography with Assistance from Use of the Image Segmentation Method. *Appl. Sci.* **2020**, *10*, 137. https://doi.org/10.3390/app10010137 and is used under the Creative Commons Attribution 4.0 International License (https://creativecommons.org/licenses/by/4.0/).

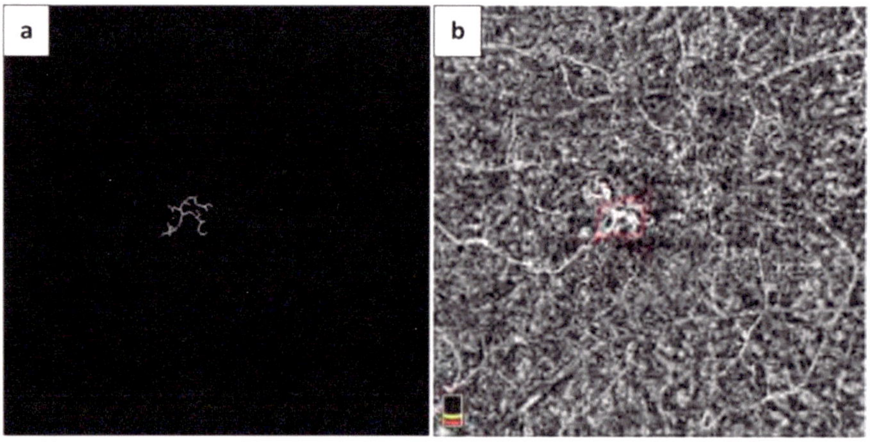

Fig. (2). Processed optical coherence tomography angiography (OCT-A) images of choroidal neovascularization (CNV). (**a**) Digitally image skeletonization of CNV branches. (**b**) The resulting digital deep CNV OCTA image. This modified copyright-free figure was obtained from Cheng; Lin; Hsiao; and Chang. Detection of Choroidal Neovascularization by Optical Coherence Tomography Angiography with Assistance from Use of the Image Segmentation Method. *Appl. Sci.***2020**, *10*, 137. https://doi.org/10.3390/app10010137 and is used under the Creative Commons Attribution 4.0 International License (https://creativecommons.org/licenses/by/4.0/).

IMAGING WITH OCTA

Several OCT-A systems are commercially available, including the popular Optovue Avanti (Optovue Inc., Fremont, California, USA; now Visonix, Chartres, France). At the simplest level, the OCTA machine obtains B-scans and uses built-in software to build a merged 3-dimensional OCT angiogram. The software was also designed to correct for background noise, which may arise from a variety of sources, including eye movements. Additional algorithms can evaluate the obtained data and calculate sets of perfusion indices for different retinal sections: superficial plexus, deep plexus, outer retina, and choriocapillaris [18]. Furthermore, perfusion indices are separately calculated in both the parafoveal and perifoveal areas, which automatically exclude the foveal avascular zone (FAZ). Separately, the FAZ area can be quantified and reported using this software.

When used in healthy subjects, OCT-A produces high-quality angiograms that are similar to conventional fluorescein angiography [24]. In a study of 52 healthy eyes, Savastano *et al.* used OCTA to observe two separate vascular networks in the inner retina (superficial and deep networks) that are connected by vertical vessels [25]. This application demonstrates OCTA's ability of OCT-A to differentiate various layers of the retinal vasculature and characterize finer details, including interconnecting vessels between layers. Another study by Samara *et al.* evaluated the FAZ area and found it to be quite variable in normal subjects, ranging from 0.071 to 0.527 mm^2 in the superficial plexus and 0.160 to 0.795 mm^2 in the deep plexus [26]. Additionally, the FAZ area in both plexuses showed inverse correlations with central macular volume and thickness, and no correlation with either age or sex. The FAZ area in the deep plexus is significantly larger than that in the superficial plexus. These applications of OCT-A demonstrate its ability to enable the visualization and qualification of the retinal vasculature at levels not previously obtainable.

VISUALIZATION OF CNV IN AMD

Neovascular AMD

Neovascular AMD accounts for approximately 15% of all AMD cases but accounts for the majority of cases with significant visual impairment. Neovascular AMD is classified into three types based on CNV location [18]. Type I CNV emerges from the choroid and resides between Bruch's membrane and the retinal pigment epithelium (RPE). Type II CNV expands between the RPE and retina, whereas Type III CNV originates from the choroid and progresses into the retina to form a retinal-choroidal anastomosis. CNV can also be classified based on their branching morphology (Fig. **3**).

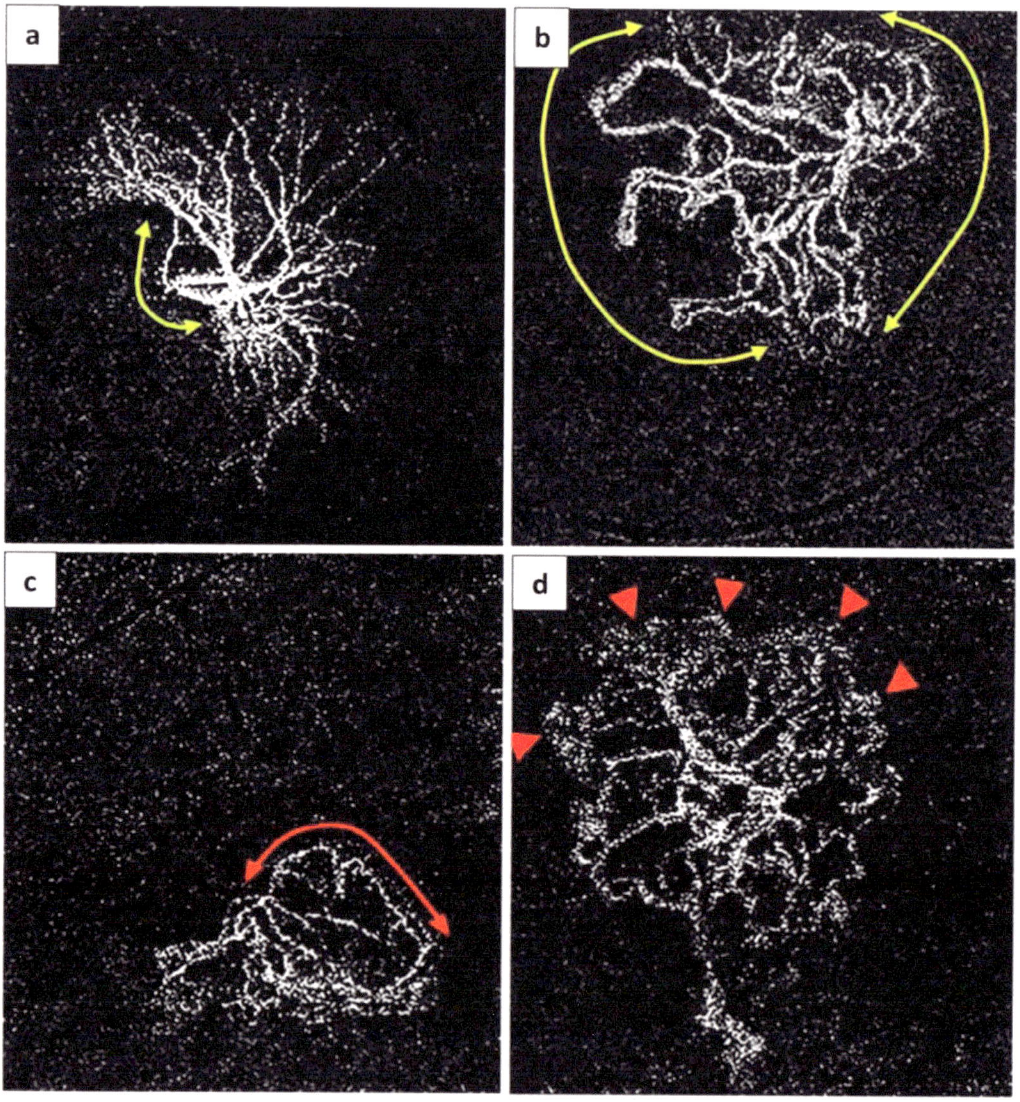

Fig. (3). Choroidal neovascularization (CNV) can be classified into two main types of the optical coherence tomography angiography (OCTA): (**a**) CNV with an open circuit and (**b**) CNV with a closed circuit. An open circuit is characterized by less anastomotic vessels bounding the exterior border of the lesion (yellow lines with arrows), while a closed circuit is the opposite. CNV can also be characterized to have either (**c**) a peripheral loop (red line with red arrows) or (**d**) capillary fringe (red arrowheads). This modified copyright-free figure was obtained from Bae, Kim, Shin, and Kang. Predictors of neovascular activity during neovascular age-related macular degeneration treatment based on optical coherence tomography angiography. Scientific reports. (2019) 9:19240 | https://doi.org/10.1038/s41598-019-55871-8 is used under the Creative Commons Attribution 4.0 International License (https://creativecommons.org/licenses/by/4.0/).

In one of the first published accounts of OCTA usage in the evaluation of CNV, Jia et al. reported that OCTA revealed more distinct patterns in the vasculature that were not obscured by coexisting subretinal hemorrhages [27]. All CNV cases in thc study had reduced choroidal flow next to the neovascularization (NV), with one case showing significantly lower flow. Additionally, the flow index computed from the en face OCT angiogram of the outer retinal layer was higher in cases with larger CNV and type II CNV.

In another study, 72 eyes (48 eyes with CNV and 24 eyes without CNV) were imaged using OCT-A and compared with conventional fluorescein angiography [20]. Among the 48 eyes with CNV, 31 had CNV associated with neovascular AMD, 71% (22/31) of which had subretinal fluid, intraretinal fluid, and poorly circumscribed vessels. Additionally, seven eyes had CNV-associated subretinal fluid buildup (central serous chorioretinopathy). Thirty eyes were imaged using both OCTA and fluorescein angiography, demonstrating a sensitivity of 50% (4/8) and a high specificity of 91% (20/22).

Ameen et al. published an early investigation of Type II CNV in patients with neovascular AMD using OCT-A [28]. In this study, 14 eyes were imaged and diagnosed with Type II CNV, which was characterized by the presence of hyperflow lesions in the outer retina. These neovascular retinas exhibited glomerulus-shaped (4/14 eyes) or medusa-shaped (10/14 eyes) lesions, surrounded by a dark halo. Interestingly, lesions were also observed in the choriocapillaris layer, which was connected to the retinal lesions via thick main branches in 10/14 eyes. No abnormal flow was detected in the superficial layer or deep retina on OCT-A images. Unlike fluorescein angiography, this study showed that OCT-A's ability to segment the retina can reveal key features of CNV that are not easily obtained with conventional techniques.

Unlike the other two types, Type III CNV expands into the retina and forms chorioretinal anastomosis. OCTA has been used to study 29 eyes with Type III CNV in neovascular AMD patients [29]. In approximately one-third of the eyes (10/29, 34%), distinct neovascular complexes appeared as small clusters of small vessels in the outer retinal layers. Intriguingly, these vessels were connected to the inner retinal vasculature via feeder vessels, demonstrating interconnected vasculature in some CNV cases. In another report by the same group, OCT-A evaluation of 18 eyes with type 3 CNV identified lesions that emerged from the deep capillary plexus and formed tuft shaped vasculature that extended to the subretinal pigment epithelium layer [30]. Lesions were also reported in the choriocapillaris layer, with some being connected to the choroid by small vessels (Fig. **4**).

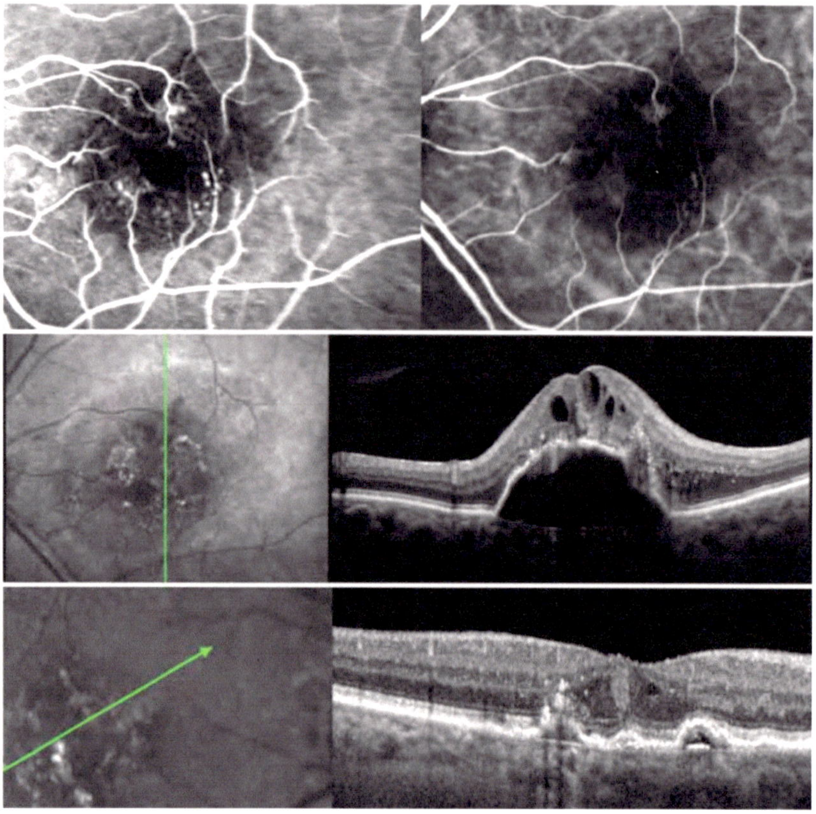

Fig. (4). Retinal angiomatous proliferation (RAP) is a unique variant of neovascular age-related macular degeneration. Up to 15% of patients with neovascular age-related macular degeneration have RAP. Clinical characteristics associated with RAP include bilateral disease, the presence of pigment epithelial detachments, and pseudodrusen. RAP is more frequently associated with the development of retinal pigment epithelial tears and geographic atrophy that can lead to severe vision loss. This unchanged composite figure depicts a stereo fluorescein angiography and ICG (upper right and left image, respectively) and OCT of the left and right eye (middle and inferior image) of a RAP choroidal neovascularization in an 89-year-old patient. This image was originally published in the Retina Image Bank® website. Author -Rafael Reis Pereira, MD. Co-authors - Andre Maya, MD and Gabriel Andrade, MD. Retina Clinic. Retina Image Bank. 51777. © The American Society of Retina Specialists.

Patients with pre-existing CNV in one eye are at a significantly higher risk of developing CNV in the fellow eye [31, 32]. Therefore, it is important to identify subclinical CNV in the fellow eye, which may progress into clinical cases. OCT-A was used to determine the presence of subclinical CNV in the fellow eyes of 34 patients with unilateral neovascular AMD [33]. OCTA revealed a notably high prevalence of subclinical CNV in the fellow eyes (5/34, 14.7%). Thus, it may be beneficial to monitor not only the affected eye but also the fellow eye to identify subclinical cases of CNV, to enable early anti-VEGF intervention and possibly better visual outcomes.

It is worth noting that different OCT-A machines may produce varying results in clinical settings. In a cohort of 27 eyes diagnosed with CNV secondary to AMD, SD-OCT-A and SS-OCT-A devices were used consecutively to quantify CNV lesion areas [8]. Between the two machines, the measured areas of CNV were significantly larger with the images captured by SS-OCT-A than with those captured by SD-OCT-A. The authors concluded that SS-OCTA imaging provided a more accurate representation of CNV using indocyanine green angiography as the ground truth. These findings suggest that OCT-A results should be evaluated in the context of the technology and machines used to obtain data.

Dry AMD

Advanced AMD manifests as either exudative AMD (wet AMD) or geographic atrophy (GA). GA is characterized by degeneration of the outer retinal segments, including the photoreceptors, RPE, and choriocapillaris, but without CNV [13]. Although the exact mechanism remains unclear, some cases of GA progress to CNV, whereas others do not, highlighting the importance of early detection in clinical intervention. Advanced degeneration typically present in the retina with GA poses a challenge for the detection of NV by conventional imaging modalities because of significant alterations in the RPE and exposure of choroidal vessels. In contrast, OCTA is very useful in this context to detect the presence of emerging CNV and evaluate the state of the choriocapillaris.

Palejwala *et al.* performed a study of 32 eyes at heightened risk for CNV development, as indicated by the presence of drusen, pigmentary changes, or CNV in the fellow eye [34]. Of the 32 eyes, two (6%) showed signs of Type I CNV on the OCT-A images. These lesions were not associated with fluid on OCT or leakage on fluorescein angiography, which would normally have missed these early signs of CNV. One of the two patients was followed for 8 months without treatment, and slight enlargement of the CNV flow area was noted without fluid buildup on OCT or vision loss.

In another study, de Oliveira Dias et al. used OCT-A to assess 160 patients with dry AMD in one eye and neovascular AMD in the other eye [35]. Of the 160 eyes, 14.4% (23/160 eyes) showed subclinical signs of NV. Furthermore, these eyes exhibited a significantly increased chance of conversion to exudation within 1 year (21.1% in eyes with subclinical NV *vs.* 3.6% in eyes without subclinical NV). Thus, the risk of exudation was significantly higher in eyes with OCT-Adetectable subclinical NV, highlighting the need for more frequent follow-up evaluations in at-risk patients. Collectively, these studies demonstrate the unique capability of OCT-A to identify the early signs of CNV before clinical presentation.

APPLICATION OF OCT-A IN THE MANAGEMENT OF CNV

Anti-VEGF therapy remains the most effective treatment option for CNV, and various groups have demonstrated the use of OCTA to track CNV during the course of anti-VEGF therapy to monitor treatment effectiveness. Spaide et al. provided one of the first reports on the use of OCT-A to monitor CNV treated with anti-VEGF [1]. In 17 eyes that received a mean of 47 intravitreal anti-VEGF injections, OCTA showed large vascular diameters in CNV, even in small lesions. The vessels also displayed few branch points and sparse capillaries but more vascular connections among the larger blood vessels. Blocking VEGF signaling appeared to regress the newly formed vascular sprouts, while sparing the more developed vessels with pericyte coverage. The remaining vessels then expanded in diameter owing to the increased flow after the closure of the newly formed channels (Fig. **5**). Furthermore, more frequent anti-VEGF injections have also been associated with mature CNV, as defined by high vessel density and branching index, capillary sprouting, and anastomosis formation [36]. In this context, mature CNV, as determined by OCT-A angiography, may influence treatment decision-making.

Xu *et al.* described a longitudinal OCT-A evaluation of 41 eyes with Type I CNV treated with anti-VEGF therapy [37]. The patients were followed up for at least one year, enabling long-term assessment of CNV over time. Despite treatment, the majority of eyes (31 eyes, 80%) showed a larger CNV area at 1 year than at baseline. Approximately one-third (11 eyes, 27%) showed a doubling of the CNV area, approximately half exhibited modest growth (19 eyes, 46%), and a marginal minority (6 eyes, 15%) showed a shrunken CNV area. Overall, the mean CNV area increased from 1.60 mm^2 to 1.80 mm^2. Anatomical features, such as the capillary fringe and immature lesion morphology, are associated with CNV doubling. Of the three CNV growth patterns observed (symmetric growth, asymmetric growth, and finger-like projections), symmetric and asymmetric growth patterns correlated with a greater frequency of CNV doubling.

Rispoli *et al.* performed another OCT-A evaluation of 51 eyes with Type I CNV treated with anti-VEGF therapy [38]. These eyes were followed for a long period of time, ranging between 31 months and 58 months (mean, 38.9 months). In this study, CNV cases were observed to follow two patterns of evolution depending on whether their conditions were stabilized (55% of eyes) or continued to progress to fibrosis, chorioretinal atrophy, hemorrhage, and RPE tears (45% of eyes). Similar to previous reports, even in cases in which the disease stabilized or became chronic (requiring repeated anti-VEGF injections), the CNV area continued to grow. In cases that continued to progress, OCT-A revealed that the new vessels also became larger, thicker, and straighter, which is consistent with earlier findings [1].

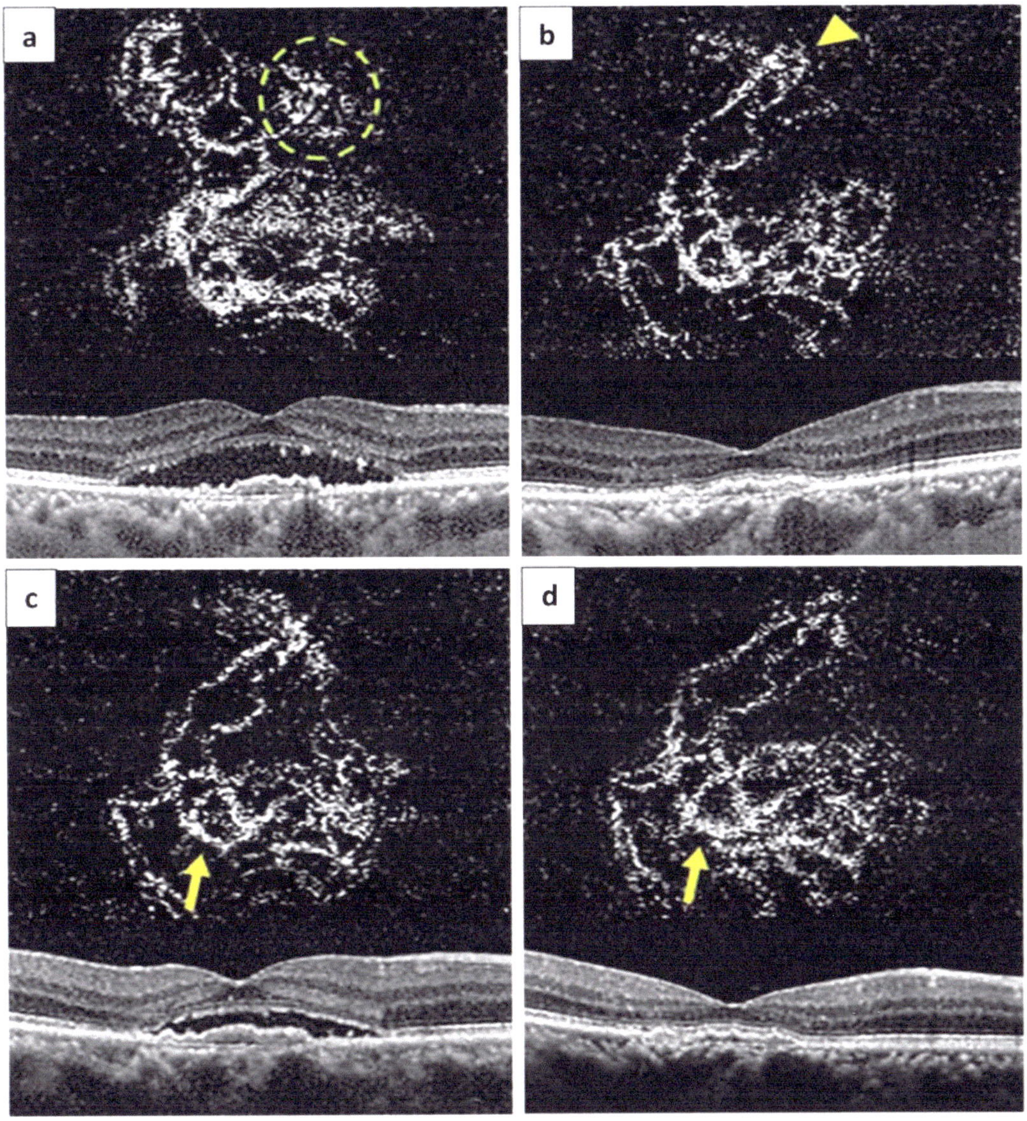

Fig. (5). Optical coherence tomography angiography (OCTA) images and corresponding OCT. Horizontal B-scans of choroidal neovascularization (CNV) in neovascular age-related macular degeneration at baseline (**a**), 8 weeks (**b**), 14 weeks (**c**), and 26 weeks (**d**) after aflibercept treatment. Anti-VEGF treatment led to the regression of immature capillaries (yellow dotted circle) and replacement with a peripheral loop (yellow arrowhead). Prolonged treatment also leads to dilation of the central vessels and the formation of anastomosing networks (yellow arrow). This modified copyright-free figure was obtained from Bae, Kim, Shin, and Kang. Predictors of neovascular activity during treatment of neovascular age-related macular degeneration based on optical coherence tomography angiography. Scientific reports. (2019) 9:19240 | https://doi.org/10.1038/s41598-019-55871-8 and was used under the Creative Commons Attribution 4.0 International License (https://creativecommons.org/licenses/by/4.0/).

Lumbroso *et al.* performed a longitudinal OCT-A evaluation of five eyes with Type II CNV treated with anti-VEGF therapy [39]. One day after the anti-VEGF injection, vessel fragmentation and NV regression were detected. The CNV area regressed with the loss of smaller vessels and pruning of thinner anastomoses. At later time points, further loss of smaller capillaries was detected, resulting in diminished CNV area and vessel narrowing. In another study, the same team reported that CNV tends to follow a 45–60-day cycle of morphological changes after anti-VEGF treatment [40]. The initial small vessel loss observed 24 h after injection reached a maximum on days 6 to 12, followed by new sprouting of vessels 20 to 50 days later. The loss of small peripheral vessel branches appeared to be accompanied by the strengthening of the vessel trunk, which manifested as increased flow after CNV reactivation.

Faatz *et al.* characterized treatment-naïve Type I and Type II CNV in 28 eyes with neovascular AMD before and after anti-VEGF therapy [41]. In this study, the total vessel length, number of individual vessel segments, and fractal dimension of CNV were significantly regressed after anti-VEGF injections (4 weeks after the first dose). These changes also corresponded to an increase in visual acuity and a reduction in retinal thickness. Here, several biomarkers measurable by OCT-A were correlated with established CNV parameters, providing additional resources for disease management. These observations were corroborated by Muakkassa et al., who tracked six treatment-naïve CNV eyes across neovascular AMD (two eyes) and one eye each with idiopathic polypoidal choroidal vasculopathy, CNV secondary to central serous chorioretinopathy and multifocal choroiditis, and macular telangiectasia Type II with subretinal neovascularization [42]. All six patients showed reduced fluid after treatment on OCT, whereas 5/6 patients demonstrated a reduction in CNV with the greatest linear dimension and CNV area at the follow-up visit (2 to 9.5 weeks after treatment).

Although a majority of studies have reported the application of OCT-A in CNV cases associated with neovascular AMD, the technique has also demonstrated the capability to image a variety of other types of CNV. When OCT-A was applied to evaluate 31 myopic CNV cases treated with anti-VEGF therapy, Wang et al. found that multiple characteristics of CNV (*e.g.,* CNV area, vessel area, vessel junction) were altered one month after the initial anti-VEGF injection [43]. In this study, vessel junctions were found to be the most sensitive biomarkers in response to anti-VEGF therapy (a reduction of approximately 50%). Consistent with earlier studies, vessel diameter significantly increased after treatment. In uveitic patients who presented with active CNV, Tang *et al.* found that OCTA exhibited 100% sensitivity for detecting inflammatory CNV across 23 CNV lesions [44]. Similar to findings from other studies, OCTA showed that the CNV area was significantly reduced as early as 1 d after anti-VEGF injection. Additionally, a rebound in capillary density and vessel size was observed approximately 14–30 days after injection. OCT-A has also been reported to track the response to treatment in patients with CNV associated with best macular dystrophy [45] and central serous chorioretinopathy [42].

The therapeutic response to anti-VEGF therapy varies among patients, so individualized approaches to dosing frequency are typically employed involving approaches such as "treat-and-extend" or "treat-as-needed." OCT-A was used to investigate CNV characteristics following the establishment of the optimal anti-VEGF treatment intervals (Fig. **6**). Uchida et al. studied 40 eyes with CNV associated with neovascular AMD as part of the AVATAR study [46]. The eyes were divided into three groups: two groups that required treatment and extension every 4-6 weeks or every 7-12 weeks and a third group that did not require injection within the last 12 months. The authors found major differences in CNV morphology between eyes that required periodic injections and those that did not. The majority of CNV cases that required active anti-VEGF therapy were irregular in shape and involved the foveal center, whereas those that did not require active intervention mostly spared the foveal center. The differences in CNV shape and location were statistically significant. In contrast, no differences were noted in several other characteristics, including CNV area and vessel density. Another report by Bae et al. found that the presence of peripheral loops and closed-circuit patterns of CNV on OCT-A were associated with the need for continuing anti-VEGF therapy [47]. Overall, OCT-A imaging revealed major differences in CNV morphology in patients who required continuous anti-VEGF therapy.

OCT-A generates valuable data on CNV vasculature that can inform treatment decisions. In a cohort of 126 eyes with neovascular AMD, Coscas et al. found that four criteria from OCT-A (presence of tiny branching vessels, anastomotic arcade, loops, and perilesional hypointense halo) had an excellent rate of predicting exudation status after anti-VEGF therapy [48]. In particular, the presence of tiny branch vessels and peripheral arcades on OCTA appeared to be particularly informative, as the two factors alone correctly predicted 71% of clinical outcomes (their presence is associated with active lesions). These case studies demonstrate the unique ability of OCTA to support the diagnosis and management of various CNV cases.

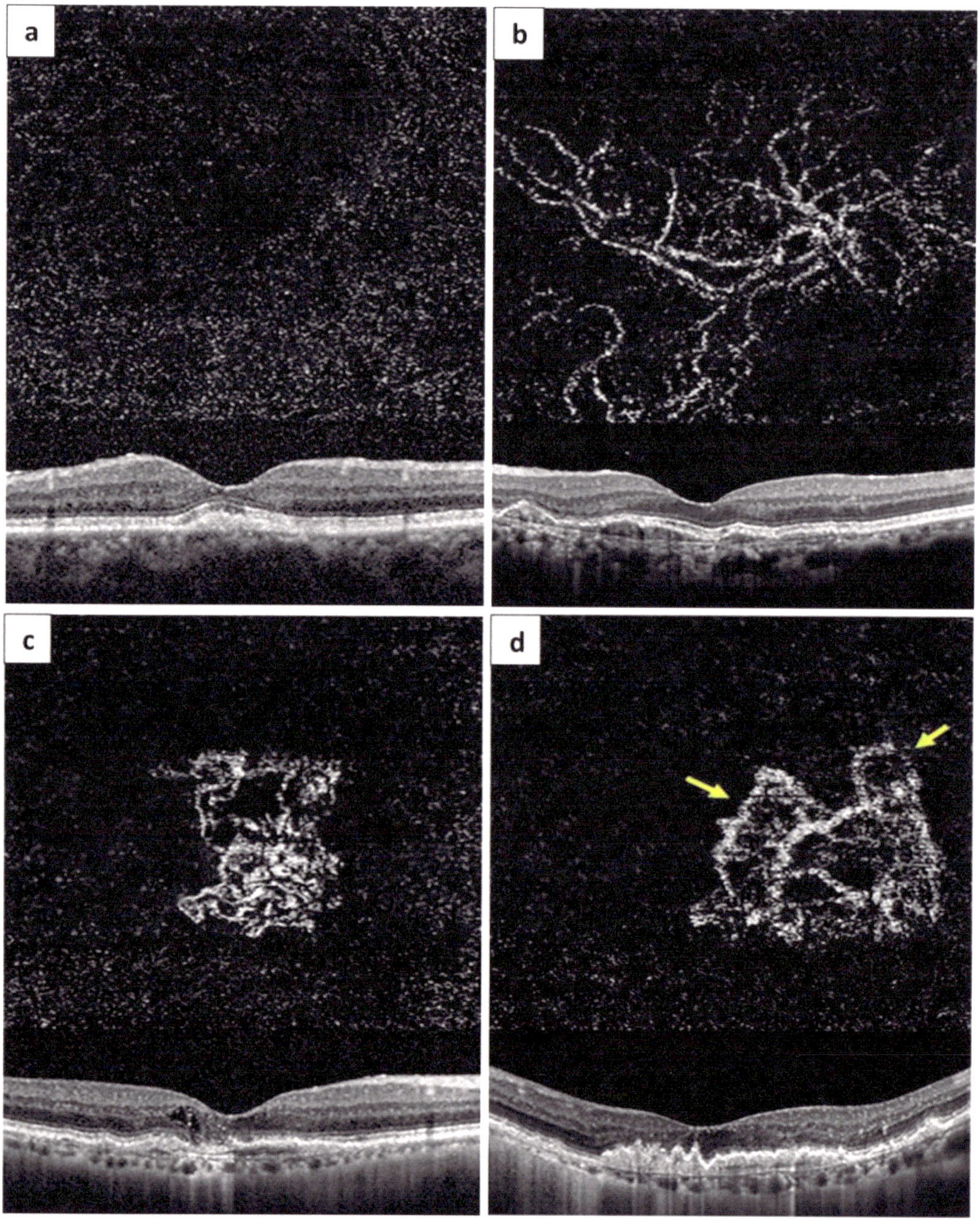

Fig. (6). Optical coherence tomography angiography (OCTA) images with corresponding OCT horizontal B-scans of age-related choroidal neovascularization. (**a**) En face OCTA image without evidence of choroidal neovascularization after 47 months of last treatment. This case received a total of 8 injections of ranibizumab. (**b**) En face OCTA image of an open-circuit pattern choroidal neovascularization 7 months after the last treatment. This case was treated with a total of 21 injections of aflibercept. (**c**) En face OCTA image of a closed-circuit pattern of age-related choroidal neovascularization 2 months after the last treatment. The patient was treated with 17 injections of ranibizumab and then the patient was switched to bevacizumab in a treat and extend protocol treatment. The inner retinal cyst was observed on horizontal OCT B-scans and the patient was maintained in antiangiogenic therapy with bevacizumab every 2 months. (**d**) Another case with a closed-circuit pattern of choroidal neovascularization. This is an en face OCTA image taken 2 months after a total of 26 injections with bevacizumab after being switched from ranibizumab. Note the peripheral loop residual choroidal neovascularization (arrows) as well as the anastomotic margin of CNV. Owing to the fact that the cyst lesion recurred at the level of inner retina layers when the treatment interval was prolonged for more than 3 months, treatment was continued every 2 months. This modified copyright-free figure was obtained from Bae, Kim, Shin and Kang. Predictors of neovascular activity during neovascular age-related macular degeneration treatment based on optical coherence tomography angiography. Scientific reports. (2019) 9:19240 | https://doi.org/10.1038/s41598-019-55871-8 and is used under the Creative Commons Attribution 4.0 International License (https://creativecommons.org/licenses/by/4.0/).

DISCUSSION

While OCTA is informative for tracking vascular changes in CNV treated with anti-VEGF therapy, these observations have not been demonstrated to significantly improve clinical outcomes [12]. Retreatment decisions are largely based on visual acuity, clinical examination, and OCT changes in exudation and retinal structure. Nonetheless, OCTA can play an important role in the decision to treat or not treat [49]. Owing to the ease of obtaining OCT-A angiograms at follow-up visits, a clinician can evaluate the changes in CNV and assess the lesion's activity status to obtain guidance on the treatment regime.

Another limitation of OCT-A is the speed of image acquisition, which limits the resolution of angiograms. Typically, the analyzed area is either a 3 × 3 mm or 6 × 6 mm square area, where visualization of a larger area results in a lower image resolution [16]. More recent wide-angle OCT-A devices can generate scans of a 12 × 12 mm area, which can compete with conventional dye-based angiography. Advances in SS-OCT-A and montage techniques can capture even larger areas of up to 31 × 27 mm, enabling the visualization of the peripheral vasculature [50]. This space is still under active development, and new and improved technologies can generate larger and higher-resolution images.

As OCT-A becomes more widely available in the clinic, clinicians can now obtain a wealth of data on retinal vasculature that was previously inaccessible. However, although the data are relatively easy to obtain, interpretation is more challenging and requires continued education and exchanges between ophthalmologists [16]. In particular, OCT-A can generate a large volume of images that are time consuming to process manually. One potential solution is the application of machine-learning algorithms that can aid in disease detection and prognosis prediction [51]. While promising, substantial issues remain with this approach owing to limited training datasets, lack of data processing standardization, low model robustness, and challenges in result interpretation [52].

Regarding imaging quality, OCT-A remains a maturing technology plagued with frequent artifacts that can lead to misinterpretation of angiograms. These artifacts arise from eye movements, eye anatomy, pathological interference, and software limitations. Although the OCT-A software is designed to minimize these errors, artifacts remain a concern and may benefit from additional technical developments. Accurate quantification of blood flow remains a challenge for OCT-A; however, this is a difficult problem that is undergoing active research [53]. Furthermore, the current lack of standardization across the field and the limited number of annotated OCT-A databases create additional constraints on the impact of this technology [14, 54]. Despite these challenges, OCT-A has been demonstrated to be a robust tool and may become widely used in a manner that is similar to that of OCT adoption by the retinal community.

CONCLUDING REMARKS

Approximately one decade after its introduction [55], OCT-A has evolved from being a tool in the academic research setting to becoming increasingly accepted in clinical practice. Compared with conventional dye-based angiography, OCT-A provides a wealth of information on the 3-dimensional structure of the retinal and choroidal vasculatures. However, angiographs derived from OCT-A contain artifacts, and a substantial amount of expertise is required to form a correct interpretation. For the time being, OCT-A may be considered a complementary option to existing dye-based angiography instead of an alternative option. Both conventional OCT and fluorescein angiography detect vascular fluid leakage, whereas OCT-A shows the source of the leak by revealing the specific vessels in the neovascular lesions. Beyond the characterization and management of CNV in neovascular AMD, OCT-A has shown promising applications in a variety of other vascular conditions, including diabetic retinopathy, central serous chorioretinopathy, uveitis, and glaucoma. As technology continues to advance and clinicians become increasingly familiar with this versatile tool, OCT-A will likely see expanded usage in both the diagnosis and management of a broad range of retinal diseases.

LIST OF ABBREVIATIONS

AMD	Age-related macular degeneration
CNV	Choroidal neovascularization
FAZ	Foveal avascular zone
GA	Geographic atrophy
NV	Neovascularization
OCT	Optical coherence tomography
OCT-A	Optical coherence tomography angiography
VEGF	Vascular endothelial growth factor.

DISCLAIMER

All scientific comments issued in this chapter are solely the responsibility of the authors and not of the institutions with which they are affiliated.

ACKNOWLEDGMENTS

We express our deep appreciation to the technical staff of the Retina Specialists Unit at Oftalmologia Integral ABC (Nonprofit Medical and Surgical Organization) affiliated with the Postgraduate Division of Studies at the National Autonomous University of Mexico.

REFERENCES

[1] Spaide RF. Optical coherence tomography angiography signs of vascular abnormalization with antiangiogenic therapy for choroidal neovascularization. Am J Ophthalmol 2015; 160(1): 6-16. [http://dx.doi.org/10.1016/j.ajo.2015.04.012] [PMID: 25887628]

[2] Jian L, Panpan Y, Wen X. Current choroidal neovascularization treatment. Ophthalmologica 2013; 230(2): 55-61. [http://dx.doi.org/10.1159/000351660] [PMID: 23949022]

[3] Khanani AM, Aziz AA, Weng CY, *et al.* Port delivery system: A novel drug delivery platform to treat retinal diseases. Expert Opin Drug Deliv 2021; 18(11): 1571-6. [http://dx.doi.org/10.1080/17425247.2021.1968826] [PMID: 34388956]

[4] Adhi M, Duker JS. Optical coherence tomography : Current and future applications. Curr Opin Ophthalmol 2013; 24(3): 213-21. [http://dx.doi.org/10.1097/ICU.0b013e32835f8bf8] [PMID: 23429598]

[5] Aumann S, Donner S, Fischer J. Optical coherence tomography (OCT): Principle and technical realization.High Resolution Imaging in Microscopy and Ophthalmology. Cham: New Frontiers in Biomedical Optics Springer International Publishing 2019; pp. 59-85. [http://dx.doi.org/10.1007/978-3-030-16638-0_3]

[6] Fujimoto J, Swanson E. The Development, commercialization, and impact of optical coherence tomography. Invest Ophthalmol Vis Sci 2016; 57(9): OCT1-OCT13. [http://dx.doi.org/10.1167/iovs.16-19963] [PMID: 27409459]

[7] Laíns I, Wang JC, Cui Y, *et al.* Retinal applications of swept source optical coherence tomography (OCT) and optical coherence tomography angiography (OCTA). Prog Retin Eye Res 2021; 84: 100951. [http://dx.doi.org/10.1016/j.preteyeres.2021.100951] [PMID: 33516833]

[8] Miller AR, Roisman L, Zhang Q, *et al.* Comparison between spectral-domain and swept-source optical coherence tomography angiographic imaging of choroidal neovascularization. Invest Ophthalmol Vis Sci 2017; 58(3): 1499-505. [http://dx.doi.org/10.1167/iovs.16-20969] [PMID: 28273316]

[9] Kostanyan T, Wollstein G, Schuman JS. New developments in optical coherence tomography. Curr Opin Ophthalmol 2015; 26(2): 110-5. [http://dx.doi.org/10.1097/ICU.0000000000000133] [PMID: 25594766]

[10] Pennington LM, Smith B. OCT: What's under the hood? Rev Ophthalmol 2022; 1: 1.

[11] Cole ED, Duker JS. OCT Technology: Will we be "swept" away? Rev Ophthalmol 2017; 1: 1.

[12] Greig EC, Duker JS, Waheed NK. A practical guide to optical coherence tomography angiography interpretation. Int J Retina Vitreous 2020; 6(1): 55. [http://dx.doi.org/10.1186/s40942-020-00262-9] [PMID: 33292740]

[13] Rocholz R, Corvi F, Weichsel J. OCT angiography (OCTA) in retinal diagnostics.High Resolution Imaging in Microscopy and Ophthalmology: New Frontiers in Biomedical Optics Springer. Cham, CH 2019. [http://dx.doi.org/10.1007/978-3-030-16638-0_6]

[14] Sampson DM, Dubis AM, Chen FK, Zawadzki RJ, Sampson DD. Towards standardizing retinal optical coherence tomography angiography: A review. Light Sci Appl 2022; 11(1): 63. [http://dx.doi.org/10.1038/s41377-022-00740-9] [PMID: 35304441]

[15] Spaide RF, Fujimoto JG, Waheed NK, Sadda SR, Staurenghi G. Optical coherence tomography angiography. Prog Retin Eye Res 2018; 64: 1-55. [http://dx.doi.org/10.1016/j.preteyeres.2017.11.003] [PMID: 29229445]

[16] Płatkowska B, Kal M, Biskup M. Optical coherence tomography angiography: Use in ophthalmological practice. Med Stud 2020; 36(3): 195-205. [http://dx.doi.org/10.5114/ms.2020.99541]

[17] Yu PK, Mehnert A, Athwal A, Sarunic MV, Yu DY. Use of the retinal vascular histology to validate an optical coherence tomography angiography technique. Transl Vis Sci Technol 2021; 10(1): 29. [http://dx.doi.org/10.1167/tvst.10.1.29] [PMID: 33520424]

[18] Chalam KV, Sambhav K. Optical coherence tomography angiography in retinal diseases. J Ophthalmic Vis Res 2016; 11(1): 84-92. [http://dx.doi.org/10.4103/2008-322X.180709] [PMID: 27195091]

[19] Coscas GJ, Lupidi M, Coscas F, Cagini C, Souied EH. Optical coherence tomography angiography versus traditional multimodal imaging in assessing the activity of exudative age-related macular degeneration: A new diagnostic challenge. Retina 2015; 35(11): 2219-28. [http://dx.doi.org/10.1097/IAE.0000000000000766] [PMID: 26398697]

[20] de Carlo TE, Bonini Filho MA, Chin AT, *et al.* Spectral-domain optical coherence tomography angiography of choroidal neovascularization. Ophthalmology 2015; 122(6): 1228-38. [http://dx.doi.org/10.1016/j.ophtha.2015.01.029] [PMID: 25795476]

[21] Soomro T, Talks J. The use of optical coherence tomography angiography for detecting choroidal neovascularization, compared to standard multimodal imaging. Eye 2018; 32(4): 661-72. [http://dx.doi.org/10.1038/eye.2018.2] [PMID: 29600987]

[22] Maesa JM, Baños-Álvarez E, Rosario-Lozano MP, Blasco-Amaro JA. Diagnostic accuracy of optical coherence tomography angiography in the detection of neovasculature in age-related macular degeneration: A meta-analysis. Acta Ophthalmol 2022; 100(2): e368-76. [http://dx.doi.org/10.1111/aos.14979] [PMID: 34309204]

[23] Ng DSC, Ho M, Chen LJ, *et al.* Optical coherence tomography angiography compared with multimodal imaging for diagnosing neovascular central serous chorioretinopathy. Am J Ophthalmol 2021; 232: 70-82. [http://dx.doi.org/10.1016/j.ajo.2021.05.029] [PMID: 34116008]

[24] Matsunaga D, Yi J, Puliafito CA, Kashani AH. OCT angiography in healthy human subjects. Ophthalmic Surg Lasers Imag Ret 2014; 45(6): 510-5. [http://dx.doi.org/10.3928/23258160-20141118-04] [PMID: 25423629]

[25] Savastano MC, Lumbroso B, Rispoli M. *IN VIVO* characterization of retinal vascularization morphology using optical coherence tomography angiography. Retina 2015; 35(11): 2196-203. [http://dx.doi.org/10.1097/IAE.0000000000000635] [PMID: 25932558]

[26] Samara WA, Say EAT, Khoo CTL, *et al.* Correlation of foveal avascular zone size with foveal morphology in normal eyes using optical coherence tomography angiography. Retina 2015; 35(11): 2188-95.
[http://dx.doi.org/10.1097/IAE.0000000000000847] [PMID: 26469536]

[27] Jia Y, Bailey ST, Wilson DJ, *et al.* Quantitative optical coherence tomography angiography of choroidal neovascularization in age-related macular degeneration. Ophthalmology 2014; 121(7): 1435-44.
[http://dx.doi.org/10.1016/j.ophtha.2014.01.034] [PMID: 24679442]

[28] El Ameen A, Cohen SY, Semoun O, *et al.* TYPE 2 neovascularization secondary to age-related macular degeneration imaged by optical coherence tomography angiography. Retina 2015; 35(11): 2212-8.
[http://dx.doi.org/10.1097/IAE.0000000000000773] [PMID: 26441269]

[29] Kuehlewein L, Dansingani KK, de Carlo TE, *et al.* Optical coherence tomography angiography of type 3 neovascularization secondary to age-related macular degeneration. Retina 2015; 35(11): 2229-35.
[http://dx.doi.org/10.1097/IAE.0000000000000835] [PMID: 26502007]

[30] Miere A, Querques G, Semoun O, El Ameen A, Capuano V, Souied EH. Optical coherence tomography angiography in early type 3 neovascularization. Retina 2015; 35(11): 2236-41.
[http://dx.doi.org/10.1097/IAE.0000000000000834] [PMID: 26457399]

[31] Silva R, Cachulo ML, Fonseca P, *et al.* Age-related macular degeneration and risk factors for the development of choroidal neovascularisation in the fellow eye: A 3-year follow-up study. Ophthalmologica 2011; 226(3): 110-8.
[http://dx.doi.org/10.1159/000329473] [PMID: 21822000]

[32] Parikh R, Avery RL, Saroj N, Thompson D, Freund KB. Incidence of new choroidal neovascularization in fellow eyes of patients with age-related macular degeneration treated with intravitreal aflibercept or ranibizumab. JAMA Ophthalmol 2019; 137(8): 914-20.
[http://dx.doi.org/10.1001/jamaophthalmol.2019.1947] [PMID: 31294771]

[33] Treister AD, Nesper PL, Fayed AE, Gill MK, Mirza RG, Fawzi AA. Prevalence of subclinical cnv and choriocapillaris nonperfusion in fellow eyes of unilateral exudative amd on oct angiography. Transl Vis Sci Technol 2018; 7(5): 19.
[http://dx.doi.org/10.1167/tvst.7.5.19] [PMID: 30280004]

[34] Palejwala NV, Jia Y, Gao SS, *et al.* Detection of nonexudative choroidal neovascularization in age-related macular degeneration with optical coherence tomography angiography. Retina 2015; 35(11): 2204-11.
[http://dx.doi.org/10.1097/IAE.0000000000000867] [PMID: 26469533]

[35] de Oliveira Dias JR, Zhang Q, Garcia JMB, *et al.* Natural history of subclinical neovascularization in nonexudative age-related macular degeneration using swept-source oct angiography. Ophthalmology 2018; 125(2): 255-66.
[http://dx.doi.org/10.1016/j.ophtha.2017.08.030] [PMID: 28964581]

[36] Faes L, Ali Z, Wagner S, *et al.* Effect of total anti-VEGF treatment exposure on patterns of choroidal neovascularisation assessed by optical coherence tomography angiography in age-related macular degeneration: A retrospective case series. BMJ Open Ophthalmol 2019; 4(1): e000244.
[http://dx.doi.org/10.1136/bmjophth-2018-000244] [PMID: 31179393]

[37] Xu D, Dávila JP, Rahimi M, *et al.* Long-term progression of type 1 neovascularization in age-related macular degeneration using optical coherence tomography angiography. Am J Ophthalmol 2018; 187: 10-20.
[http://dx.doi.org/10.1016/j.ajo.2017.12.005] [PMID: 29269100]

[38] Rispoli M, Savastano MC, Lumbroso B, Toto L, Di Antonio L. Type 1 choroidal neovascularization evolution by optical coherence tomography angiography: Long-term follow-up. BioMed Res Int 2020; 2020: 1-8.

[http://dx.doi.org/10.1155/2020/4501395] [PMID: 32382551]

[39] Lumbroso B, Rispoli M, Savastano MC. Longitudinal optical coherence tomography–angiography study of type 2 naive choroidal neovascularization early response after treatment. Retina 2015; 35(11): 2242-51.
[http://dx.doi.org/10.1097/IAE.0000000000000879] [PMID: 26457401]

[40] Lumbroso B, Rispoli M, Savastano MC, Jia Y, Tan O, Huang D. Optical coherence tomography angiography study of choroidal neovascularization early response after treatment. Dev Ophthalmol 2016; 56: 77-85.
[http://dx.doi.org/10.1159/000442782] [PMID: 27022967]

[41] Faatz H, Farecki ML, Rothaus K, *et al.* Optical coherence tomography angiography of types 1 and 2 choroidal neovascularization in age-related macular degeneration during anti-VEGF therapy: Evaluation of a new quantitative method. Eye 2019; 33(9): 1466-71.
[http://dx.doi.org/10.1038/s41433-019-0429-8] [PMID: 30971814]

[42] Muakkassa NW, Chin AT, de Carlo T, *et al.* Characterizing the effect of anti-vascular endothelial growth factor therapy on treatment-naive choroidal neovascularization using optical coherence tomography angiography. Retina 2015; 35(11): 2252-9.
[http://dx.doi.org/10.1097/IAE.0000000000000836] [PMID: 26457400]

[43] Wang Y, Hu Z, Zhu T, *et al.* Optical coherence tomography angiography-based quantitative assessment of morphologic changes in active myopic choroidal neovascularization during anti-vascular endothelial growth factor therapy. Front Med 2021; 8: 657772.
[http://dx.doi.org/10.3389/fmed.2021.657772] [PMID: 34026789]

[44] Tang W, Guo J, Liu W, Xu G. Optical coherence tomography angiography of inflammatory choroidal neovascularization early response after Anti-VEGF treatment. Curr Eye Res 2020; 45(12): 1556-62.
[http://dx.doi.org/10.1080/02713683.2020.1767790] [PMID: 32394732]

[45] Murro V, Mucciolo DP, Giorgio D, *et al.* OCTA imaging of choroidal neovascularization treated using photodynamic therapy in a young patient with best macular dystrophy. Ophthalmic Surg Lasers Imaging Retina 2018; 49(12): 969-73.
[http://dx.doi.org/10.3928/23258160-20181203-10] [PMID: 30566705]

[46] Uchida A, Hu M, Babiuch A, *et al.* Optical coherence tomography angiography characteristics of choroidal neovascularization requiring varied dosing frequencies in treat-and-extend management: An analysis of the AVATAR study. PLoS One 2019; 14(6): e0218889.
[http://dx.doi.org/10.1371/journal.pone.0218889] [PMID: 31237929]

[47] Bae K, Kim HJ, Shin YK, Kang SW. Predictors of neovascular activity during neovascular age-related macular degeneration treatment based on optical coherence tomography angiography. Sci Rep 2019; 9(1): 19240.
[http://dx.doi.org/10.1038/s41598-019-55871-8] [PMID: 31848438]

[48] Coscas F, Lupidi M, Boulet JF, *et al.* Optical coherence tomography angiography in exudative age-related macular degeneration: a predictive model for treatment decisions. Br J Ophthalmol 2019; 103(9): 1342-6.
[http://dx.doi.org/10.1136/bjophthalmol-2018-313065] [PMID: 30467129]

[49] Coscas F. Managing CNV With OCTA Retina Today 2017. Bryn Mawr Communications 2017.

[50] Zheng F, Deng X, Zhang Q, *et al.* Advances in swept-source optical coherence tomography and optical coherence tomography angiography. Adv Ophthal Prac Res 2023; 3(2): 67-79.
[http://dx.doi.org/10.1016/j.aopr.2022.10.005]

[51] Le D, Son T, Yao X. Machine learning in optical coherence tomography angiography. Exp Biol Med 2021; 246(20): 2170-83.
[http://dx.doi.org/10.1177/15353702211026581] [PMID: 34279136]

[52] Ran A, Cheung CY. Deep learning-based optical coherence tomography and optical coherence

tomography angiography image analysis: An updated summary. Asia Pac J Ophthalmol 2021; 10(3): 253-60.
[http://dx.doi.org/10.1097/APO.0000000000000405] [PMID: 34383717]

[53] Richter D, Fard AM, Straub J, Wei W, Zhang Q, Wang RK. Relative retinal flow velocity detection using optical coherence tomography angiography imaging. Biomed Opt Express 2020; 11(11): 6710-20.
[http://dx.doi.org/10.1364/BOE.408481] [PMID: 33282519]

[54] Coscas F, Sellam A, Glacet-Bernard A, *et al.* Normative data for vascular density in superficial and deep capillary plexuses of healthy adults assessed by optical coherence tomography angiography. Invest Ophthalmol Vis Sci 2016; 57(9): OCT211-23.
[http://dx.doi.org/10.1167/iovs.15-18793] [PMID: 27409475]

[55] Jia Y, Tan O, Tokayer J, *et al.* Split-spectrum amplitude-decorrelation angiography with optical coherence tomography. Opt Express 2012; 20(4): 4710-25.
[http://dx.doi.org/10.1364/OE.20.004710] [PMID: 22418228]

CHAPTER 7

Epiretinal Membrane Formation and Macular Perfusion Findings in Rhegmatogenous Retinal Detachment Treated with Vitrectomy or Scleral Buckling

Miguel A. Quiroz-Reyes, MD[1,*], Erick A. Quiroz-Gonzalez[1,2], Miguel A. Quiroz-Gonzalez[1], Jorge Morales-Navarro[2], Felipe Esparza-Correa[2], Jorge E. Aceves-Velazquez[2], Jennifer H. Kim-Lee[2], Alejandra Nieto-Jordan[2], Margarita Montano[1], Sanjay Marasini[3] and **Virgilio Lima-Gomez, MD[4]**

[1] *Oftalmologia Integral ABC, Retina Department, Medical and Surgical Assistance Institution (Nonprofit Organization), Affiliated with the Postgraduate Studies Division, National Autonomous University of Mexico, Mexico City, Mexico*

[2] *Institute of Ophthalmology, Fundacion Conde de Valenciana, Private Assistance Institution (Nonprofit Organization), Mexico City, Mexico*

[3] *Department of Ophthalmology, The University of Auckland, Auckland, New Zealand*

[4] *Ophthalmology Service, Hospital Juarez de Mexico, Public Assistance Institution (Nonprofit Organization), Mexico City, Mexico*

Abstract: Despite the abundant literature on management options for noncomplicated macula-off rhegmatogenous retinal detachment (RRD) repair, the role of the corresponding long-term postoperative macular perfusion indices and their correlation with the postoperative epiretinal membrane (ERM) formation remain vaguely understood. In this chapter, we have analyzed the incidence of postoperative ERM proliferation and the differences in the corresponding postoperative macular perfusion indices in patients who underwent two well-known surgical approaches for noncomplicated macula-off RRD. Postoperative microstructural and perfusional findings were compared, and their correlation with best-corrected visual acuity (BCVA), postoperatively, was assessed. Two study groups based on the surgical procedures performed for noncomplicated macula-off RRD were analyzed. The postoperative incidence of ERM was 23.2% and 23.63% in the buckle vitrectomy groups, respectively ($p>0.05$). The RRD recurrence rates in the buckle and vitrectomy groups were 8.8% and 1.82%, respectively ($p>0.001$). The mean BCVA values before ERM removal in the buckle and vitrectomy groups were 0.40±0.33 log of the minimum

* **Corresponding author Miguel A. Quiroz-Reyes, MD:** Oftalmologia Integral ABC, Retina Department, Medical and Surgical Assistance Institution (Nonprofit Organization), Affiliated with the Postgraduate Studies Division, National Autonomous University of Mexico, Mexico City, Mexico; Tel: +52 55 5217 2732; Fax: +52 55 1664 7180; E-mails: drquiroz@prodigy.net.mx and drquirozreyes7@gmail.com

angle of resolution (logMAR) and 0.47±0.19 logMAR, respectively ($p<0.05$). The final mean postoperative BCVA in the buckle and vitrectomy groups were 0.43±0.14 logMAR and 0.28±0.19 logMAR, respectively ($p<0.05$). When the retinal perfusional indices of the buckle and vitrectomy groups were compared with the normal control group, all the perfusional indices differed significantly ($p<0.01$).

Keywords: Additional surgery rate, Brilliant blue dye, Choriocapillaris flow area, Deep vascular plexus, Ellipsoid zone, Epiretinal membrane, External limiting membrane, Internal limiting membrane, Macula-off retinal detachment, Noncomplicated rhegmatogenous retinal detachment, Primary vitrectomy, Scleral buckle, Superficial vascular plexus, Vessel density.

INTRODUCTION

Several complications may occur during scleral buckle surgery to manage primary noncomplicated macula-off rhegmatogenous retinal detachment (RRD) [1]. These complications may include vitreoretinal complications, retinal perforation with vitreoretinal entrapment, choroidal hemorrhage, and subretinal bleeding [1]. One of the most commonly observed postoperative complications after scleral buckling and cryotherapy surgery is macular ectopia due to vitreomacular traction and proliferative vitreoretinopathy (PVR) with recurrent and complicated RRD along with epiretinal membrane (ERM) proliferation [1, 2].

Data from a recent (2022) meta-analysis of 7212 eyes showed that the scleral buckle offers a slightly higher final reattachment rate and a reduced risk of macular edema and cataract in cases of RRD [3]. However, the historical data reveal that primary vitrectomy is the preferred procedure for noncomplicated RRD as it reduces complications. Poulsen *et al.* [4] reported that approximately 36% macular attachment was achieved after pars plana vitrectomy (PPV) in primary RRD, and most of the patients achieved a reasonable long-term visual outcome. However, the incidence of ERM is high. To prevent the development of ERM and the requirement of additional surgeries, many surgeons opt to remove the internal limiting membrane (ILM) at the time of PPV while managing RRD. However, the removal of the ILM may lead to the proliferation of glial and Müller cells, which exert a tangential contraction over the macula [5, 6]. Therefore, the potential benefits of prophylactic ILM removal are controversial [7 - 11].

Over the last decade, retinal imaging has progressed significantly, facilitating an accurate assessment of anatomical, vascular and functional outcomes before and after retinal surgery. Recent studies have shown that after vitreoretinal surgeries, early microvascular alterations in the retina can be observed and quantified to monitor and predict surgical outcomes. Optical coherent tomography angiography (OCT-A) devices have allowed a detailed analysis of the retina and choriocapillaris in the macular retina in different pathologic conditions and highlighted distinct changes [12]. Therefore, assessing perfusional indices after vitreoretinal surgeries, including primary scleral buckle placement and primary vitrectomy, would allow us to make future surgical decisions for better anatomical and functional outcomes.

Methodology and Chapter Design

This chapter aims to elaborate on the postoperative outcomes in two surgical groups. The objectives were to 1) determine the postoperative comparative incidence of ERM proliferation, 2) analyze the long-term final postoperative structural findings using optical coherence tomography (OCT), 3) correlate the final postoperative best-corrected visual acuity (BCVA) with the two types of surgical procedures in cases of uncomplicated macula-off RRD, and 4) compare the perfusional indices between the buckling group and vitrectomy group to those of the control emmetropic group to explore potential microvascular alterations (Table **1**).

To analyze structural and perfusional findings, complications were identified associated with scleral buckle and vitrectomy with a complementary buckle. All vitrectomy eyes on which a complementary scleral buckle was placed were not included in this analysis.

Table 1. Study groups. The anatomical and functional outcomes of the groups were compared to evaluate trans- and postoperative complications [7].

Study groups	Group characteristics
Buckle group	Noncomplicated primary RRD eyes without preoperative ERM proliferation and that were managed using 360° scleral buckle surgery, and rhegmatogenous lesions limited cryotherapy retinopexy or additional subretinal fluid exo-drainage
Vitrectomy group	Noncomplicated primary RRD eyes without evidence of preoperative ERM proliferation that underwent primary vitrectomy with no ILM removal

The SD-OCT and OCT-A findings were compared with the emmetropic control groups to identify any potential alterations after the surgeries. The dataset analyzed was taken from a previous report by the authors [7] (Figs. **1** and **2**).

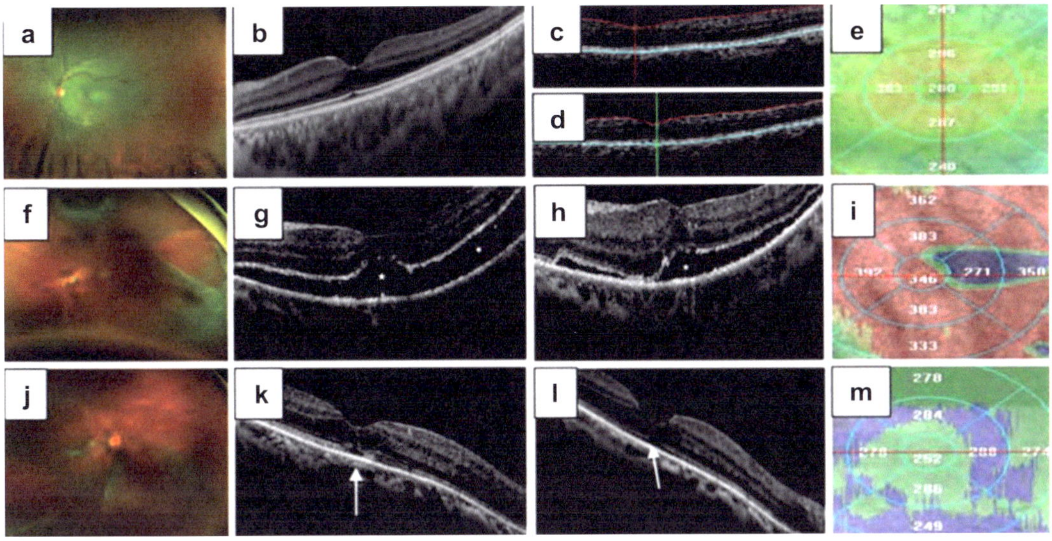

Fig. (1). ***Normal control and abnormal findings.*** (**a**) to (**e**) Multimodal tomographic and topographic evaluation images depict a healthy normal control eye. (**f**) An Optos fundus color photo of a primary rhegmatogenous retinal detachment (RRD) with a large posterior rolled edge retinal tear at the 2.00 o'clock meridian in a -3.00 myopic eye managed with primary vitrectomy and a complemental scleral buckle technique. (**g**) Image depicts a SD-OCT horizontal scan with a small postoperative amount of subretinal fluid (SRF) 3 weeks after the buckle procedure (white asterisk). (**h**) Image depicts a shallow residual amount of SRF 12 weeks postoperatively (white asterisk). (**i**) Image shows an abnormal topographic thickness retinal map on Ret-vue SD-OCT with diffuse retinal thickening. (**j**) Image depicts a wide-field Optos fundus color photo that shows a primary RRD involving the macula, and some evidence of preoperative epiretinal membrane (ERM) proliferation was noted. (**k**) SD-OCT horizontal B-scan image obtained at 8 weeks postoperatively depicts a small defect in the external layers of the subfoveal central macula consistent with subfoveal ellipsoid and external limiting membrane (ELM) disruption (white arrow). (**l**) Image depicts a horizontal B-scan through the central macula, and ellipsoid and ELM biomarkers revealed an almost normal microstructural appearance at the end of follow-up (white arrow). (**m**) Image depicts a postoperative normal topographic thickness macula map of this successful case of primary vitrectomy after undergoing a successful ERM proliferation removal technique. This modified figure was adapted from [7] and GJMR 2021 vol 21 Issue 6. ISSN: 2249-4618. Print ISSN:0975-5888vol 21 Issue 6 and is used under the Creative Commons Attribution 4.0 International License (https://creativecommons.org/licenses/by/4.0/).

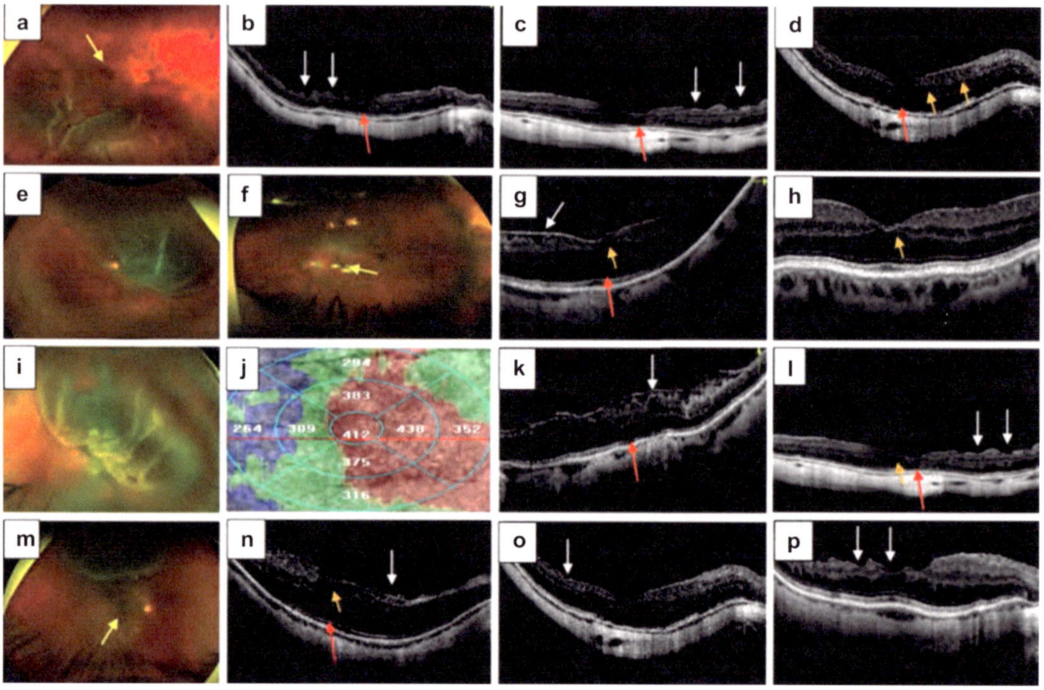

Fig. (2). ***Postoperative structural findings.*** (**a**) A postoperative wide-angle Optos color photo of a failed primary gas-vitrectomy in a case of primary RRD, wherein some submacular bleeding (yellow arrow) is noted. (**b**) to (**d**) Horizontal B-scan images from a case of the vitrectomy group that depicts an attached macula with evidence of postoperative ERM proliferation in a symptomatic patient with a best corrected visual acuity (BCVA) of 20/200 (1.00 logMAR unit equivalent). This eye underwent a second surgical procedure, epiretinal membrane removal, wherein the final BCVA after the ERM was 20/100 (0.70 logMAR units equivalent). Spectralis horizontal and vertical crossline images through the foveal center depict diffuse retinal thinning and dimpling of the superficial nerve fiber layer defects due to dissociated optic nerve fiber layer (DONFL) defects (white arrows). Some loss of normal foveal contour is mainly noted in the horizontal scan and the vertical scan through the center of the fovea. However, the ELM line and the ellipsoid zone (EZ) biomarker did not show full structural recovery (red arrows). Some irregularity of the inner layers of the retina were also detected (yellow arrows). (**e**) An Optos wide-angle color fundus photo with an acute and very bullous-elevated macula-off RR. This pseudophakia due to exchange refractive IOL eye surgery seven years prior is noted a 56-year-old low myope and symptomatic male patient who underwent successful primary vitrectomy. Eight weeks after the first surgery, the eye remains symptomatic with some distorted vision. ERM proliferation over the central macula was also detected and depicted on the cross line horizontal and vertical scans through the foveal center. (**f**) Image depicts that after ERM removal, the macula remains attached with no ERM proliferation. (**g**) and (**h**) Long-term crossline postoperative B-scans depict a regular macular profile with outer biomarkers recuperated (red arrow) and inner retina layers with retinal cystic and discrete fluid accumulation (yellow arrows). (**i**) An Optos wide-angle photo that depicts a macula-off primary RRD that underwent an uneventful 360-degree 503 scleral round Lincoff sponge buckling technique and cryotherapy of the superotemporal degenerative open lattice-associated rhegmatogenous retinal lesions with uncomplicated trans-scleral SRF drainage. Six weeks after the surgical buckling procedure, the patient exhibited postoperative macular thickening associated with ERM proliferation. (**j**) Image shows diffuse retinal thickening. (**k**) Image shows a corresponding postoperative SD-OCT slightly inferior to the center of the fovea horizontal scan depicting irregular and diffuse macular thickening associated with ERM proliferation with wrinkling of the inner superficial retina layers (white arrow). In addition, countless deep cystic spaces and residual submacular fluid (yellow arrow) are noted. However, the EZ appears preserved, whereas the ELM line (red arrow) does not with a BCVA of 20/160 (0.90 logMAR units equivalent). Image show ERM proliferation along with severe wrinkling of the superficial retinal layers (white arrow). At this stage, the ELM line appears attenuated and discontinuous, and the EZ exhibits some disruption (red arrow). The final follow-up BCVA was 20/60 (0.48 logMAR units). (**l**) Image shows post-ERM removal in the last follow-up evaluation with a BCVA of 20/100 (0.70 logMAR units equivalent). The macula appears moderately atrophic. The Spectralis horizontal scan through the central fovea depicts recuperation of the foveal contour with a very thin central fovea (yellow arrow). Some dimpling of the superficial retinal layers (white arrows) is noted. The ELM line appears well defined, and the EZ (red arrow) exhibited irregular hyporeflectivity (red arrow). (**m**) An Optos wide-angle color fundus image of the right eye with a superior primary RRD and shallow macular involvement with preoperative evidence of primary ERM macular proliferation (yellow arrow). (**n**) Image depicts a horizontal B-scan through the foveal center with evidence of macular thickening, limited evidence of submacular fluid macular accumulation, and conspicuous evidence of ERM proliferation (white arrow). Foveal thinning and loss of the ELM line with preserved EZ reflectivity are depicted. (**o**) Spectralis horizontal scan through the central fovea depicts recuperation of the foveal contour with a very thin central fovea. Some DONFL (dimples) of the superficial retinal layers (white arrow) are noted. The ELM line appears discontinuous with the EZ exhibiting irregular hyporeflectivity (red arrow). A disrupted EZ is noted. (**p**) Spectralis vertical scan through the central fovea depicts normal macular neuroretinal thickness. Some loss of the normal foveal contour is noted over the temporal side of the macula. In addition, accentuation and more evidence of the DONFL (dimples) of the superficial retinal layers (white arrows) are noted. The ELM line and EZ reflectivity looked normal and preserved at the end of the follow-up. This modified figure was adopted from [7] and GJMR 2021 vol 21 Issue 6. ISSN: 2249-4618. Print ISSN:0975-5888vol 21 Issue 6 and is used under the Creative Commons Attribution 4.0 International License (https://creativecommons.org/licenses/by/4.0/).

Ancillary Examinations

The ancillary methods were recommended to acquire cross-sectional images of the macular region using SD-OCT. The presence of a noncomplicated macula-off RRD should be confirmed by indirect ophthalmoscopy and B-scan ultrasonography. The postoperative microstructural evaluation should be performed using SD-OCT (Spectralis OCT Heidelberg Engineering. Heidelberg, Germany) or a swept-source (SS)-OCT device (Topcon Medical Systems, Inc., Oakland, NJ, USA). The long-term postoperative perfusion evaluation method has been described in detail in Chapter 7. Briefly, we performed postoperative perfusion and quantitative VD and choroidal flow evaluations using an OCT-A device (RTVue XR OCT Avanti with AngioVue Software; OptoVue, Inc., Fremont, CA, USA). We used default retinal imaging settings and built-in projection artifact removal tools to perform image adjustment and segmentation. Segmentation for the superficial vascular plexus, deep vascular plexus, outer retina layer, and choriocapillaris flow area (CFA) evaluation should be performed in AngioVue software (Figs. **3 to 5**).

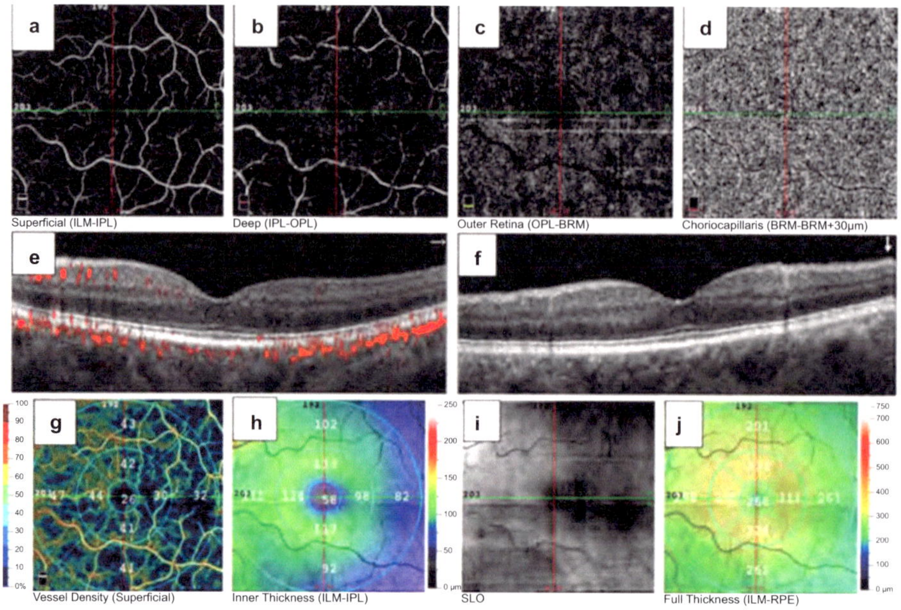

Fig. (3). ***Normal control optical coherent tomography biomarkers.*** (**a**) Normal macular superficial vascular plexus. (**b**) Normal macular deep vascular plexus. (**c**) En-face outer retina slab appearance. (**d**) to (**f**) Automated red and blue segmentation lines in crossline B-scan images with normal inner and outer layers of the macula. (**g**) Superficial vessel density slab at the different macula subregions with the ETDRS grid overlay. (**h**) Superficial regular normal inner macula topography. (**i**) En-slab solo image of the superficial macula. (**j**) Image depicts full-thickness regular and normal macular topography, and the values are presented in the key to the right.

Surgical Procedures Recommended for Noncomplicated RRD

Scleral Buckling Procedures

The surgical methods described in this chapter have been published previously [7]. In brief, in the buckling group analyzed, a methodical, standardized, classical scleral buckle surgical procedure was performed by an experienced vitreoretinal surgeon (MAQR). According to the morphological appearance of the RRD, transscleral subretinal fluid (SRF) drainage assisted with a 7-0 Vicryl polyglactin suture (needle P-1, 3/8 c, reverse cutting; ETHICON) was performed through the scleral wall on the selected meridian site based on previous visualization and location of large choroidal vessels to avoid potential subretinal or choroidal bleeding, which was prevented or treated by diathermy, if necessary, after SRF drainage. The eye volume and pressure lost were recovered with sterilized air. Only in the buckling group, before or after the retina was reattached, limited transscleral cryotherapy was applied over or around the suspected rhegmatogenous lesions, preferably after retina reattachment, to avoid retinal pigment epithelium (RPE) cell dispersion with the assistance of a binocular indirect ophthalmoscope and a 20-diopter condenser lens. The tenon capsule and conjunctival tissue were repositioned, carefully sutured, and fixed to the episcleral tissue with the same 7-0 Vicryl polyglactin to protect the explant and prevent infections, conjunctival erosions, and explant extrusions [7].

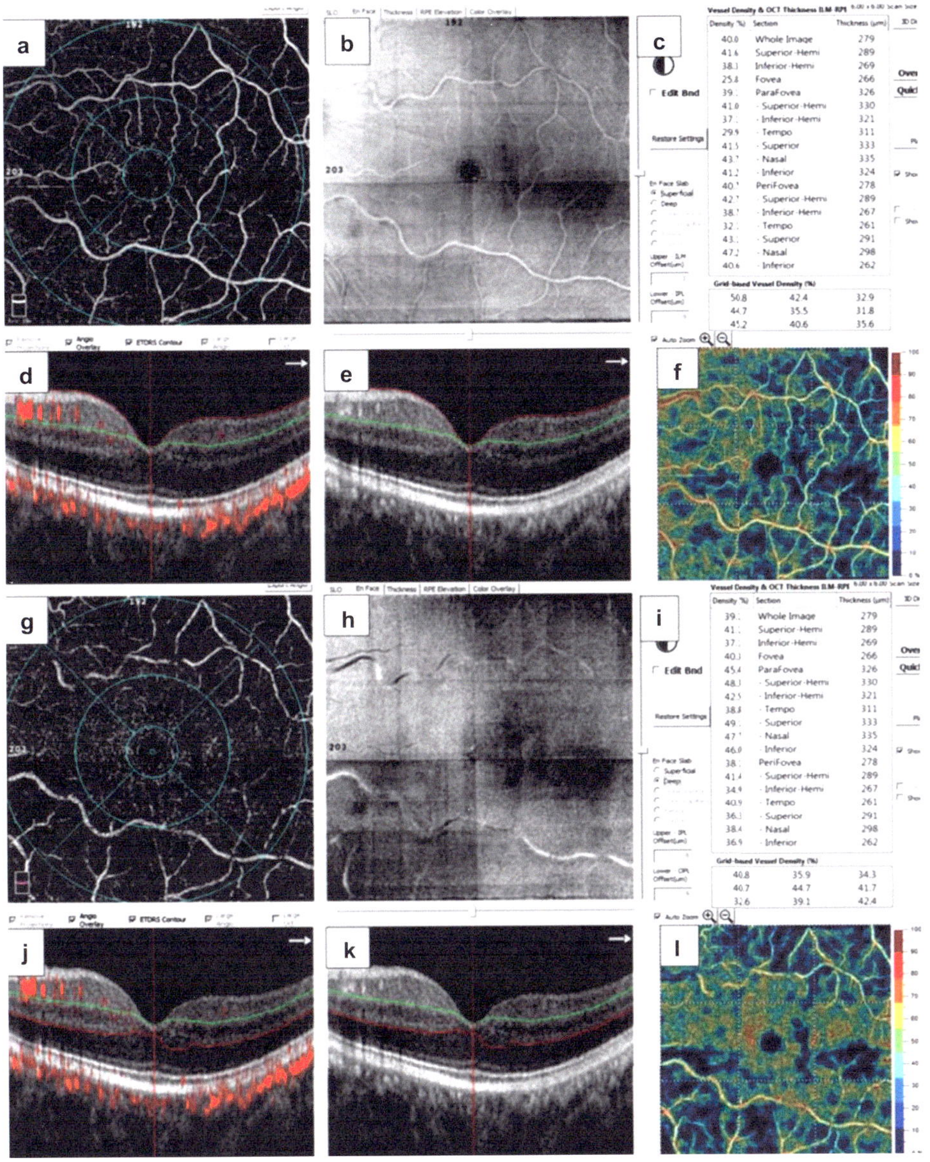

Fig. (4). ***Normal control optical coherent tomography biomarkers.*** (**a**) Normal superficial vascular plexus slab. (**b**) Image depicts an en face normal superficial aspect of the macula. (**c**) Table with the mean values of vessel density and macula thickness at the different subfields of the macula, and grid-based vessel density at the bottom of the table. (**d**) and (**e**) Horizontal B-scan images with automated red and blue segmentation lines through the center of the fovea with normal inner and outer normal biomarkers. The red dots indicate choroidal flow. (**f**) Color overlays on the optical coherence tomography angiography (OCT-A) images indicate normal superficial VD values according to the key to the right. (**g**) Normal deep vascular plexus at the different subregions of the macula on the ETDRS-like grid overlay. (**h**) Image depicts the en face deep aspect of the retina showing a heterogeneous normal RPE. (**i**) Table with the comparative mean value of vessel density and macula thickness at the different subfield of the macula. (**j**) and (**k**) Horizontal B-scan images with automated red and green segmentation lines through the center of the fovea with normal inner and outer normal biomarkers. (**l**) Color overlays on the OCT-A images indicate normal deep VD values (value key presented on the right).

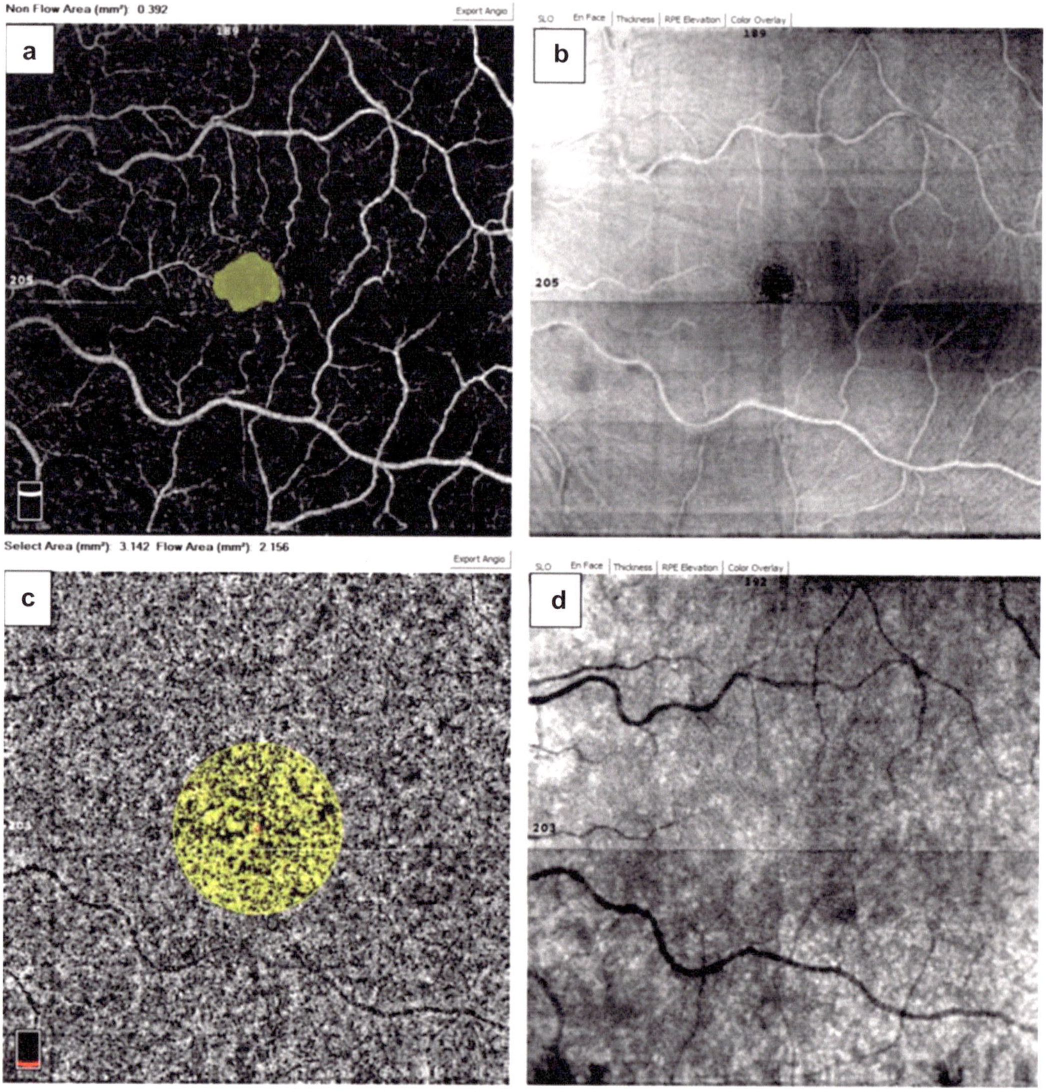

Fig. (5). ***Normal control optical coherent tomography.*** (**a**) Normal, nonperfused foveal avascular zone with normal diameter and shape. (**b**) En face normal aspect of the inner layers of the retina. (**c**) Normal choriocapillaris flow at the selected area of 3.142 mm^2. (**d**) En face normal aspect of the deep retina with normal heterogeneous retinal pigment epithelium.

Vitrectomy Techniques

The methods used here have been described in the author's previous publications [7]. In the vitrectomy group, a standard 23- or 25-gauge three-port pars plana vitrectomy (Alcon Constellation Vision System. Alcon Labs, Fort Worth, TX, USA) with a total vitreous release of the retina was performed in all eyes under local anesthesia plus sedation by one of the authors (MAQR). Vitrectomy was performed using a contact wide-angle viewing precorneal lens system (ROLS reinverted system, Volk Medilex, Miami, FL, USA), a wide-angle viewing system with a noncontact lens (Insight Instruments, Inc. Stuart, FL, USA), or recently in the last cases, the Zeiss ARTEVO 800 digital ophthalmic 3-D head-up microscope with the Resight noncontact lens system (Carl Zeiss Meditec AG, Jena, Germany); this new digital microscope with a hybrid mode (coaxial and 3-d HD 4K monitor) and integrated transoperative OCT allowed for real-time retinal structural analysis and detection of ERM proliferation, thus enabling more precise membrane stripping. In addition to central vitrectomy, our standard technique used a diluted triamcinolone acetonide adjuvant (Kenalog 40 mg/mL; Bristol-Myers Squibb, New York, NY, USA) to identify and better visualize the vitreous and its base and to safely perform necessary removal of its cortical face from the surface of the retina using a silicone-tipped cannula with active suction prior to perfluorocarbon liquid (PFCL) infusion and reattachment of the retina, focusing on achieving a free and mobile posterior hyaloid face. The retina was reattached by a PFCL-assisted technique to effectively perform hydropneumatic retinal manipulation and assisted SRF endodrainage in all the vitrectomy eyes. The vitreous base was shaved 360°, assisted with scleral depression in all eyes. This scleral depression allowed the removal of the vitreous traction completely from flap tears and the careful shaving and debulking of the vitreous base using a mostly closed port duty cycle and low infusion pressure, even in areas of a detached retina, without producing iatrogenic retinal tears. Our young patients generally showed vitreous that was attached or only partially detached, and removal of the core vitreous was relatively straightforward; however, separation of the posterior hyaloid and other areas of adherent vitreous in the periphery with a very mobile retina was technically intricate, especially when concurrent lattice degeneration was present. Once the retina was reattached and in the absence of a scleral buckle, performing a meticulous peripheral vitrectomy and ensuring that all retinal tears were identified and laser-treated was crucial. A benefit of vitrectomy in these groups was that it allowed the removal of all vitreous opacities, treated the opacified lens capsules [7].

We performed SRF endodrainage by creating a tiny site-selected drainage retinotomy or using preexisting endodiathermy-marked retinal breaks. First, fluid-to-fluid exchange was performed over the retinal break to remove viscous proteinaceous SRF, reduce the extent of SRF and minimize the chance of trapped SRF before proceeding to an air-fluid exchange continuing with SRF drainage. Once the retina was completely free of vitreous traction and completely reattached, argon laser endophotocoagulation around the rhegmatogenous lesions and suspected retina areas was thoroughly performed; to completely dry out the subretinal space, a second air-fluid exchange was performed, and as the last surgical step, a nonexpandable bubble containing 15% perfluoropropane (C_3F_8) or 20% sulfur hexafluoride (SF_6) gas mixture was used as a long-acting tamponade at the end of the procedure in all cases.

SUMMARIZED ANALYSIS AMONG GROUPS

The baseline characteristics of the two study groups that have been previously published [7] are presented in Table **2**.

Table 2. Baseline characteristics of the two groups previously published by the authors [7].

Variable	Buckle Group	Vitrectomy Group	p Value
Age, mean±SD	44.3±15.9	50.4±13.5	0.054
Sex	-	-	-
Female	75 (60%)	19 (34.5%)	1.00
Male	50 (40%)	36 (65.5%)	-
Preop lens status	-	-	-
Phakic	48 (78.4%)	31 (36.4%)	0.068
Pseudophakic	27 (21.6%)	24 (43.6%)	-
Preop macula-off (weeks), mean± SD	3.6±2.5	4.52±2.4	0.425
Postop follow-up (months), mean±SD	26.12±13.4	25.62±12.4	0.131
Preop BCVA, mean ±SD	1.03±0.28	1.036±0.258	0.386

BCVA, best-corrected visual acuity; Postop, postoperative; Preop, preoperative; SD, standard deviation

Buckle Group

In the buckling group, additional surgeries not studied in this chapter were needed to correct for complications, such as recurrent RRD (11 eyes) with an additional surgery rate (ASR) of 8.8%, ERM removal (27 eyes; ASR of 21.6%), buckled revision (4 eyes; ASR of 3.2%), phakovitrectomy (3 eyes; ASR of 2.4%), vitrectomy (2 eyes; ASR of 1.6%), phakovitrectomy ERM removal (1 eye; ASR of 0.8%), and vitrectomy ERM removal (1 eye; ASR of 0.8%). Additionally, other serious surgical complications were treated conservatively and without further surgeries, such as thorough complication drainage (8 eyes; 6.4%), retinal perforation (7 eyes; 5.6%), trans-operative presence of submacular blood as a complication of SRF drainage or full-thickness scleral perforations (5 eyes; 4.0%) handled with pneumatic displacement, and noncomplex vitreoretinal entrapment released with surgical maneuvers in the first surgery (3 eyes; 2.4%) with a general ASR of 37.6% in the buckling group (Fig. **6**). A description of the consequent perfusion abnormalities observed is also presented (Fig. **7**).

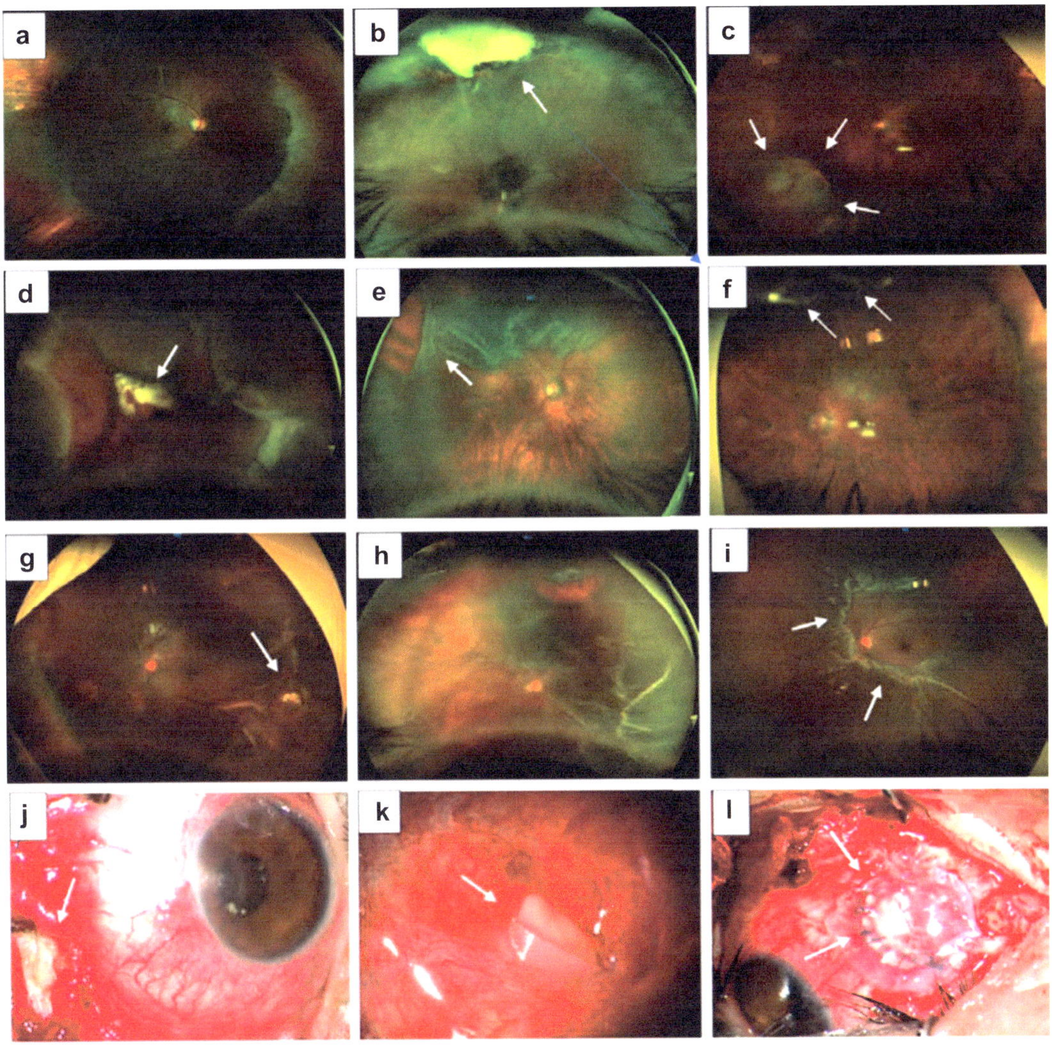

Fig. (6). ***Transoperative and postoperative buckle complications.*** (**a**) Image depicts an example of nicely buckled postoperative primary RRD that underwent an uneventful 360-degree 504 round Lincoff scleral sponges. No transoperative complications developed, and no evidence of ERM proliferation was noted with a final BCVA at the end of the follow-up of 20/30 (0.18 logMAR units). (**b**) An Optos wide-field color fundus photo of the left eye in the buckling group showed condensation and the initial appearance of a superior dense whitish vitreous hemorrhage (white arrow). In this case, a recurrent RRD was detected, and the eye underwent a vitrectomy procedure and endolaser retinopexy. Six weeks after the vitrectomy procedure, the total retina remained attached with evidence of ERM proliferation at the macula level; thus, the patient was unable to undergo a surgical ERM/ILM removal procedure. The BCVA at the end of follow-up was 20/80 (0.60 logMAR units equivalent). (**c**) Optos wide-field color image of a fundus 6 weeks after the buckling surgical procedure, wherein the eye continued to exhibit low-grade inflammation with some vitreous cells and the presence of a postoperative dome-shaped granuloma lesion (white arrows) at the 7 o'clock meridian, which resolved with anti-inflammatory and periocular antibiotics. The final BCVA at the end of the follow-up was 20/30 (0.18 logMAR units). (**d**) An image depicting a 360-degree severe nonkissing postoperative hemorrhagic choroidal detachment as a complication of massive choroidal bleeding after unintentional scleral perforation in the buckling procedure. However, the retina remains attached over the choroidal, and the macula and posterior pole appear attached. Retinal whitening is observed due to the presence of myelinated nerve fibers (white arrow). (**e**) Image of a right phakic eye in the vitrectomy group with a failed buckling procedure and no evidence of cryotherapy with nontreated rolled posterior edges retinal tear at the 10 o'clock meridian (white arrow). Another operculated retinal tear is present at the 11 o'clock meridian with a rolled posterior edge. The retinal indentation is very shallow, and the macula appears flat. Five days after the first surgical procedure, the eye underwent uneventful phakovitrectomy. Sixteen weeks after the phakovitrectomy procedure, the patient became symptomatic, and ERM proliferation over the macula was observed. The aforementioned eye underwent an uneventful ERM removal procedure, and the final BCVA at the end of the follow-up was 20/50 (0.40 logMAR units). (**f**) A buckle eye with some superior retinal scarring from excessive cryotherapy (white arrows), and the retina remained with a normal macula. The 360-degree scleral buckle and retina indentation appear regular and smooth. (**g**) Image from a 32-year-old phakic female who underwent a complicated scleral buckling procedure of her left eye. Two weeks after surgery, a mild vitreoretinal entrapment (white arrow) is noted with shallow evidence of SRF as well as a full-thickness retinal fold (red arrow) running from the entrapment site towards the posterior pole along the inferotemporal vascular arcade. In addition, blood remains on the preretinal space, and the BCVA at this level was 20/100 (0.70 logMAR units). The same eye also developed ERM proliferation and underwent phakovitrectomy with ERM removal. Summarizing the findings of this patient's eye, we noticed that she suffered from several complications: subretinal blood, retinal perforation, vitreoretinal entrapment and ERM proliferation over the macula at the end of follow-up. The final BCVA was 20/70 (0.54 logMAR units) at the end of the follow-up. (**h**) An Optos wide-angle view of the fundus of the left eye with a primary phakic non-complicated macula-off rhegmatogenous retinal detachment managed initially with a failed 360-degree oval 505 style S Labtician sponge buckling procedure. At the 1 o'clock meridian, there is a nontreated active leaking retinal tear along the posterior edge of lattice degeneration. One week after the first procedure, the eye underwent an uneventful phakovitrectomy, and the final BCVA at the end of follow-up was 20/40 (0.30 logMAR units). (**i**) Optos wide-field color fundus image depicts a recurrent RRD detected at 6 weeks after a buckling procedure with evidence of retinal rigidity, superficial epiretinal proliferation forming partial-thickness retinal folds around the optic nerve (white arrows). The macula appeared attached, and the eye underwent vitrectomy and ERM proliferation removal. After this second procedure, the retina remained attached with a final BCVA of 20/80 (0.60 logMAR units) at the end of follow-up. (**j**) Image depicts a long-term scleral buckling complication consistent with conjunctival erosion and exposition of the Lincoff sponge with some degree of infection after 32 months of the initial surgical procedures (white arrow). After sponge removal without sponge exchange, the retina remained attached, and the final BCVA was 20/50 (0.40 logMAR units). (**k**) and (**l**) Images from case #12 of the buckling dataset show the eye of a 48-year-old patient 4 years after the buckling surgical procedure. The eye had a long-term scleral complication consistent with severe scleral thinning erosion due to the use of exoplant in the hard silicon sleeve and exoplant intrusion into the globe. The eye was treated with scleral bank patch and amnios grafting over the debilitated scleral wall (white arrows), and the perforated retina remained attached with a final BCVA at the end of follow-up of 20/25 (0.10 logMAR units). This modified figure was adapted from [7] and GJMR 2021 vol 21 Issue 6. ISSN: 2249-4618. Print ISSN:0975-5888vol 21 Issue 6 and is used under the Creative Commons Attribution 4.0 International License (https://creativecommons.org/licenses/by/4.0/).

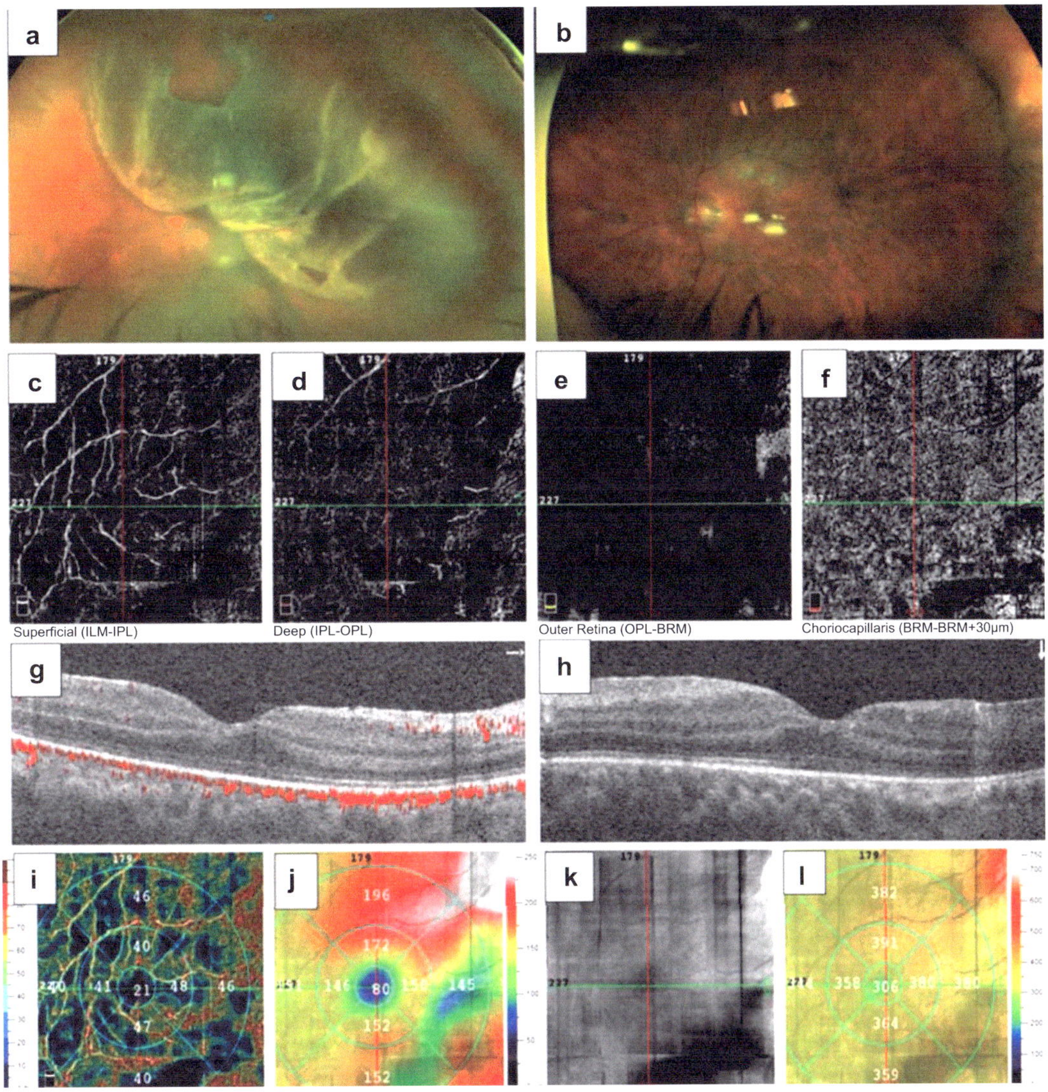

Fig. (7). Perfusion findings in a buckled eye. (**a**) Optos photo of bullous rhegmatogenous retinal detachment with a retinal tear is observed at the 12 o'clock meridian, and involvement of the macula is noted. The patient underwent an uneventful scleral buckle procedure with transscleral subretinal fluid drainage and satisfactory postoperative evolution. The postoperative BCVA was 20/40 (**a**) and (**b**) noncopyrighted images previously published [7] by the authors). (**c**) Image depicts the macular superficial vascular plexus slab with microcirculatory perfusion deficiencies. (**d**) The macular deep vascular plexus slab showed profound vascular perfusion deficiencies that were quantified as very low compared with that of control eyes. (**e**) and (**f**) Images depict abnormal outer retina and choriocapillaris slabs with some regions lacking choriocapillaris flow. (**g**) and (**h**) Images depict horizontal and vertical crossline structural evaluation through the fovea, an irregular postoperative foveal profile, and some abnormalities at the level of a layer of Henle. The scarcity of red dots indicates deficiencies in vascular flow intraretinally and at the level of choriocapillaris. (**i**) An abnormally deep vascular plexus at the different subregions of the macula on the ETDRS-like grid overlay when quantified and compared with the mean of that of normal controls. (**j**) Long-term postoperative irregular full-thickness macular topography. (**k**) En face deep retina layer aspect. (**l**) En face superficial retina aspect.

Vitrectomy Group

The baseline characteristics and a summary of postoperative outcomes of the vitrectomy group are presented in Tables **2** and **3**.

Table 3. Summary of postoperative outcomes in two groups.

Variables	Buckle group	Vitrectomy group	p value
Mean preop BCVA, mean±SD	1.03±0.2	1.036±0.25	0.386
Mean postop BCVA, mean ± SD before ERM removal	0.40±0.33	0.47±0.19	<0.05
ERM detection (weeks), mean±SD	11.9±4.54	18.0±6.45	0.009
RRD recurrence rate	8.8%	1 (1.82%)	0.001
Mean final BCVA after ERM removal, mean±SD	0.43±0.14	0.28±0.19	<0.05
Foveal contour abnormalities	19 eyes (15.2%)	Six eyes (11.3%)	<0.05
Mean CSFT (microns), mean±SD	243.57±41.95	266.71±32.75	0.173
DONFL defects present	31 eyes (24.8%)	Five eyes (11.36%)	<0.05
IS/OS (ellipsoid zone) integrity	Disrupted=25 eyes (20%) Normal=86 eyes (68.8%)	Disrupted=16 eyes (29.09%) Normal=39 eyes (70.40%)	0.002
ELM line appearance	Abnormal=24 eyes (19.2%) Normal=86 eyes (68.8%)	Disrupted=16 eyes (29.09%)	0.654
Follow-up period (months), mean ± SD	26.11±13.42	24.80±12.34	0.133

BCVA, best-corrected visual acuity; CSFT, central subfoveal thickness; DONFL, diffuse optic fiber layer; ERM, epiretinal membrane; IS/OS, internal segment/external segment; Preop, preoperative; RRD, rhegmatogenous retinal detachment; SD, standard deviation.

The GLM for the preoperative BCVA was not associated with the preoperative BCVA when adjusting for cofounders in the multivariate analyses. It was also found that postoperative BCVA was positively associated with the presence of significant ERM proliferation in the postoperative ERM proliferation analysis (rho=0.45, $p<0.01$). Additionally, there was a significant negative association when only vitrectomy was performed in the first surgery variable (rho=-0.23, $p<0.01$) and was significantly negatively associated with the variable preoperative period of macula-off in weeks (rho=-0.02, $p<0.05$).

The general prevalence of preoperative primary ERM proliferation was 4.78%. However, this prevalence should not be statistically considered due to the heterogeneity of criteria used to define preoperative primary or postoperative secondary ERM proliferation and because the eyes without evidence of preoperative ERM proliferation were intentionally selected.

The structural results are summarized in Table **2**. The correlation of some study variables with structural and visual outcomes was analyzed. In brief, no correlation was noted between postoperative BCVA and DONFL defects ($p>0.05$). Similarly, poor BCVA was associated with more CSFT alterations (rho=0.13, $p<0.05$). Additionally, better BCVA was associated with a lower incidence of ELM line alterations (rho=0.102, $p<0.05$). The mean postoperative BCVA in the eyes without dimples was 0.52±0.14 logMAR, and the mean postoperative BCVA in the eyes with dimples was 0.59±0.16 logMAR ($p>0.05$). The postoperative BCVA in some eyes that underwent ILM removal was not analyzed in this chapter, and the changes consistent with EZ disruptions ($p>0.05$) or ELM line abnormalities are shown ($p>0.05$) (Fig. **8**).

In the vitrectomy group, poor BCVA was associated with more EZ disruptions ($p<0.001$). Additionally, CSFT correlated with postoperative BCVA (rho=0.403, $p<0.05$), signifying that poor BCVA was associated with increased CSFT abnormalities. Similarly, poor BCVA was also associated with higher chances of ELM line abnormalities (rho=0.192, $p<0.05$). No eyes developed dimples (DONFL defects) regardless of their BCVA. In the eyes that developed ERM proliferation, BCVA did not correlate with the presence of EZ or ELM line abnormalities ($p>0.05$) (Fig. **9**).

The ASR rate in the vitrectomy group was 9.6%. Although not analyzed in this chapter, vitrectomy revision and ILM removal were performed in nine eyes (8.6%), vitrectomy in two eyes (1.9%), and phakovitrectomy ERM peeling in one eye (1.0%). The comparative incidence of early or short-term postoperative complications between the buckling and vitrectomy groups requiring additional surgical procedures was statistically significant ($p<0.05$) (Figs. **6** and **10**).

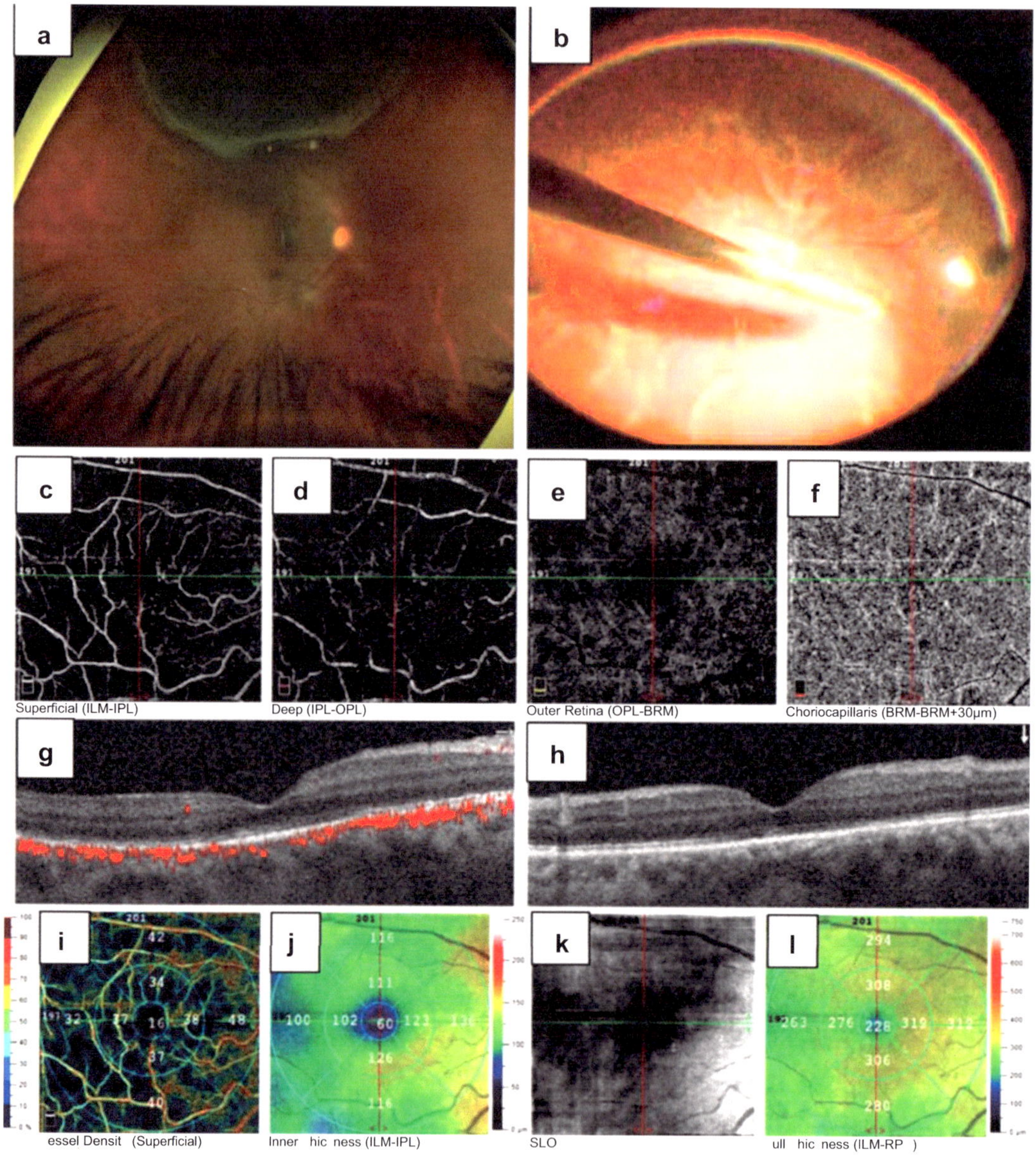

Fig. (8). ***Perfusion findings in a vitrectomy eye.*** (**a**) Optos wide-field color photo of a primary rhegmatogenous retinal detachment with superficial macular involvement that underwent uneventful primary vitrectomy. (**b**) Transoperative image of the primary vitrectomy endoillumination and peripheral vitreous trimming (**a**) and (**b**) noncopyrighted images previously published [7] by the authors). (**c**) (**d**) and (**f**) Images of the four vascular plexus slabs of the full-thickness retina and choriocapillaris depicting normal circulation pattern and perfusion indices compared with those of the control group. (**g**) and (**h**) Horizontal and vertical crossline structural B-scan evaluation depicting a normal foveal profile and normal outer retinal biomarkers. (**i**) Normal superficial vascular plexus at the different subregions of the macula on the ETDRS-like grid overlay when quantified and compared with the mean of that of normal controls. (**j**) The inner thickness topography of the macula was normal. (**k**) The SLO en face image was normal at the level of the superficial macula. (**l**) The full-thickness macula topography and values on the key to the right were between the normal range. This modified figure was adapted from [7] and GJMR 2021 vol 21 Issue 6. ISSN: 2249-4618. Print ISSN:0975-5888vol 21 Issue 6 and is used under the Creative Commons Attribution 4.0 International License (https://creativecommons.org/licenses/by/4.0/).

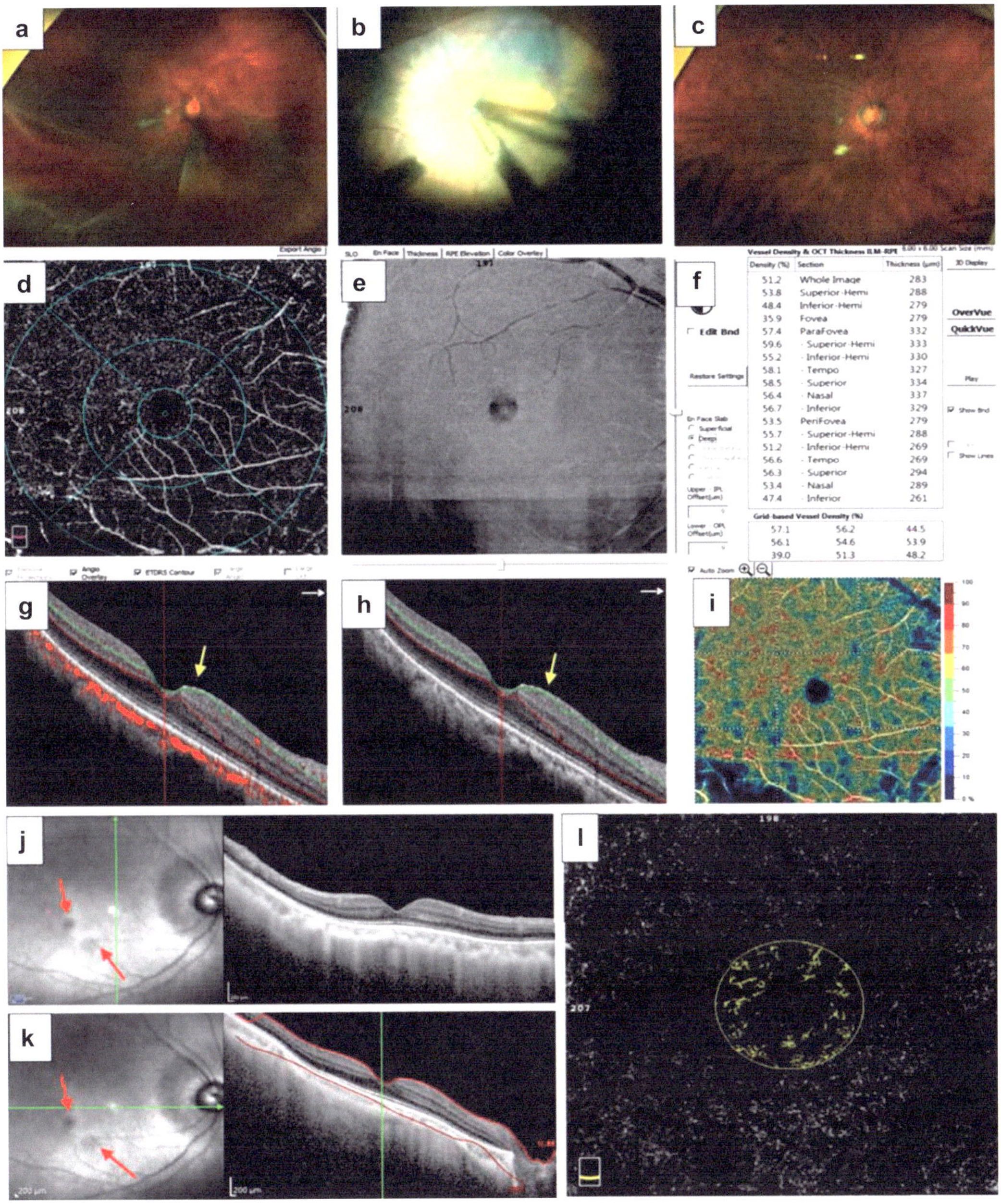

Fig. (9). ***Perfusion findings in an ERM peeling eye.*** (**a**) Optos wide-field color photo of a primary rhegmatogenous retinal detachment with evidence of epiretinal membrane (ERM) proliferation. (**b**) Surgical image of removal of the epiretinal membrane proliferation. (**c**) Corresponding long-term postoperative image (**a**) (**b**) and (**c**) noncopyrighted images previously published [7] by the authors). (**d**) Quantified superficial vascular plexus with important flow deficiencies in the different subregions of the macula based on the ETDRS-like grid overlay. (**e**) SLO en face image of the superficial macula. (**f**) The table presents the vessel densities and the macular thickness in microns at the different subregions of the macula. The grid-base vessel density exhibits at the bottom of the table. (**g**) and (**h**) Structural B-scans through the fovea depicting well preserved and recovered outer retinal biomarkers. However, well-documented retinal thinning is noted mainly over the temporal side of the macula, as demonstrated by the automated red and green segmentation lines (yellow arrows). (**i**) and (**k**) Abnormal en face superficial aspect of the retina with some dimpling noted in the corresponding vertical and horizontal crossline structural evaluation (red arrows). The foveal profile is preserved, and the outer retinal biomarkers are present. (**l**) Postoperative deep outer retina deficient choroidal values are noted compared with the control. This modified figure was adapted from [7] and GJMR 2021 vol 21 Issue 6. ISSN: 2249-4618. Print ISSN:0975-5888vol 21 Issue 6 and is used under the Creative Commons Attribution 4.0 International License (https://creativecommons.org/licenses/by/4.0/).

Retinal perfusional data on a reduced number of post operated patients evaluated is shown in Table **4**. Except for superficial foveal VD, all other perfusional indices differed significantly ($p<0.01$) from the control emmetropic groups. Deep foveal VD and choriocapillaris flow area were similar between the buckle group and vitrectomy group, whereas all other perfusional findings differed between the two groups. Pearson's correlation (Table **5**) showed that none of the perfusional indices correlated with the final BCVA in the vitrectomy and buckle groups, whereas superficial whole macula VD and deep whole macula VD in control emmetropic groups negatively correlated with the final BCVA ($p<0.05$) (Figs. **7-9**).

Table 4. Comparison of the retinal perfusional findings in the normal emmetropic, buckle, and vitrectomy groups.

Study groups	Superficial FAZ area (mm^2, mean ± SD)	Superficial foveal VD (%, mean ± SD)	Deep foveal VD (%, mean ± SD)	Superficial parafoveal VD (%, mean ± SD)	Deep parafoveal VD (%, mean ± SD)	Superficial whole macula VD (%, mean ± SD)	Deep whole macula VD (%, mean ± SD)	Choriocapillaris flow area (mm^2, mean ± SD)
Control emmetropic (n=25)	0.33 ± 0.04	27.17 ± 3.40	31.39 ± 3.06	58.76 ± 3.03	59.17 ± 2.60	56.93 ± 4.27	58.5 ± 3.6	2.53±0.27
Buckle group (n=51)	0.68± 0.12*	27.94±3.22	34.63±42.02*	50.90± 5.24*	52.63± 4.96*	50.11± 3.60*	49.38±7.92*	1.88±0.20*
Vitrectomy group (n=52)	0.68± 0.29*	27.4±3.4	29.19±3.19*	49.58± 5.76*	51.82± 5.38*	48.34± 4.01*	49.5± 4.38*	1.88±0.42*
Comparison with control emmetropic (p value)	0.0001	NS	0.01	0.0001	0.0001	0.0001	0.0001	0.0001

(Table 4) cont.....

Study groups	Superficial FAZ area (mm^2, mean ± SD)	Superficial foveal VD (%, mean ± SD)	Deep foveal VD (%, mean ± SD)	Superficial parafoveal VD (%, mean ± SD)	Deep parafoveal VD (%, mean ± SD)	Superficial whole macula VD (%, mean ± SD)	Deep whole macula VD (%, mean ± SD)	Choriocapillaris flow area (mm^2, mean ± SD)
Comparison between buckle group and vitrectomy group (t-test p value)	0.039*	0.0001	0.053	0.0001	0.0001	0.0001	0.0001	0.28

Table 5. Pearson's correlation statistics of final BCVA among the two study groups and control group.

-	Superficial FAZ area	Superficial foveal VD	Deep foveal VD	Superficial parafoveal VD	Deep parafoveal VD	Superficial whole macula VD	Deep whole macula VD	Choriocapillaris flow area
Control emmetropic	0.58	0.08	0.81	0.75	0.81	0.01*	0.01*	0.88
Buckle group	0.34	0.32	0.18	0.12	0.12	0.06	0.08	0.6
Vitrectomy group	0.13	0.47	0.51	0.17	0.28	0.50	0.28	0.22

LITERATURE REVIEW AND DISCUSSION

The analysis of the authors' experience in this chapter results showed functionally satisfactory outcomes in the vitrectomy group compared with those in the buckling group. We found a significant percentage of postoperative ERM proliferation in the buckling and vitrectomy groups. We also observed multiple structural alterations and perfusional abnormalities in the long-term postoperative biomarkers. Eyes that developed secondary postoperative ERM proliferation in the buckling group and the vitrectomy group showed statistically significant improvements in BCVA once the macular ERM proliferation was removed, but the abnormalities in the status of the biomarkers did not disappear.

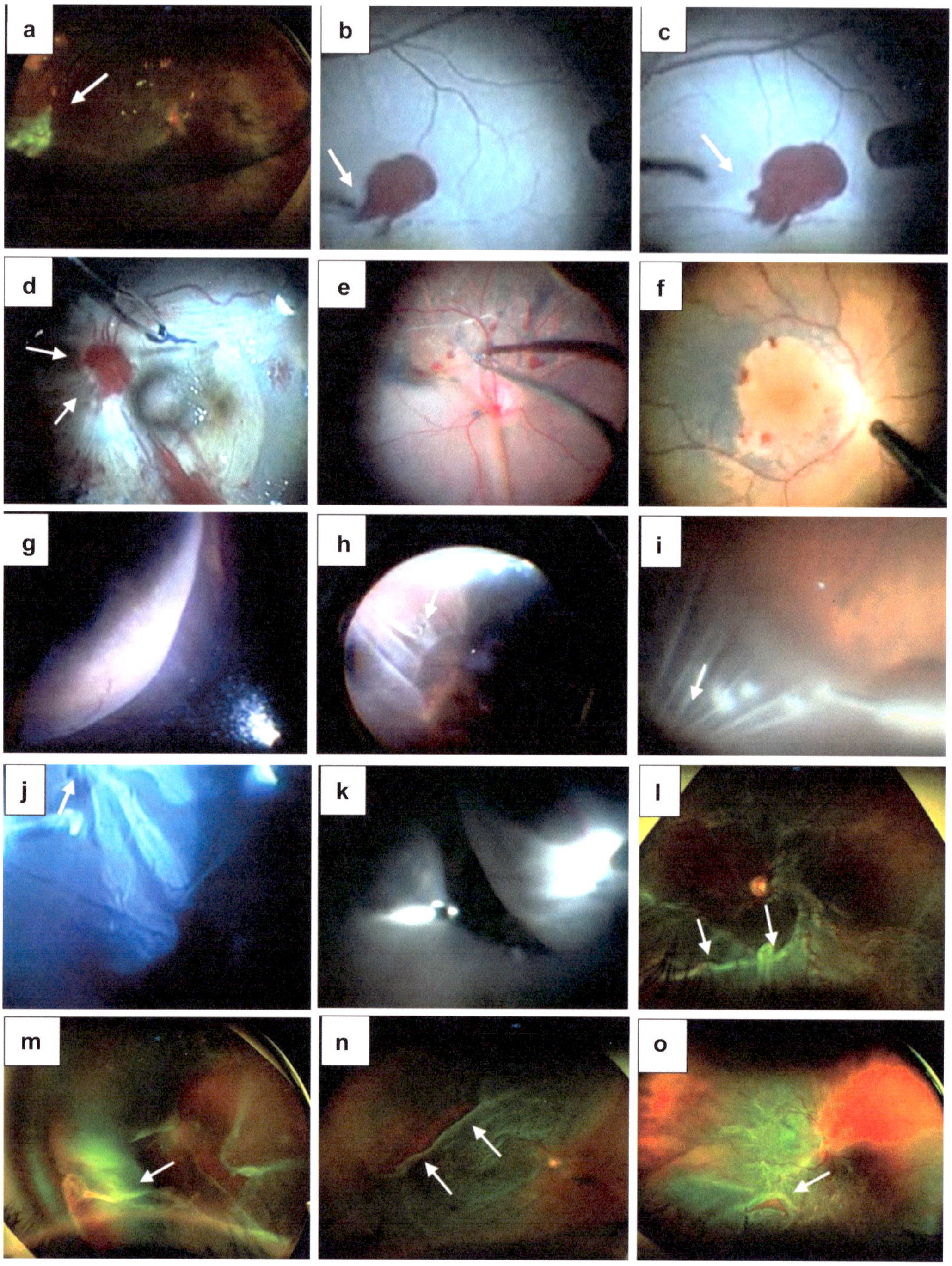

Fig. (10). ***Transoperative and postoperative vitrectomy and internal limiting membrane peeling complications.*** (**a**) Image shows a case of a failed buckle procedure with a recurrent RRD that underwent vitrectomy complement with ERM/ILM complex removal due to the presence of significant ERM proliferation. Recent argon laser spots (white arrow) and 70% residual SF_6 gas bubble with evidence of inferior, shallow recurrent retinal detachment are shown. (**b**) and (**c**) Sequential images depict a rather dim brilliant blue (BBG) ILM staining with arterial bleeding at the time of pulling the ILM in a case with a shallow macula-off retinal detachment (white arrows). (**d**) Image depicts bleeding from the papilla as the ILM is peeled off in this macula-off RRD case (white arrows). In this case, BBG ILM staining-perfluorocarbon heavy liquids to reapply the retina-ILM three-step removal technique was used. (**e**) Image depicts tractional bleeding as the ILM was being pulled to release the macula. (**f**) Image depicts spot bleeding due to inner retinal punctate retinopathy-related ILM peeling. (**g**) Image depicts a hydraulic choroidal and pars plana detachment caused by a mispositioning of the infusion vitrectomy line trocar entry site. (**h**) Transoperative image with vitreoretinal entrapment at the level of the vitrectomy entry site, along with a tiny peripheral retinal tear (white arrow). (**i**) Transoperative image depicts vitreoretinal entrapment at the level of the vitrectomy entry site (white arrow). (**j**) Image depicts a vitreoretinal entrapment (white arrow) at the moment of transoperative transient ocular hypotony. (**k**) Image depicts a hydraulic choroidal and pars plana detachment caused by a mispositioning of the infusion vitrectomy line trocar entry site. (**l**) Image depicts Optos wide-angle color photo 6 weeks after primary vitrectomy of a very complex PVR complicated RRD. Membrane subretinal membrane proliferation is noted around the optic nerve and beneath the detached inferior retina (white arrows). (**m**) Image depicts a complex hemorrhagic choroidal and rhegmatogenous RRD (white arrow). (**n**) Image depicts Optos wide-angle color photo 6 weeks after primary vitrectomy of a very complex PVR complicated RRD, and a large retinal tear is shown supertemporally (white arrows). (**o**) Image depicts a subtotal complicated RRD after primary vitrectomy, and an active leaking retinal tear with rolled-back borders is noted between 6 and 7 o'clock meridians (white arrow). The posterior pole retina appears stiff. The functional results in the selected groups of patients with ERM/ILM complex removal were not functional or statistically analyzed in this chapter. The modified figure was adapted from [7] and GJMR 2021 vol 21 Issue 6. ISSN: 2249-4618. Print ISSN:0975-5888vol 21 Issue 6 and is used under the Creative Commons Attribution 4.0 International License (https://creativecommons.org/licenses/by/4.0/).

The placement of a scleral buckle is the most established technique for treating primary RRD [8]. There has been a plethora of information supporting this procedure's short-term efficacy; however, there is a relative paucity of long-term data. Scleral buckle surgery and primary PPV techniques are the most common surgical techniques used in treating RDs [9]. These procedures are performed alone or in combination with other surgeries. Several authors suggest that vitrectomy techniques alone should be used to manage a primary, noncomplicated macula-off RRD. However, the literature suggests that while some cases can be managed successfully with vitrectomy, an important subset of noncomplicated, macula-off RRD will benefit from buckling techniques [10]. Recent reports propose that the total proportions of surgical failures in the PPV group were higher than those in the scleral buckling group [11]. Therefore, we conducted the analysis of selected patients in this study to gain insight into a better surgical technique to manage RRD through retrospective cohort data and related postoperative perfusional markers across the groups. We reported long-term anatomical and visual outcomes and perfusional outcomes after two different types of surgeries in our patient cohort.

The narrative in this chapter shows that placing a scleral buckle adds additional risks and possible undesirable postoperative complications. The management of noncomplicated RRD with scleral buckling achieved good anatomic outcomes.

However, this procedure can be associated with transoperative and postoperative complications, which require additional surgeries. In our cohort, 39.2% of eyes [7] required different additional interventions in the buckling group. To manage macula-off RRD with vitrectomy, we placed a complementary 360° scleral buckle only in complex or complicated cases involving diffuse tractional membranes, such as RRDs complicated with significant PVR, failed prior RRD surgery, extensive peripheral vitreoretinal adhesions with multiple retinal tears, RRD associated with penetrating globe injury and/or retained intraocular foreign bodies and selected RRD associated with giant retinal tears.

The selective use of a complementary scleral buckle can achieve good visual outcomes in noncomplicated cases [13]. However, in complex clinical cases, such as those with total RRD, better anatomical outcomes are achieved through vitrectomy when complemented with scleral buckling [14].

Peeling the ILM off during surgery has been dependent on several factors, including preexisting ERM proliferation in the macula and a surgeon's personal choice [15]. There have been reports of no functional or structural benefits of ILM peeling after primary vitrectomy for noncomplicated RRD [16]. In patients in whom ILM remains unpeeled and ERM proliferation occurs, additional surgeries are required, complicating the disease management process and the visual prognosis [14, 15]. The incidence of postoperative ERM proliferation has been reported to range from 27.6% to 38.4% after cryoretinopexy and from 21.5% to 58% after vitrectomy without ILM removal [17 - 19]. We observed a postoperative ERM proliferation rate of 23.2% in the buckling group, and 23.63% in the vitrectomy group. These findings are concurrent with the literature. In a retrospective analysis of 89 eyes with primary macula-involved retinal detachment, Garweg *et al.* [20] reported a lower redetachment rate, incidence of secondary epiretinal membranes, and revitrectomy rates in the ILM-peeled group. This clinical variable was not analyzed in the present chapter.

In the vitrectomy group, we found that some variables, such as first surgery, BCVA before ERM, recurrence of ERM, additional surgery, ERM proliferation detection in weeks, final postoperative BCVA, foveal contour abnormalities, and DONFL defects, were significantly more common. However, functional analysis of these structural abnormalities in SD-OCT considered categorical variables, such as EZ disruptions, CSFT abnormalities, and ELM line discontinuities; however, these variables were not directly correlated with the final BCVA due to a lack of statistical significance.

Tabandeh *et al.* [18] reported the role of prophylactic ILM removal in reducing the incidence of postoperative ERM proliferation. They reported that case selection based on the complexity of RD might be decisive in obtaining a good visual outcome. ILM removal avoids the necessity for additional surgeries; however, the procedure can cause several transoperative complications, mainly related to mechanical trauma (e.g., retinal tears, retinal edema, papillary hemorrhage, retinal hemorrhage, iatrogenic punctuate hemorrhagic retinopathy, vitreous hemorrhage, and subretinal hemorrhage) [21]. Such clinical conditions may lead to decreased final visual acuity. Moreover, structural sequelae such as DONFL defects may occur due to a diffuse loss of Müller cell end-feet [22 - 24]. We observed the DONFL defects in the form of concentric macular dark spots, known as retinal dimples, in the vitrectomy group. In some eyes, a modified and improved appearance of the external layer of the retina was observed without a total recovery of the normal tomographic pattern. This superficial dimpling finding has been reported as a consequence of ILM removal and was first described by Alkabes *et al.* [24] as a subclinical finding. Its effect on macular function as measured by microperimetry and mfERG [22] remains controversial; patients undergoing ILM removal techniques were not functionally analyzed in this chapter. However, an improvement in the final BCVA was documented in the selected group of eyes once the ERM proliferation was removed.

We observed that tiny DONFL defects without ILM removal in the limited number of eyes that underwent ERM removal did not affect final BCVA, as previously described by other authors [25].

Few studies [26] have shown that the final BCVA correlates better with the period the photoreceptors remain detached from the RPE. This possible deleterious complication might be correlated with the appearance of the EZ, and this strong SD-OCT biomarker was found to be serially abnormal and disrupted in our study. Schuman *et al.* [27] correlated the retinal cleavage plane of the ILM using transmission electron microscopy with the functional results with histopathological data. There were no conclusive remarks regarding whether the presence and amount of retinal cell fragments in ILM specimens correlate with functional deficits.

Furthermore, only one eye (1.8%) in the vitrectomy group in our study was found to harvest long-term residual SRF. However, advanced age is considered a significant risk factor for developing postoperative SRF, especially in patients where a buckle is placed. A gradual decrease in RPE pumping due to aging after reattachment to the neurosensory retina could explain this finding [28, 29]. The median age in our study was 51±14 years, and only one eye with chronic residual SRF was reported. Consequently, this variable was not considered a cause for poor visual results.

In this study using SD-OCT, we documented multiple structural alterations, such as diffuse thinning of the neurosensory macula, morphological alterations in the foveal contour, a significant decrease in the mean CSFT, and EZ and ELM line disruptions and reflectivity discontinuities, in the two groups. A statistically nonsignificant predominance of these alterations was observed in the vitrectomy group (Table **2**). Retinal perfusional data showed that all other perfusional indices differed significantly ($p<0.01$) from the control emmetropic groups except for superficial foveal VD. As the superficial FAZ area enlarged, deep foveal VD increased in the buckle group but decreased in the vitrectomy group, and deep parafoveal, superficial whole macula VD, deep whole macula VD, and CFA decreased in both the buckle and vitrectomy groups compared with the control emmetropic group (all $p<0.01$). Retinal perfusional data is shown in Table **4**. Except for superficial foveal VD, all other perfusional indices differed significantly ($p<0.01$) from the control emmetropic groups. Similarly, deep foveal VD and CFA were similar between the buckle only and vitrectomy only groups whereas all other perfusional findings differed between the two groups. Pearson's correlation demonstrated that better macular perfusion could predict a better visual outcome. In the buckle group, the superficial FAZ area correlated with the final visual acuity.

A recently published meta-analysis [30] reported a recurrence RRD rate between 28% and 21% after scleral buckling and primary vitrectomy, respectively, and Deiss *et al.* [31] reported a recurrence RRD rate of 25.55% after vitrectomy with ILM peeling in the treatment of primary macula involving RRD. We observed a high rate of recurrence of detachment in the vitrectomy group (24.0%) and considered that perhaps the ERM removal maneuvers were intimately associated with the risk of producing tiny subclinical iatrogenic rhegmatogenous lesions, which significantly increased the incidence of such condition.

How the removal of ILM affects functional recovery is still unclear, and further studies are required to understand this question [32]. We consider that the only indication for ILM removal in the management of a noncomplicated macula-off RRD is to relieve or prevent postoperative macular traction caused by a well-documented pre- or trans-operative ERM proliferation. Therefore, a noncomplicated macula-off RRD should be managed with vitrectomy and macular surgery involving the removal of the ERM/ILM complex and additional scleral buckling performed at the surgeon's discretion. When the ILM was removed, the incidence of ERM was 0.003% [16] to 2.0% (Table **2**) and ranged from 21.5% to 58% when the ILM was not removed. A prophylactic approach to prevent the formation of ERM proliferation over the macula is not currently justified in our experience and should be reserved for complicated cases; thus, this

ILM removal approach was not functionally nor statistically analyzed in this chapter.

Znaor *et al.* [30] reported that the duration of RRD prior to primary vitrectomy is not a significant risk factor for postoperative BCVA. However, we found a strong positive correlation between the final BCVA and the mean period of macular detachment before surgery (3.6±2.5 weeks in the buckling group and 4.4±2.6 weeks in the vitrectomy group). This factor possibly contributed to the poor functional result in the buckling group. The same authors reported a greater subfoveal thickness and lower final vision, which should be interpreted carefully since the thickness is also related to a patient's age, and choroidal structure deterioration and photoreceptor loss with aging could explain this finding [33]. While highly effective, scleral buckling techniques involve the permanent insertion of a buckle device around the eye, which may alter the normal physiology of the vascular tissue, including restricting circulation. Indeed, previous studies have shown that scleral buckling is associated with reduced tissue blood velocity in the retina and choroid [34, 35]. The choroid is a highly vascularized tissue that provides an essential blood supply to the RPE and outer retina [36]. A restricted blood supply to the choroid may adversely affect the outer retina, including photoreceptors, potentially disrupting tissue homeostasis and causing chorioretinal tissue damage. The choroidal vascularity index (CVI) is a recently introduced quantification parameter that represents the vascular status of the choroid based on OCT high quality images [37]. CVI was developed as a more precise and robust measurement of choroidal vascularity than previous measurements (such as choroidal vessel diameter and choroidal thickness), which have important limitations [38]. Variations in CVI can be used as an indicator of choroidal vasculature changes, but it cannot capture choriocapillaris flow, an important characteristic of choroidal vasculature [39].

The partial report analyzed in the present chapter has several strengths, including a long-term design that helps generalize the findings to evaluate structural and perfusional retinal and choroidal values and assess complications. The retrospective design is the main limitation of the study, and due to the limited sample size, mainly reflected in the reduced perfusional analysis dataset, real-life conclusions cannot be obtained based on a few cases. Notwithstanding these limitations, we have reported several interesting structural and perfusional findings that will stimulate further studies in the field.

CONCLUDING REMARKS

The removal of the ERM/ILM complex to avoid postoperative ERM reproliferation or postoperative ERM proliferation is not justified, as it may potentially lead to future complications and poor visual outcomes. Although no significant difference in ERM proliferation was noted between the two groups, there were significant functional, structural and perfusional differences between the buckling group and the vitrectomy group. Therefore, further studies are required to better establish the role of ILM removal in postoperative ERM proliferation and the role of buckling surgery on the macular perfusion indices and final correlated BCVA. Further investigation evaluating the CVI and the role of long-term scleral buckling is needed. Additionally, we observed that at long-term follow-up, a microstructurally and functionally abnormal macula was visible in the two groups but predominantly in the buckling group; long-term lower macular perfusional indices were observed mainly in the buckling group, but additional results with CVI evaluation are needed. The anatomical and functional results of this comparative, retrospective, long-term structural and perfusional study indicated significant visual damage at the clinical level when a noncomplicated macula-off RRD is associated with the placement of a scleral buckle as reflected in lower postoperative perfusional indices or associated with a primary ERM proliferation that must be resolved by performing vitrectomy complemented with ERM proliferation removal techniques as described in this report. It remains to be resolved in future studies how the 360° scleral buckling procedures or postoperative presence of ERM proliferation or its surgical removal together with the ILM affects the macular retinal perfusion and CVI indices and consequently the final BCVA.

PATIENT CONSENT

Written informed consent was obtained from all patients in accordance with institutional guidelines.

SUPPLEMENTARY MATERIAL

Table S1: Shapiro–Wilk normality test results.

Table S2: Descriptive statistics for the numeric variables.

Table S3: Summary statistics for the categorical variables.

Table S4: Correlations between the numeric variables.

Table S5: Mann–Whitney U test results. (**A**) Preoperative best corrected visual acuity (BCVA). (**B**) Postoperative BCVA. (**C**) BCVA after epiretinal membrane surgery.

Table S6: A. Kruskal–Wallis test results of the preoperative best-corrected visual acuity (BCVA) with the categorical variables. B. Kruskal–Wallis test results of the postoperative BCVA with the categorical variables. C. Kruskal–Wallis test results of BCVA after epiretinal membrane surgery with the categorical variables.

Table S7: Generalized linear model results of preoperative best-corrected visual acuity (BCVA), postoperative BCVA, and BCVA after epiretinal membrane surgery.

Table S8: Shapiro–Wilk normality test results.

Table S9: Descriptive statistics for the numeric variables.

Table S10: Summary statistics for the categorical variables.

Table S11: Descriptive statistics with respect to the peeling (preoperative epiretinal membrane proliferation) groups.

Table S12: Correlations among the numeric variables.

Table S13: Mann–Whitney U test results. (**A**) Preoperative best corrected visual acuity (BCVA). (**B**) Postoperative BCVA. (**C**) Final BCVA.

Table S14: Kruskal–Wallis test results. (**A**) Preoperative best corrected visual acuity (BCVA). (**B**) Postoperative BCVA. (**C**) Final BCVA.

Table S15: Generalized linear model results. (**A**) Preoperative best corrected visual acuity (BCVA). (**B**) Postoperative BCVA. (**C**) Final BCVA.

Additional Figure S1: Spearman's rank correlation coefficient test showed that there was a moderate to strong positive correlation (rho= 0.57, $p<0.01$) of the postoperative BCVA in logMAR units with the BCVA after ERM surgery. In addition, there was a weak negative correlation (rho = -0.2, $p<0.05$) between postoperative BCVA in logMAR units and the follow-up period in months.

Additional Figure S2: Spearman's rank correlation coefficient test showed a weak positive correlation (rho= 0.32, $p<0.05$) between the preoperative period with the macula-off in weeks and the CSFT findings in microns; it also showed a weak negative correlation (rho= -0.29, $p<0.05$) between the preoperative BCVA in logMAR units and ERM detection in weeks.

Additional Figure S3: Postoperative BCVA was significantly negatively associated when only vitrectomy (nonpeeling group) was performed in the first surgery variable (coefficient = -0.23, $p<0.01$) and significantly negatively associated with the variable preoperative period of macula-off in weeks (coefficient= -0.02, $p<0.05$).

Additional Figure S4: The GLM for the final BCVA in log MAR units after ERM proliferation removal showed that it was significantly positively associated ($p>0.01$) with the postoperative.

Additional Figure S5: It shows when only vitrectomy was the first surgery variable and with the preoperative BCVA.

LIST OF ABBREVIATIONS

ASR	Additional surgery rate
BBG	Brilliant Blue G
BCVA	Best-corrected visual acuity
CFA	Choriocapillaris flow area
CVI	Choroidal vascularity index
CSFT	Central subfoveal thickness
DONFL	Dissociated optic nerve fiber layer
ELM	External limiting membrane
ERM	Epiretinal membrane
FAZ	Foveal avascular area
ILM	Internal limiting membrane
logMAR	Logarithm of the minimum angle of resolution
OCT	Optical coherence tomography
OCT-A	Optical coherent tomography angiography
PFCL	Perfluorocarbon liquid
PVR	Proliferative vitreoretinopathy
RD	Retinal detachment
RPE	Retinal pigment epithelium
RRD	Rhegmatogenous retinal detachment
SD-OCT	Spectral-domain optical coherence tomography
SS	Swept source
VD	Vessel density

DISCLAIMER

All the scientific comments issued in this chapter are solely the responsibility of the authors and not of the institutions with which they are affiliated. This chapter is an extended and modified version of the article published by the same author(s) in the following journal. J Clin Exp Ophthalmol 2021, Vol.12 Iss.S18 No:1000005.

ACKNOWLEDGMENTS

We express our deep appreciation to the technical staff of the Retina Specialists Unit at Oftalmologia Integral ABC (Nonprofit Medical and Surgical Organization) affiliated with The Postgraduate Division Studies at the National Autonomous University of Mexico.

REFERENCES

[1] La Heij EC, Derhaag PFJM, Hendrikse F. Results of scleral buckling operations in primary rhegmatogenous retinal detachment. Doc Ophthalmol 2000; 100(1): 17-25. [http://dx.doi.org/10.1023/A:1001733602965] [PMID: 11117407]

[2] Chronopoulos A, Schutz J, Varga Z, Souteyrand G, Thumann G. Complications of encircling bands-prevention and management. J Clin Exp Ophthalmol 2015; 6(3): 2. [http://dx.doi.org/10.4172/2155-9570.1000440]

[3] Nichani PAH, Dhoot AS, Popovic MM, *et al.* Scleral buckling alone or in combination with pars plana vitrectomy for rhegmatogenous retinal detachment repair: A meta-analysis of 7212 eyes. Ophthalmologica 2022; 245(4): 296-314. [http://dx.doi.org/10.1159/000524888] [PMID: 35533652]

[4] Poulsen CD, Green A, Grauslund J, Peto T. Long-term outcome of patients operated with pars plana vitrectomy for primary rhegmatogenous retinal detachment. Ophthalmic Res 2020; 63(1): 25-33. [http://dx.doi.org/10.1159/000499130] [PMID: 31013505]

[5] Halfter W, Willem M, Mayer U. Basement membrane-dependent survival of retinal ganglion cells. Invest Ophthalmol Vis Sci 2005; 46(3): 1000-9. [http://dx.doi.org/10.1167/iovs.04-1185] [PMID: 15728558]

[6] Almony A, Nudleman E, Shah GK, *et al.* Techniques, rationale, and outcomes of internal limiting membrane peeling. Retina 2012; 32(5): 877-91. [http://dx.doi.org/10.1097/IAE.0b013e318227ab39] [PMID: 22105502]

[7] Quiroz-Reyes MA, Quiroz-Gonzalez EA, Morales-Navarro J. A critical analysis of non-complicated macula-off rhegmatogenous retinal detachment with and without internal limiting membrane peeling. J Clin Exp Ophthalmol 2021; 12: 19.

[8] Schwartz SG, Kuhl DP, McPherson AR, Holz ER, Mieler WF. Twenty-year follow-up for scleral buckling. Arch Ophthalmol 2002; 120(3): 325-9. [http://dx.doi.org/10.1001/archopht.120.3.325] [PMID: 11879136]

[9] Popovic MM, Muni RH, Nichani P, Kertes PJ. Pars plana vitrectomy, scleral buckle, and pneumatic retinopexy for the management of rhegmatogenous retinal detachment: A meta-analysis. Surv Ophthalmol 2022; 67(1): 184-96. [http://dx.doi.org/10.1016/j.survophthal.2021.05.008] [PMID: 34043984]

[10] Klaas JE, Siedlecki J, Steel DH, Laidlaw DAH, Priglinger S. How should we report the foveal status in eyes with *macula-off* retinal detachment? Eye 2022. [http://dx.doi.org/10.1038/s41433-022-02074-7] [PMID: 35505112]

[11] Kawano S, Imai T, Sakamoto T. Scleral buckling versus pars plana vitrectomy in simple phakic macula-on retinal detachment: A propensity score-matched, registry-based study. Br J Ophthalmol 2022; 106(6): 857-62. [http://dx.doi.org/10.1136/bjophthalmol-2020-318451] [PMID: 33514527]

[12] Cacciamani A, Cosimi P, Ripandelli G, Di Nicola M, Scarinci F. Epiretinal membrane surgery: Structural retinal changes correlate with the improvement of visual function. J Clin Med 2020; 10(1): 90.

[http://dx.doi.org/10.3390/jcm10010090] [PMID: 33383922]

[13] Tabandeh H, Khachaturov A, Rezaei KA, Boyer DS. Supplemental scleral buckle in the era of small incision vitrectomy and wide-angle viewing systems. Retina 2020; 40(10): 1894-9. [http://dx.doi.org/10.1097/IAE.0000000000002706] [PMID: 31834132]

[14] Tan HS, Mura M, Lesnik Oberstein SY, de Smet MD. Primary retinectomy in proliferative vitreoretinopathy. Am J Ophthalmol 2010; 149(3): 447-52. [http://dx.doi.org/10.1016/j.ajo.2009.10.017] [PMID: 20172071]

[15] Schneider EW, Geraets RL, Johnson MW. Pars plana vitrectomy without adjuvant procedures for repair of primary rhegmatogenous retinal detachment. Retina 2012; 32(2): 213-9. [http://dx.doi.org/10.1097/IAE.0b013e3182278b29] [PMID: 21811205]

[16] Eissa MGAM, Abdelhakim MASE, Macky TA, Khafagy MM, Mortada HA. Functional and structural outcomes of ILM peeling in uncomplicated macula-off RRD using microperimetry & en-face OCT. Graefes Arch Clin Exp Ophthalmol 2018; 256(2): 249-57. [http://dx.doi.org/10.1007/s00417-017-3875-7] [PMID: 29299741]

[17] Nam KY, Kim JY. Effect of internal limiting membrane peeling on the development of epiretinal membrane after pars plana vitrectomy for primary rhegmatogenous retinal detachment. Retina 2015; 35(5): 880-5. [http://dx.doi.org/10.1097/IAE.0000000000000421] [PMID: 25545479]

[18] Tabandeh H, London NJS, Boyer DS, Flynn HW Jr. Outcomes of small-gauge vitreoretinal surgery without scleral-depressed shaving of the vitreous base in the era of wide-angle viewing systems. Br J Ophthalmol 2019; 103(12): 1765-8. [http://dx.doi.org/10.1136/bjophthalmol-2018-313626] [PMID: 30770355]

[19] Bovey EH, Uffer S, Achache F. Surgery for epimacular membrane: Impact of retinal internal limiting membrane removal on functional outcome. Retina 2004; 24(5): 728-35. [http://dx.doi.org/10.1097/00006982-200410000-00007] [PMID: 15492626]

[20] Garweg JG, Deiss M, Pfister IB, Gerhardt C. Impact of inner limiting membrane peeling on visual recovery after vitrectomy for primary rhegmatogenous retinal detachment involving the fovea. Retina 2019; 39(5): 853-9. [http://dx.doi.org/10.1097/IAE.0000000000002046] [PMID: 29394235]

[21] Abdullah ME, Moharram HEM, Abdelhalim AS, Mourad KM, Abdelkader MF. Evaluation of primary internal limiting membrane peeling in cases with rhegmatogenous retinal detachment. Int J Retina Vitr 2020; 6(1): 8. [http://dx.doi.org/10.1186/s40942-020-00213-4] [PMID: 32411388]

[22] Schwartz SG, Flynn HW. Primary retinal detachment: Scleral buckle or pars plana vitrectomy? Curr Opin Ophthalmol 2006; 17(3): 245-50. [http://dx.doi.org/10.1097/01.icu.0000193097.28798.fc] [PMID: 16794436]

[23] Haritoglou C, Gass CA, Schaumberger M, Ehrt O, Gandorfer A, Kampik A. Macular changes after peeling of the internal limiting membrane in macular hole surgery. Am J Ophthalmol 2001; 132(3): 363-8. [http://dx.doi.org/10.1016/S0002-9394(01)01093-5] [PMID: 11530049]

[24] Alkabes M, Salinas C, Vitale L, Burés-Jelstrup A, Nucci P, Mateo C. En face optical coherence tomography of inner retinal defects after internal limiting membrane peeling for idiopathic macular hole. Invest Ophthalmol Vis Sci 2011; 52(11): 8349-55. [http://dx.doi.org/10.1167/iovs.11-8043] [PMID: 21862645]

[25] Tari SR, Vidne-Hay O, Greenstein VC, Barile GR, Hood DC, Chang S. Functional and structural measurements for the assessment of internal limiting membrane peeling in idiopathic macular pucker. Retina 2007; 27(5): 567-72. [http://dx.doi.org/10.1097/IAE.0b013e31802ea53d] [PMID: 17558317]

[26] Spaide RF. "Dissociated optic nerve fiber layer appearance" after internal limiting membrane removal is inner retinal dimpling. Retina 2012; 32(9): 1719-26. [http://dx.doi.org/10.1097/IAE.0b013e3182671191] [PMID: 23007669]

[27] Schumann RG, Gandorfer A, Priglinger SG, Kampik A, Haritoglou C. Vital dyes for macular surgery: a comparative electron microscopy study of the internal limiting membrane. Retina 2009; 29(5): 669-76. [http://dx.doi.org/10.1097/IAE.0b013e318196b1c8] [PMID: 19174722]

[28] Balducci N, Morara M, Veronese C, Torrazza C, Pichi F, Ciardella AP. Retinal nerve fiber layer thickness modification after internal limiting membrane peeling. Retina 2014; 34(4): 655-63. [http://dx.doi.org/10.1097/IAE.0000000000000004] [PMID: 24670998]

[29] Chen H, Lukas TJ, Du N, Suyeoka G, Neufeld AH. Dysfunction of the retinal pigment epithelium with age: Increased iron decreases phagocytosis and lysosomal activity. Invest Ophthalmol Vis Sci 2009; 50(4): 1895-902. [http://dx.doi.org/10.1167/iovs.08-2850] [PMID: 19151392]

[30] Znaor L, Medic A, Binder S, Vucinovic A, Marin Lovric J, Puljak L. Pars plana vitrectomy versus scleral buckling for repairing simple rhegmatogenous retinal detachments. Cochrane Libr 2019; 2019(3): CD009562. [http://dx.doi.org/10.1002/14651858.CD009562.pub2] [PMID: 30848830]

[31] Deiss M, Kaya C, Pfister IB, Garweg JG. Impact of vitreal tamponade on functional outcomes in vitrectomy with ILM peeling in primary macula-involving retinal detachment: A retrospective analysis. Clin Ophthalmol 2020; 14: 4493-500. [http://dx.doi.org/10.2147/OPTH.S287107] [PMID: 33380783]

[32] Ripandelli G, Scarinci F, Piaggi P, *et al.* Macular pucker: To peel or not to peel the internal limiting membrane? A microperimetric response. Retina 2015; 35(3): 498-507. [http://dx.doi.org/10.1097/IAE.0000000000000330] [PMID: 25158943]

[33] Fitzgerald MC, Tolley E, Frase S, *et al.* Functional and morphological assessment of age-related changes in the choroid and outer retina in pigeons. Vis Neurosci 2001; 18(2): 299-317. [http://dx.doi.org/10.1017/S0952523801182143] [PMID: 11417804]

[34] Nagahara M, Tamaki Y, Araie M, Eguchi S. Effects of scleral buckling and encircling procedures on human optic nerve head and retinochoroidal circulation. Br J Ophthalmol 2000; 84(1): 31-6. [http://dx.doi.org/10.1136/bjo.84.1.31] [PMID: 10611096]

[35] Regillo CD, Sergott RC, Brown GC. Successful scleral buckling procedures decrease central retinal artery blood flow velocity. Ophthalmology 1993; 100(7): 1044-9. [http://dx.doi.org/10.1016/S0161-6420(93)31541-1] [PMID: 8321526]

[36] Borrelli E, Sarraf D, Freund KB, Sadda SR. OCT angiography and evaluation of the choroid and choroidal vascular disorders. Prog Retin Eye Res 2018; 67: 30-55. [http://dx.doi.org/10.1016/j.preteyeres.2018.07.002] [PMID: 30059755]

[37] Agrawal R, Gupta P, Tan KA, Cheung CMG, Wong TY, Cheng CY. Choroidal vascularity index as a measure of vascular status of the choroid: Measurements in healthy eyes from a population-based study. Sci Rep 2016; 6(1): 21090. [http://dx.doi.org/10.1038/srep21090] [PMID: 26868048]

[38] Betzler BK, Ding J, Wei X, *et al.* Choroidal vascularity index: A step towards software as a medical device. Br J Ophthalmol 2022; 106(2): 149-55. [http://dx.doi.org/10.1136/bjophthalmol-2021-318782] [PMID: 33514528]

[39] Singh RB, Perepelkina T, Testi I. Imaging-based assessment of choriocapillaris: A comprehensive review. Semin Ophthal Taylor Fran 2022; 0(0): 1-22. [PMID: 35982638]

CHAPTER 8

OCT-A Findings and Usefulness in Alzheimer's Disease, Parkinson's Disease, and Systemic Lupus Erythematosus

Sanjay Marasini[1] and **Miguel A. Quiroz-Reyes, MD**[2,*]

[1] *Department of Ophthalmology, The University of Auckland, Auckland, New Zealand*

[2] *Oftalmologia Integral ABC, Retina Department, Medical and Surgical Assistance Institution (Nonprofit Organization), Affiliated with the Postgraduate Studies Division, National Autonomous University of Mexico, Mexico City, Mexico*

Abstract: The eye is a window to the brain because of its inherent connection to the central nervous system (CNS). Several brain disorders manifest as ophthalmic abnormalities and can be detected through a detailed assessment of the eyes. In the last decade, extensive evaluation of retinal microvascular changes using optical coherence tomography angiography (OCT-A) has been performed for several diseases, such as Parkinson's disease, Alzheimer's disease, and systemic lupus erythematosus. Although the results from the available studies are conflicting (mainly due to heterogeneous study populations), they agree on the applicability of this technology for the early identification of these diseases. This chapter summarizes the OCT-A screening and monitoring uses for these diseases and hypotheses for the potential identification of disease characteristics.

Keywords: Alzheimer's disease, Autoimmune diseases, Binarization, Cognitive impairment, Foveal avascular zone, Fundus fluorescein angiography, Hydroxychloroquine, Macular perfusion, Neurodegenerative diseases, Optical Coherent Topography, Optical Coherence Tomography Angiography, Parkinson's disease, Perfusion density, Retinal vessel density, Perfusion density, Retinal thinning, Skeletonization, Systemic Lupus Erythematosus, Vascular perfusion indices, Vessel density.

* **Corresponding author Miguel A. Quiroz-Reyes, MD:** Oftalmologia Integral ABC, Retina Department, Medical and Surgical Assistance Institution (Nonprofit Organization), Affiliated with the Postgraduate Studies Division, National Autonomous University of Mexico, Mexico City, Mexico; Tel.: +52 55 217 2732; Fax: +52 55 1664 7180; E-mails: drquiroz@prodigy.net.mx and drquirozreyes7@gmail.com

INTRODUCTION

The eye is referred to as a window to the brain because of its inherent connection to the central nervous system. Several brain disorders (*e.g.,* brain tumors) affect eye function; therefore, a detailed anatomical and physiological assessment of the eyes can help diagnose these disorders. The correct diagnosis of neurodegenerative brain diseases, such as Parkinson's disease and Alzheimer's disease, is especially challenging. Approximately 25% of the cases are diagnosed incorrectly, even in developed countries [1]. Expanding the knowledge base for these conditions' heterogeneous clinical presentations has helped identify newer methods to diagnose these conditions. Genetic testing, histopathological testing, olfactory testing, magnetic resonance imaging (MRI), and computed tomography imaging are currently used to diagnose most brain disorders. However, these methods are invasive, costly, and time consuming. Therefore, non-invasive cost-effective methods that can help diagnose such diseases are currently under investigation. One such emerging technique is optical coherence tomography angiography (OCT-A), which provides noninvasive detailed numerical quantification of microvascular perfusion of the retina (which is known to be affected by neurodegenerative diseases). Optical coherence tomography (OCT) measurements of the retina have revealed several valuable diagnostic findings in neurodegenerative diseases. However, their diagnostic power is limited because of the overlap in OCT changes seen in neurodegenerative diseases and prevalent ophthalmological diseases such as glaucoma, diabetic retinopathy, and age-related macular degeneration [2]. Therefore, the integration of vascular perfusion parameters, such as microvascular perfusion density, vessel calibers, and alterations in vascular network organization, may increase the diagnostic accuracy of these conditions. Therefore, these parameters can be measured using OCT-A and have the potential to be developed as indicators of brain disease [2].

First used to image the retina in 1991 [3], OCT-A technology has made a significant leap in disease diagnosis in recent years, especially for its use in en face visualization of the retinal circulation into anatomic slabs of the superficial and deep vascular networks that supply the various retinal layers [4]. OCT-A essentially captures the backscattering of light between constantly moving red blood cells and a static neurosensory retina without the use of a dye. These images approach histology-level resolution, which shows the potential of detecting early microvascular pathological changes in patients *in vivo* [5]. Vascular pathology in retinal diseases (such as diabetic retinopathy, uveitis, retinal arterial occlusion, and retinal venous occlusions) can be assessed through quantitative analysis of anatomical markers using OCT-A, which makes it easier to compare pathologies. These analyses included vessel and perfusion densities, representing the percentage of blood vessels occupying a given area following image binarization and skeletonization. OCT-A also allows the mapping of important clinical findings such as macular telangiectasia, impaired perfusion, microaneurysms, and capillary modelling [5]. OCT-A has been extensively used to evaluate its effectiveness in diagnosing the clinical and subclinical stages of several brain diseases and monitoring their progression.

OCT-A Technology

Detailed descriptions of the types and uses of OCT-A systems are beyond the scope of this book chapter, and readers are referred to a recent review by Lains *et al.* [6] for a more extensive understanding of OCTA application for retinal conditions. For practical guidance on OCT-A interpretations, readers are referred to the publication by Greig *et al.* [7] and the assessment of the anterior segment by Lee *et al.* [8].

Conventional structural OCT aids clinicians in visualizing the anatomical changes that affect vision, but it does not offer information on the differences between small blood vessels and static tissue in most retinal layers [9]. As a result, OCT does not provide important information regarding vascular changes, such as capillary dropout or pathologic blood vessels in the retina [9]. In contrast, OCT-A employs motion contrast imaging to generate high-resolution volumetric blood flow information to generate angiographic images within seconds that provide both structural and functional information. This method aims to contrast blood vessels from static tissues by assessing the change in the OCT signal caused by flowing blood cells [9]. OCT-A compares the decorrelation signal (differences in the backscattered OCT signal intensity or amplitude) between sequential OCT b-scans taken at precisely the same cross-section to construct a map of blood flow. Axial bulk motion from patient movement is eliminated; therefore, sites of motion between repeated OCT b-scans represent strict erythrocyte movement in retinal blood vessels [10]. Each three-dimensional scan takes approximately six seconds to obtain. OCT angiograms can then scroll outward from the internal limiting membrane to the choroid to visualize the individual vascular plexus and segment the inner retina, choriocapillaris, or other areas of interest [10]. With developments in OCT system speeds owing to better hardware, methods for OCT-A have shifted from comparing adjacent A-scans to sequential cross-sectional B-scans. This ensured that a slower flow in the microvasculature could be detected [9]. However, leakage information cannot be appreciated, and the exact size and location can be measured for pathologies, such as choroidal neovascularization.

This chapter focuses on the use of OCT-A technology for neurological diseases.

Systemic lupus erythematosus (SLE), a chronic autoimmune inflammatory disease, is of interest to ophthalmologists owing to its association with the eye.

Immune complex vasculopathy and inflammatory mediators have been implicated in the pathogenicity of SLE [11]. Approximately 35% of these patients are treated with hydroxychloroquine, which is known to cause drug-related retinopathy [12]. Research has shown that hydroxychloroquine causes retinopathy after prolonged SLE treatment (> 5 years) [11]. The most common ocular manifestation of SLE is keratoconjunctivitis sicca, followed by retinopathy. Retinal associations of SLE include retinal hemorrhage, vasculitis, cotton wool spots, and hard exudates [13]. Symptomatic retinopathy in SLE has been reported in 0.66% of patients, and almost 10% of asymptomatic patients have lupus retinopathy [14, 15]. Historically, fundus fluorescein angiography (FFA) has been used to investigate vascular abnormalities during the therapeutic treatment of SLE. However, in recent years, the use of noninvasive imaging technology, OCT-A, has been increasingly used to assess cases of SLE, as it has the potential to detect subclinical diseases.

OCT-A could be a sensitive and specific procedure to help identify disease parameters to screen for early-stage diseases. Identifying disease-specific anatomic markers of retinal structural and microvascular changes may help improve the diagnostic accuracy of various neurodegenerative diseases and drug-induced retinopathies. Therefore, in this chapter, OCT-A findings in Parkinson's disease, Alzheimer's disease, and SLE are discussed to summarize the literature for potential clinical applications and explore new research questions.

OCT-A in Alzheimer's Disease

Alzheimer's disease is a degenerative neurological condition and a leading cause of dementia in the United States [3]. Approximately 5.8 million people aged 65 years and older had Alzheimer's disease as of 2020. Since the life expectancy of people is increasing worldwide, the prevalence of Alzheimer's disease will continue to grow, especially in low- and middle-income countries. Owing to similarities to other neurodegenerative conditions that cause a decline in cognitive function, the condition is difficult to diagnose clinically, particularly among elderly groups, and is characterized by impaired executive functioning, which progresses slowly and ultimately causes severe cognitive impairment. This affects multiple domains of the daily living activities of patients, and eventually, severe disease, leading to death. Since clinical symptoms appear much earlier than appreciable neuropathological changes, early screening and diagnosis are warranted in patients with subclinical diseases.

There is strong evidence of a correlation between clinical Alzheimer's disease and retinal vascular changes. Therefore, it is believed that a careful analysis of these alterations can help identify the pathology in earlier stages when combined with other existing investigations that include histopathologic examination of the brain through invasive biopsy. Other definitive diagnostic methods for Alzheimer's include cerebrospinal fluid testing and positron emission tomography of the brain, which are costly techniques for many patients. Since the retina and brain share many neuronal and vasculature characteristics, OCT-A findings may serve as biomarkers for preclinical Alzheimer's disease. These relatively affordable noninvasive methods, if they can screen for diseases such as Alzheimer's disease, would be widely used, and other costly and invasive tests such as cerebral spinal fluid (CSF) analysis or neuroimaging would not be required on an urgent basis [16]. The results are easy to interpret and provide rapid high-resolution images, thereby improving clinical accuracy and efficiency. Additionally, there has been a strong correlation between OCT-A findings and cortical atrophy, immunohistochemical staining, and the results of neurocognitive testing, which are objective methods for Alzheimer's disease diagnosis [17, 18]. Therefore, OCT-A findings can be complementary in strengthening the diagnosis and/or screening of preclinical diseases, and further research in this area is warranted.

Studies have shown that patients with Alzheimer’s disease exhibit narrowed vessel caliber, reduced blood flow, increased blood oxygen saturation, and tortuosity in histopathological observations [4]. Other findings reported in the retina of patients with Alzheimer's disease include islet amyloid polypeptide levels, pericyte number, and vessel length compared to normal subjects [4]. Relative to the control groups, these patients had significantly enlarged foveal avascular zone (FAZ) and decreased vascular density in all retinal zones of the superficial vascular complex [19]. Several previous studies have compared retinal thinning between patients with Alzheimer's disease and normal control subjects using OCT-A. Most of these studies reported that retinal thinning is mostly observed in the retinal nerve fiber layer (RNFL) and ganglion cell-inner plexiform layer (GC-IPL). However, it has been demonstrated that the thickness of the outer retinal layers is not associated with Alzheimer's disease or other forms of dementia [20].

Studies have reported that the overall mean RNFL thickness tends to be lower in Alzheimer's disease. Retinal thinning is restricted to the superior quadrant [32]. The variation in retinal thickness is also attributed to genetic variation between individuals [33]. Interestingly, a large prospective cohort study (n = 3300) found that RNFL thinning was associated with an increased risk of dementia, particularly dementia due to Alzheimer's disease [34]. However, some studies could not detect any differences in retinal thickness between patients with Alzheimer’s disease and healthy controls [35] (Table **1**).

Table 1. Summary of the most recent literature on OCT-A findings in Alzheimer's disease, Parkinson's disease, and systemic lupus erythematosus.

Disease	OCT-A findings
Alzheimer's disease	Decreased superficial vascular density [21], OCT and OCT-A measurements correlate with established measures of Alzheimer's disease such as neuropsychological testing or neuroimaging [3], significantly greater retinal thinning when compared to both healthy controls and patients with mild cognitive impairment [22, 23], superficial vascular density is significantly lower than that in normal subjects and there is a significant decrease in parafoveal superficial capillary plexus [21, 24], enlarged foveal avascular zone and decreased choroidal thickness [19], parafoveal flow and vessel density could be used as early disease biomarkers in Alzheimer's disease [24].
Parkinson's disease	Decreased retinal vessel density and perfusion density as well as choroidal structural changes are seen when compared with the controls [25], increased peripapillary microvascular density and flux relative to normal subjects [26], decreased vascular perfusion indices, and significantly declined FAZ areas that correlated with the increasing severity of the disease [27].
Systemic lupus erythematosus	Significantly lower mean macular thickness and GC-IPL thicknesses, vessel density, and perfusion density [28], lower superficial vessel densities are seen than healthy controls in the upper and lower macular regions, and the deep plexus and vessel density loss was detected in all sectors [29]. Inner retinal thickness was reduced in the outer superior and temporal regions, and full retinal thickness was reduced in the outer temporal regions [30]. Vessel density in the superficial capillary plexus was significantly reduced in patients taking hydroxychloroquine for more than five years [31].

Recent literature indicates that retinal thinning in patients with Alzheimer’s may represent a non-specific decline in cognitive function. Most of the published literature has reported significantly reduced RNFL thickness in patients with mild cognitive impairment (MCI) compared to healthy controls [22, 36]. Interestingly, when retinal thinning is compared between Alzheimer's and MCI or healthy subjects, Alzheimer's has significantly greater retinal thinning [22, 23]. Although most studies suggest a significant correlation between retinal thickness changes and Alzheimer's disease, some published studies contradict this finding, especially in mild diseases [37]. It is possible that these observational differences could be due to differences in sample sizes between studies. Additionally, MCI is a more general, nonspecific clinical diagnosis than Alzheimer's disease, and all patients with MCI do not develop Alzheimer's disease, and there is a chance that clinical findings may be different between these two conditions.

It has been demonstrated that microvascular and structural changes in the retina occur much earlier than symptoms in patients with Alzheimer's disease. Therefore, OCT-A may be useful for detecting Alzheimer's disease in its early stages [38]. Wang *et al.* [21]. explored retinal vascular density changes in Alzheimer's disease and MCI patients using OCT-A in a set of 62 Alzheimer's disease patients, 47 MCI patients, and 49 cognitively healthy controls. They found that the superficial groups had significantly lower scores than the control group. However, there was no difference in the FAZ among the three groups. The ganglion cell complex, inner parafoveal, and peripapillary retinal nerve fiber layer (p-RNFL) thicknesses were associated with superficial vascular density. They did not find a significant correlation between global cognition scores or the Fazekas score and retinal OCT-A flow density. The authors concluded that retinal microvascular dysfunction is common in patients with MCI and Alzheimer's disease.

In a systematic review, Song *et al.* [3] evaluated whether certain OCT and OCT-A parameters were significantly associated with Alzheimer's and MCI. They included seventy-one studies representing 6757 patients, of which 2350 had Alzheimer's disease, 793 had MCI, 2902 were healthy controls, and 841 had a range of other neurodegenerative diseases. Their review suggested that OCT and OCT-A measurements correlate with established measures of Alzheimer's disease, such as neuropsychological testing or neuroimaging.

Zabel *et al.* [39] compared OCT-A findings (retinal microvasculature within the macula and optic nerve head) in Alzheimer's disease, primary open-angle glaucoma, and healthy controls. They found that the density of vessels in the deep vascular plexus of the retina was significantly reduced and that the FAZ was higher in the Alzheimer's disease group than in the glaucoma and control groups. They concluded that in patients with Alzheimer's disease, deeper retinal layers are affected, which is different from glaucoma, in which superficial vessels are affected.

Bulut *et al.* [19] compared the OCT-A findings in Alzheimer's disease and control groups. All participants underwent a detailed neurological examination, including the Mini-Mental State Examination (MMSE), to evaluate cognitive function. They found that the MMSE scores and retinal vascular density were much lower in the Alzheimer's group. Similarly, the foveal avascular zone was significantly enlarged compared with that in the control group, and the choroidal thickness was significantly lower. Therefore, the authors concluded that retinal and choroidal vascular pathologies can be detected through OCT-A imaging and can be used as new biomarkers in early disease diagnosis.

Similarly, Zhang *et al.* [24] investigated whether OCT-A findings can identify early Alzheimer's disease with MCI. They observed that cognitively impaired participants had significantly decreased parafoveal superficial capillary plexus. These results suggest that parafoveal flow and vessel density could be used as early disease biomarkers in Alzheimer’s disease.

Although there is convincing evidence that OCT-A findings correlate with Alzheimer's disease, several discrepancies exist between reported studies regarding vessel density (VD). Some studies report changes mainly in the inner retinal layer supplied by the superficial plexus [40], whereas others [39] claim that retinal vascular changes occur in the deep plexus. However, Chua *et al.* [41] found that the eyes of patients with Alzheimer's disease had significantly reduced macular VD in both plexuses, whereas patients with mild cognitive impairment showed a reduction in the superficial plexus.

Yoon *et al.* [42] showed that patients with Alzheimer's disease have significantly reduced macular VD, perfusion density (PD), and macular GC-IPL thickness compared with MCI and healthy controls (Fig. **1**).

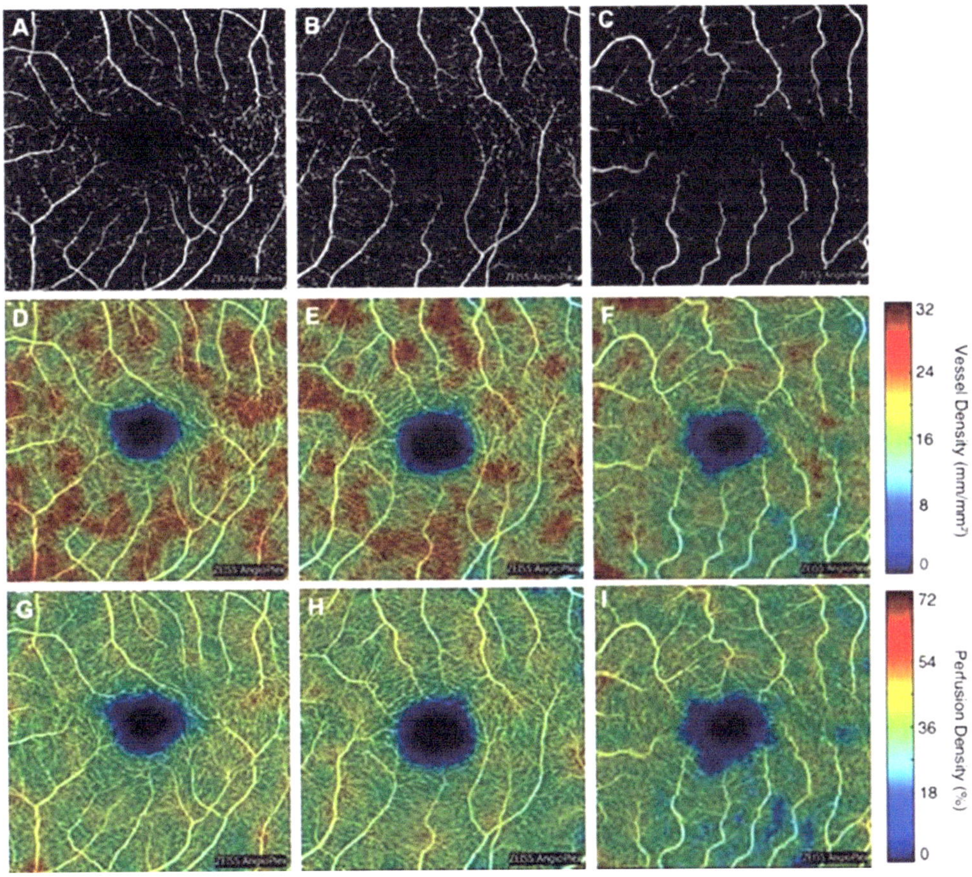

Fig. (1). Representative OCT angiography images of the superficial capillary plexus in control (**a**), mild cognitive impairment (**b**), and Alzheimer's disease (**c**) patients. Quantitative color maps of vessel density (**d–f**) and perfusion density (**g–i**) are shown. Images show decreased vessel density and perfusion density in (**f**, i) AD compared with the control participant (**d**, **g**) and the participant with mild cognitive impairment (**e**, **h**). This modified figure was adapted from a previous publication by Yoon *et al.* [42].

OCT-A in Parkinson's Disease

Parkinson's disease is a debilitating neurodegenerative disease caused by the progressive death of dopaminergic neurons in the substantia nigra [43]. The disease has a characteristic clinical triad of bradykinesia, rigidity, resting tremor, and other symptoms such as olfactory loss, sleep dysfunction, and cognitive impairment. The disease was diagnosed based on the patient's medical history and clinical examination. History includes prodromal features (*e.g.*, rapid eye movements and sleep disorders), characteristic movement difficulties (*e.g.*, tremor and stiffness), and psychological or cognitive problems (*e.g.*, cognitive decline, depression, and anxiety) [44]. Commonly followed clinical diagnostic criteria for Parkinson's are the Movement Disorder Society clinical diagnostic criteria [43]. Imaging tools used to diagnose Parkinson's disease include dopamine transporter single-photon emission computed tomography (DaT SPECT), which is highly accurate (98% to 100% sensitivity and specificity) for detecting nigrostriatal cell loss in individuals with Parkinsonism [44]. Despite well-developed diagnostic criteria and tools, approximately 20% of patients with Parkinson's remain undiagnosed at the community level [45]. This is due to difficulties related to atypical features, which complicate diagnostic procedures. Therefore, the development of objective tools (biomarkers) that can help diagnose the disease is highly desirable.

Several studies have reported characteristic alterations in the structure and microvasculature of the retina and choroid in the eyes of patients with Parkinson's [25]. Patients with Parkinson's disease display characteristic visual impairments related to visual acuity, color discrimination, motion perception, and contrast sensitivity [46]. Therefore, ophthalmic and neuro-ophthalmic evaluation is evolving as an important early diagnosis and management tool in these patients, especially focusing on ocular biomarkers using imaging tools such as OCT-A [47]. Therefore, in this chapter, we summarize the most pertinent findings of OCT-A for potential clinical application in the early diagnosis of Parkinson's disease.

Zhang *et al.* [48] performed Swept-Source OCT and SS-OCT-A to assess the retinas of patients with Parkinson's and matched healthy controls. They reported decreased superficial and deep flow densities in most regions of the retina in Parkinson's. Investigators have suggested that decreasing retinal flow density provides greater diagnostic power than retinal thickness measurements in the early stages of Parkinson's disease, potentially serving as imaging biomarkers in its diagnosis and staging. Similarly, Robbins *et al.* [25] characterized OCT and OCT-A findings in the microvasculature perfusion in the retina and choroid of patients with Parkinson's disease and compared the data with age- and sex-matched healthy controls. Using vigorous statistical techniques, they found that individuals with Parkinson's disease had decreased retinal vessel density (VD), perfusion density, and choroidal structural changes compared with healthy controls. They concluded that the observed differences may represent novel biomarkers for disease detection.

Robbins *et al.* [49] compared radial peripapillary capillary plexus vascular parameters and RNFL thickness between patients with Parkinson's disease and controls in a prospective control study. They reported that peripapillary microvascular density and flux increased in the majority of patients with Parkinson's disease when compared with controls after adjusting for age and sex, but RNFL thickness did not differ between groups. They also reported that the peripapillary OCT-A parameters did not correlate with disease severity, but the OCT-A findings may indicate early disease [26]. Xu *et al.* [27] evaluated microvascular perfusion indices at different stages of Parkinson's disease (Hoehn-Yahr (H-Y) stages) using OCT-A and correlated these parameters with clinical findings. They found that most of the vascular perfusion indices decreased in patients with Parkinson's disease compared to those in the control groups (Fig. **2**). The FAZ areas also declined significantly with increasing severity in patients with Parkinson's. The authors concluded that OCT-A may have significant value in identifying microvascular changes in patients with Parkinson's disease at different clinical stages and may also be useful for monitoring disease progression [27].

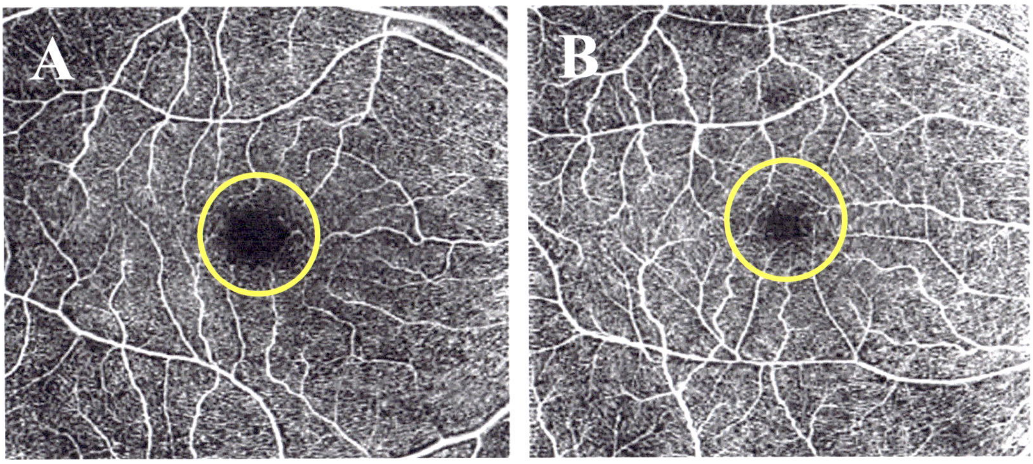

Fig. (2). The foveal avascular zone (FAZ) area (marked with a yellow circle) was found to be significantly decreased in patients with Parkinson's disease (**b**) compared to healthy controls (**a**). The image was modified from the publication of Xu *et al.* [50].

Patients with Parkinson's disease exhibit several microvascular changes in the retina that are often correlated with disease severity and may harbor preclinical disease. A gap in the current literature seems to be found in the variation of the study protocols, which has caused diversity in the study findings. An important step forward is the development of a uniform protocol to investigate potential clinical markers by categorizing study populations based on disease severity, age groups, and other study variables (*e.g.*, demographics, sex, and OCT-A parameters) that have shown variability within studies. Therefore, the assessment of patients with Parkinson's using OCT-A and the correlation of currently existing diagnostic criteria (history and clinical assessments) may help identify the disease early.

OCT-A in Systematic Lupus Erythematosus

SLE is an inflammatory autoimmune connective tissue disease that affects multiple ocular structures, including the retina and choroid [28]. In SLE, detecting posterior segment diseases, such as optic neuritis, ischemic optic neuropathy, retinal vasculitis, occlusive retinopathies, and choroidopathy, is important for evaluating disease activity and preventing permanent visual loss [31]. The disease is treated with hydroxychloroquine, which may cause toxic retinopathy and paracentral visual field defects [51]. It is suggested that due to early damage to ganglion cells and their photoreceptors in the parafoveal region, retinal sensitivity is reduced [52]. Multifocal electroretinography (mfERG) can detect early parafoveal toxicity in these patients [53]. However, the sensitivity of the test depends on the stage of the disease (most useful in the early stages or to confirm bull's eye damage), and its diagnostic value decreases as the disease becomes more obvious on SD-OCT, FFA, and fundus examination. Other tests to screen patients taking hydroxychloroquine include spectral-domain OCT and fundus autofluorescence. SD-OCT is particularly useful at the very early toxicity stage, as it shows parafoveal thinning [53].

Piñero *et al.* [52] reported a patient with SLE who was treated with hydroxychloroquine. They showed that multichannel perimetry could detect sensitivity losses in the parafoveal area at a much earlier stage with no OCT or 10-2 automated perimetry alterations [52]. Using OCT, several retinal changes have been reported in SLE, including degenerative foveal thinning, incomplete posterior vitreous detachment, and epiretinal membranes [11]. Almost 70% of patients receiving hydroxychloroquine are known to exhibit OCT changes [11].

In recent years, there has been strong support for the use of OCT-A to monitor SLE patients on treatment regimens. OCT-A is a fast and noninvasive method for visualizing vascular alterations in small vessels and capillaries of the retina and choriocapillaris, and can be useful for monitoring the ocular consequences of SLE treatment. Since the use of hydroxychloroquine is widespread and almost 10% of patients with SLE have asymptomatic visual disorders, asymptomatic retinopathy can be easily identified using OCT-A [15].

Işık *et al.* [28] evaluated the choroidal and retinal layers using OCT and retinal microvascular structures with OCT-A in patients with SLE and compared the findings with those of healthy controls. They found that the mean macular and GC-IPL thicknesses were lower in the patient group. Similarly, the VD and PD were significantly lower in the patient group. Moreover, central foveal thickness and foveal avascular zone parameters were negatively correlated, whereas VD and GC-IPL thickness were positively correlated. The authors concluded that OCT-A evaluation of patients with SLE may be useful in detecting subclinical changes [28].

Retinal vascular abnormalities are associated with renal involvement in SLE [15]. Using OCT-A, Mizuno *et al.* [15]. were able to diagnose asymptomatic retinal vasculitis using OCT-A during ophthalmological examination. This highlights the importance of OCT-A screening in ophthalmology clinics, as it may help detect earlier retinal changes in patients with SLE. Similarly, Arfeen *et al.* [29] evaluated retinal microvascular density in patients with SLE using OCT-A and correlated VD with disease activity and damage risk in 20 patients, each in the SLE and control groups. They found that SLE patients had lower superficial vessel densities in the upper and lower macular regions than normal patients. VD loss was detected in all sectors of the deep plexus. The authors recommended that VD should be included in the assessment of SLE activity and damage scores.

More recently, using OCT-A, Liu *et al.* [30] investigated the differences in retinal thickness and superficial vascular density between SLE patients and healthy controls. They observed that inner retinal thickness was reduced in the outer superior and temporal regions, and full retinal thickness was reduced in the outer temporal regions, compared to the control group. Thinning of retinal thickness was negatively correlated with erythrocyte sedimentation rate in the inner retina at the outer temporal and outer superior retina, and the full retina in the outer temporal regions. The authors concluded that OCT-A measurement of retinal thickness may be a potential marker for the diagnosis of SLE and an indicator of its inflammatory activity.

Mihailovic *et al.* [31] evaluated retinal microvascular density using OCT-A in SLE patients treated with hydroxychloroquine. They categorized the treated patients into high- and low-risk groups in terms of the duration of medication as more than or less than five years. They found that VD in the superficial capillary plexus was significantly reduced in the high-risk and low-risk groups compared to that in the healthy control group. Additionally, the VD was lower in the high-risk group than in the low-risk group. They also found that FAZ areas were larger in hydroxychloroquine-treated patients than in the control group (Fig. **3**). They concluded that hydroxychloroquine might have a protective effect on the retinal microvasculature, and the assessment of individuals with SLE using OCT-A could be useful in diagnosing and monitoring vascular alterations.

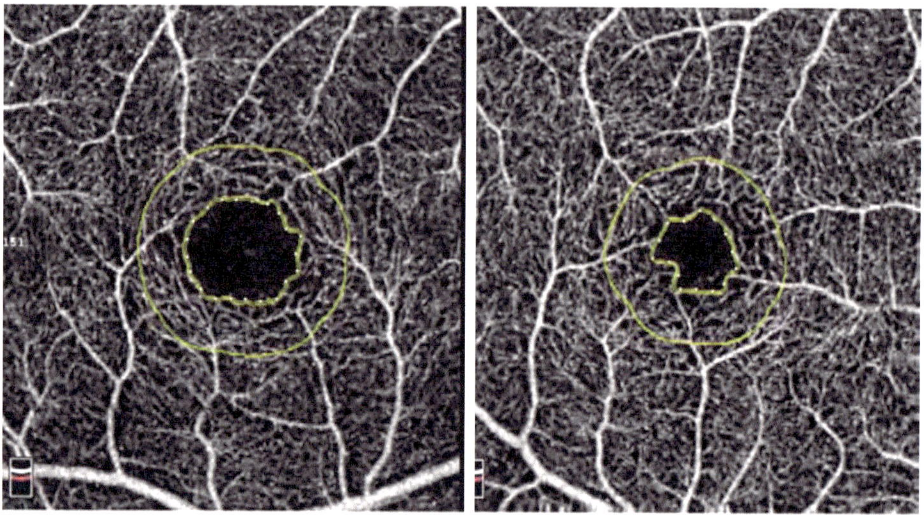

Fig. (3). The FAZ area (marked with a central yellow circle) of SLE patients treated with hydroxychloroquine for two months (**a**) was found to be larger than that of the normal controls (**b**). This modified figure was adapted from the publication of Mihailovic [31].

As with neurodegenerative diseases, OCT-A can be an important tool for monitoring pathology and treatment outcomes in patients with SLE. Although studies have indicated several changes in the retinal vasculature, there is a lack of consensus regarding the specific signs of this disease. A likely sign of SLE could be VD quantification in different subregions of the retina. However, its usefulness in monitoring pathology in both treated and untreated SLE patients requires further investigation. The literature stresses that patients with SLE receiving hydroxychloroquine will benefit from OCT-A assessments, as they may remain asymptomatic despite having retinopathy. The clinical correlation of available tests, such as chromatic perimetry, ERG, SD-OCT, and OCT-A, for their sensitivity and specificity in detecting early stage disease can be an important research question for developing OCT-A as a specific diagnostic tool in SLE monitoring [11].

CONCLUDING REMARKS

OCT-A has revolutionized ophthalmology practice over the last two decades and has been widely used to evaluate a spectrum of retinal vascular diseases, including diabetic retinopathy and retinal occlusive disorders. Owing to the high resolution of the technology, which is often at the histological level, the technique demonstrates early clinical findings such as microaneurysms, capillary remodelling, and neovascularization. As it facilitates the quantitative and qualitative measurement of tissue structures, it has become an important tool in routine disease diagnosis and management. Interestingly, because of the current understanding of microvascular changes in several brain and other diseases that affect the health of the retina, there has been a large amount of literature on the use of OCT-A as a potential biomarker for these diseases. This chapter reviews the most pertinent and recent data on Alzheimer's, Parkinson's, and SLE. It was observed that these three conditions show and share several characteristic retinal and microvascular perfusional changes, which often appear much earlier than the clinical symptoms. Although most of the current literature supports OCT-A findings as potential biomarkers in these disease groups, there are contradictory findings, largely due to heterogeneity in the included population and different stages of the diseases studied (*e.g.,* mild, moderate, or severe disease). Further exploration of OCT-A as a screening tool for neurodegenerative conditions is required. Similarly, the current literature suggests that all patients with SLE, regardless of their ophthalmic symptoms, should be evaluated using OCT-A, as it can detect earlier microvascular changes in the retina [15]. Increasing evidence suggests a correlation between OCT-A findings and renal involvement in SLE patients.

FUTURE DIRECTIONS

Although the current literature on the use of OCT-A to identify biomarkers for specific diseases is very diverse, with overlapping findings, and is therefore non-specific, there is a consensus regarding its applicability in identifying preclinical brain diseases and connective tissue diseases that affect the retina. Categorizing diseases by severity, age, patient history, and clinical signs and correlating them with different OCT-A parameters should be the next research question to identify specific biomarkers for these conditions. Therefore, it is important to develop protocols for disease severity and OCT-A measurements so that proper diagnostic criteria can be established to help screen/diagnose neurodegenerative diseases and connective tissue disorders and their potential multiorgan involvement. Additionally, most studies have presented retrospective cross-sectional data, which have concurrently provided evidence of perfusional changes in the diseases discussed above. However, to obtain more robust evidence, it is important to develop long-term prospective studies to compare the differences in the observed changes between the control and disease groups. These data will help to solidify the current understanding of OCT-A findings in these diseases and potentially develop specific biomarkers for these conditions. Moreover, it is important to note that several retinal structures, such as foveal avascular zones, vary significantly within the normal population. Therefore, the long-term evaluation of individual changes in OCT-A markers over time may be a better indicator of disease pathology.

LIST OF ABBREVIATIONS

CSF	Cerebral spinal fluid
DaT SPECT	Single-photon emission computed tomography
FAZ	Foveal avascular zone
FFA	Fundus fluorescein angiography
GC-IPL	Ganglion cell-inner plexiform layer
MCI	Mild cognitive impairment
mfERG	Multifocal electroretinography
MMSE	Mini-mental state examination;
MRI	Magnetic resonance imaging
OCT	Optical coherent tomography
OCT-A	Optical coherent tomography angiography
PF	Perfusion density
p-RNFL	Peripapillary retinal nerve fiber layer
SD-OCT	Spectral-domain optical coherence tomography
SS-OCT-A	Swept-source optical coherence tomography angiography
SLE	Systemic lupus erythematosus
VD	Vessel density.

DISCLAIMER

All scientific comments issued in this chapter are solely the responsibility of the authors and not of the institutions with which they are affiliated.

ACKNOWLEDGMENTS

We express our deep appreciation to the technical staff of the Retina Specialists Unit at the Oftalmologia Integral ABC (Nonprofit Medical and Surgical Organization) affiliated with Postgraduate Division Studies at the National Autonomous University of Mexico.

REFERENCES

[1] Tolosa E, Wenning G, Poewe W. The diagnosis of Parkinson's disease. Lancet Neurol 2006; 5(1): 75-86.
[http://dx.doi.org/10.1016/S1474-4422(05)70285-4] [PMID: 16361025]

[2] Moons L, De Groef L. Multimodal retinal imaging to detect and understand Alzheimer's and Parkinson's disease. Curr Opin Neurobiol 2022; 72: 1-7.
[http://dx.doi.org/10.1016/j.conb.2021.07.007] [PMID: 34399146]

[3] Song A, Johnson N, Ayala A, Thompson AC. Optical coherence tomography in patients with Alzheimer's disease: What can it tell us? Eye Brain 2021; 13: 1-20.
[http://dx.doi.org/10.2147/EB.S235238] [PMID: 33447120]

[4] Asanad S, Mohammed I, Sadun AA, Saeedi OJ. OCTA in neurodegenerative optic neuropathies: Emerging biomarkers at the eye–brain interface. Ther Adv Ophthalmol 2020; 12.
[http://dx.doi.org/10.1177/2515841420950508] [PMID: 32923939]

[5] Kashani AH, Chen CL, Gahm JK, *et al.* Optical coherence tomography angiography: A comprehensive review of current methods and clinical applications. Prog Retin Eye Res 2017; 60: 66-100.
[http://dx.doi.org/10.1016/j.preteyeres.2017.07.002] [PMID: 28760677]

[6] Laíns I, Wang JC, Cui Y, *et al.* Retinal applications of swept source optical coherence tomography (OCT) and optical coherence tomography angiography (OCTA). Prog Retin Eye Res 2021; 84: 100951.
[http://dx.doi.org/10.1016/j.preteyeres.2021.100951] [PMID: 33516833]

[7] Greig EC, Duker JS, Waheed NK. A practical guide to optical coherence tomography angiography interpretation. Int J Retina Vitreous 2020; 6(1): 55.
[http://dx.doi.org/10.1186/s40942-020-00262-9] [PMID: 33292740]

[8] Lee WD, Devarajan K, Chua J, Schmetterer L, Mehta JS, Ang M. Optical coherence tomography angiography for the anterior segment. Eye Vis 2019; 6(1): 4.
[http://dx.doi.org/10.1186/s40662-019-0129-2] [PMID: 30775387]

[9] Gao SS, Jia Y, Zhang M, *et al.* Optical coherence tomography angiography. Invest Ophthalmol Vis Sci 2016; 57(9): OCT27-36.
[http://dx.doi.org/10.1167/iovs.15-19043] [PMID: 27409483]

[10] Kim DY, Fingler J, Zawadzki RJ, *et al.* Optical imaging of the chorioretinal vasculature in the living human eye. Proc Natl Acad Sci 2013; 110(35): 14354-9.
[http://dx.doi.org/10.1073/pnas.1307315110] [PMID: 23918361]

[11] Fouad SA, Esmat Mahmoud Ali SM, Rezk Alnaggar ARL, Mahfouz S, Essam M, El-Gendy H. Structural retinal assessment using optical coherence tomography and fundus fluorescein angiography in systemic lupus erythematosus patients. J Clin Rheumatol 2021; 27(1): 34-9.
[http://dx.doi.org/10.1097/RHU.0000000000001162] [PMID: 31688343]

[12] Petri M. Hydroxychloroquine use in the Baltimore Lupus Cohort: effects on lipids, glucose and thrombosis. Lupus 1996; 5(1) (1): 16-22.
[http://dx.doi.org/10.1177/0961203396005001051] [PMID: 8803905]

[13] Ushiyama O, Ushiyama K, Koarada S, *et al.* Retinal disease in patients with systemic lupus erythematosus. Ann Rheum Dis 2000; 59(9): 705-8.
[http://dx.doi.org/10.1136/ard.59.9.705] [PMID: 10976084]

[14] Gao N, Li MT, Li YH, *et al.* Retinal vasculopathy in patients with systemic lupus erythematosus. Lupus 2017; 26(11): 1182-9.
[http://dx.doi.org/10.1177/0961203317698050] [PMID: 28355986]

[15] Mizuno Y, Nishide M, Wakabayashi T, Nishida K, Kumanogoh A. OCTA, a sensitive screening for asymptomatic retinopathy, raises alarm over systemic involvements in patients with SLE. Ann Rheum

Dis 2020; 79(2): e17-7.
[http://dx.doi.org/10.1136/annrheumdis-2018-214751] [PMID: 30487146]

[16] Ibne Mokbul M. Optical coherence tomography: Basic concepts and applications in neuroscience research. J Med Eng 2017; 2017: 3409327.
[http://dx.doi.org/10.1155/2017/3409327]

[17] Asanad S, Fantini M, Sultan W, *et al.* Retinal nerve fiber layer thickness predicts CSF amyloid/tau before cognitive decline. PLoS One 2020; 15(5): e0232785.
[http://dx.doi.org/10.1371/journal.pone.0232785] [PMID: 32469871]

[18] Lee EJ, Kim TW, Lee DS, *et al.* Increased CSF tau level is correlated with decreased lamina cribrosa thickness. Alzheimers Res Ther 2016; 8(1): 6.
[http://dx.doi.org/10.1186/s13195-015-0169-3] [PMID: 26857246]

[19] Bulut M, Kurtuluş F, Gözkaya O, *et al.* Evaluation of optical coherence tomography angiographic findings in Alzheimer's type dementia. Br J Ophthalmol 2018; 102(2): 233-7.
[http://dx.doi.org/10.1136/bjophthalmol-2017-310476] [PMID: 28600299]

[20] Uchida A, Pillai JA, Bermel R, *et al.* Outer retinal assessment using spectral-domain optical coherence tomography in patients with Alzheimer's and Parkinson's disease. Invest Ophthalmol Vis Sci 2018; 59(7): 2768-77.
[http://dx.doi.org/10.1167/iovs.17-23240] [PMID: 29860463]

[21] Wang X, Zhao Q, Tao R, *et al.* Decreased retinal vascular density in Alzheimer's disease (AD) and mild cognitive impairment (MCI): An optical coherence tomography angiography (OCTA) study. Front Aging Neurosci 2021; 12: 572484.
[http://dx.doi.org/10.3389/fnagi.2020.572484] [PMID: 33519415]

[22] Liu D, Zhang L, Li Z, *et al.* Thinner changes of the retinal nerve fiber layer in patients with mild cognitive impairment and Alzheimer's disease. BMC Neurol 2015; 15(1): 14.
[http://dx.doi.org/10.1186/s12883-015-0268-6] [PMID: 25886372]

[23] Gao L, Liu Y, Li X, Bai Q, Liu P. Abnormal retinal nerve fiber layer thickness and macula lutea in patients with mild cognitive impairment and Alzheimer's disease. Arch Gerontol Geriatr 2015; 60(1): 162-7.
[http://dx.doi.org/10.1016/j.archger.2014.10.011] [PMID: 25459918]

[24] Zhang YS, Zhou N, Knoll BM, *et al.* Parafoveal vessel loss and correlation between peripapillary vessel density and cognitive performance in amnestic mild cognitive impairment and early Alzheimer's Disease on optical coherence tomography angiography. PLoS One 2019; 14(4): e0214685.
[http://dx.doi.org/10.1371/journal.pone.0214685] [PMID: 30939178]

[25] Robbins CB, Thompson AC, Bhullar PK, *et al.* Characterization of retinal microvascular and choroidal structural changes in Parkinson disease. JAMA Ophthalmol 2021; 139(2): 182-8.
[http://dx.doi.org/10.1001/jamaophthalmol.2020.5730] [PMID: 33355613]

[26] Robbins CB, Grewal DS, Thompson AC, *et al.* Identifying peripapillary radial capillary plexus alterations in Parkinson's disease using OCT angiography. Ophthalmol Retina 2022; 6(1): 29-36.
[http://dx.doi.org/10.1016/j.oret.2021.03.006] [PMID: 33713852]

[27] Xu B, Wang X, Guo J, *et al.* Retinal microvascular density was associated with the clinical progression of parkinson's disease. Front Aging Neurosci 2022; 14: 818597.
[http://dx.doi.org/10.3389/fnagi.2022.818597] [PMID: 35250544]

[28] Işık MU, Akmaz B, Akay F, *et al.* Evaluation of subclinical retinopathy and angiopathy with OCT and OCTA in patients with systemic lupus erythematosus. Int Ophthalmol 2021; 41(1): 143-50.
[http://dx.doi.org/10.1007/s10792-020-01561-8] [PMID: 32851556]

[29] Arfeen SA, Bahgat N, Adel N, Eissa M, Khafagy MM. Assessment of superficial and deep retinal vessel density in systemic lupus erythematosus patients using optical coherence tomography

angiography. Graefes Arch Clin Exp Ophthalmol 2020; 258(6): 1261-8. [http://dx.doi.org/10.1007/s00417-020-04626-7] [PMID: 32162113]

[30] Liu R, Wang Y, Xia Q, *et al.* Retinal thickness and microvascular alterations in the diagnosis of systemic lupus erythematosus: A new approach. Quant Imaging Med Surg 2022; 12(1): 823-37. [http://dx.doi.org/10.21037/qims-21-359] [PMID: 34993121]

[31] Mihailovic N, Leclaire MD, Eter N, Brücher VC. Altered microvascular density in patients with systemic lupus erythematosus treated with hydroxychloroquine—an optical coherence tomography angiography study. Graefes Arch Clin Exp Ophthalmol 2020; 258(10): 2263-9. [http://dx.doi.org/10.1007/s00417-020-04788-4] [PMID: 32533282]

[32] Cunha JP, Proença R, Dias-Santos A, *et al.* OCT in Alzheimer's disease: Thinning of the RNFL and superior hemiretina. Graefes Arch Clin Exp Ophthalmol 2017; 255(9): 1827-35. [http://dx.doi.org/10.1007/s00417-017-3715-9] [PMID: 28643042]

[33] van de Kreeke JA, Nguyen HT, Konijnenberg E, *et al.* Optical coherence tomography angiography in preclinical Alzheimer's disease. Br J Ophthalmol 2020; 104(2): 157-61. [http://dx.doi.org/10.1136/bjophthalmol-2019-314127] [PMID: 31118186]

[34] Mutlu U, Colijn JM, Ikram MA, *et al.* Association of retinal neurodegeneration on optical coherence tomography with dementia: A population-based study. JAMA Neurol 2018; 75(10): 1256-63. [http://dx.doi.org/10.1001/jamaneurol.2018.1563] [PMID: 29946702]

[35] den Haan J, Csinscik L, Parker T, *et al.* Retinal thickness as potential biomarker in posterior cortical atrophy and typical Alzheimer's disease. Alzheimers Res Ther 2019; 11(1): 62. [http://dx.doi.org/10.1186/s13195-019-0516-x] [PMID: 31319885]

[36] Choi SH, Park SJ, Kim NR. Macular ganglion cell-inner plexiform layer thickness is associated with clinical progression in mild cognitive impairment and Alzheimers disease. PLoS One 2016; 11(9): e0162202. [http://dx.doi.org/10.1371/journal.pone.0162202] [PMID: 27598262]

[37] Paquet C, Boissonnot M, Roger F, Dighiero P, Gil R, Hugon J. Abnormal retinal thickness in patients with mild cognitive impairment and Alzheimer's disease. Neurosci Lett 2007; 420(2): 97-9. [http://dx.doi.org/10.1016/j.neulet.2007.02.090] [PMID: 17543991]

[38] O'Bryhim BE, Apte RS, Kung N, Coble D, Van Stavern GP. Association of preclinical Alzheimer disease with optical coherence tomographic angiography findings. JAMA Ophthalmol 2018; 136(11): 1242-8. [http://dx.doi.org/10.1001/jamaophthalmol.2018.3556] [PMID: 30352114]

[39] Zabel P, Kaluzny JJ, Wilkosc-Debczynska M, *et al.* Comparison of retinal microvasculature in patients with Alzheimer's disease and primary open-angle glaucoma by optical coherence tomography angiography. Invest Ophthalmol Vis Sci 2019; 60(10): 3447-55. [http://dx.doi.org/10.1167/iovs.19-27028] [PMID: 31408108]

[40] Lahme L, Esser EL, Mihailovic N, *et al.* Evaluation of ocular perfusion in Alzheimer's disease using optical coherence tomography angiography. J Alzheimers Dis 2018; 66(4): 1745-52. [http://dx.doi.org/10.3233/JAD-180738] [PMID: 30507577]

[41] Chua J, Hu Q, Ke M, *et al.* Retinal microvasculature dysfunction is associated with Alzheimer's disease and mild cognitive impairment. Alzheimers Res Ther 2020; 12(1): 161. [http://dx.doi.org/10.1186/s13195-020-00724-0] [PMID: 33276820]

[42] Yoon SP, Grewal DS, Thompson AC, *et al.* Retinal microvascular and neurodegenerative changes in Alzheimer's disease and mild cognitive impairment compared with control participants. Ophthalmol Retina 2019; 3(6): 489-99. [http://dx.doi.org/10.1016/j.oret.2019.02.002] [PMID: 31174670]

[43] Lin JB, Apte RS. Seeing Parkinson disease in the retina. JAMA Ophthalmol 2021; 139(2): 189-90. [http://dx.doi.org/10.1001/jamaophthalmol.2020.5719] [PMID: 33355611]

[44] Armstrong MJ, Okun MS. Diagnosis and treatment of Parkinson disease: A review. JAMA 2020; 323(6): 548-60.
[http://dx.doi.org/10.1001/jama.2019.22360] [PMID: 32044947]

[45] Schrag A, Ben-Shlomo Y, Quinn N. How valid is the clinical diagnosis of Parkinson's disease in the community? J Neurol Neurosurg Psychiatry 2002; 73(5): 529-34.
[http://dx.doi.org/10.1136/jnnp.73.5.529] [PMID: 12397145]

[46] Bodis-Wollner I, Kozlowski PB, Glazman S, Miri S. α-synuclein in the inner retina in parkinson disease. Ann Neurol 2014; 75(6): 964-6.
[http://dx.doi.org/10.1002/ana.24182] [PMID: 24816946]

[47] Douglas VP, Douglas KAA, Cestari DM. Ophthalmic manifestations of dementing disorders. Curr Opin Ophthalmol 2021; 32(6): 515-20.
[http://dx.doi.org/10.1097/ICU.0000000000000807] [PMID: 34494975]

[48] Zhang Y, Zhang D, Gao Y, *et al.* Retinal flow density changes in early-stage parkinson's disease investigated by swept-source optical coherence tomography angiography. Curr Eye Res 2021; 46(12): 1886-91.
[http://dx.doi.org/10.1080/02713683.2021.1933054] [PMID: 34348531]

[49] Robbins CB, Grewal DS, Thompson AC, *et al.* Identifying peripapillary radial capillary plexus alterations in Parkinson's disease using OCT angiography. Ophthalmol Retina 2022; 6(1): 29-36.
[http://dx.doi.org/10.1016/j.oret.2021.03.006] [PMID: 33713852]

[50] Xu B, Wang X, Guo J, *et al.* Retinal microvascular density was associated with the clinical progression of Parkinson's disease. Front Aging Neurosci 2022; 14: 818597.
[http://dx.doi.org/10.3389/fnagi.2022.818597] [PMID: 35250544]

[51] Farid M. Reduction in mean deviation values in automated perimetry in eyes with multifocal compared to monofocal intraocular lens implants. Am J Ophthalmol 2014; 158(2): 227-31.
[http://dx.doi.org/10.1016/j.ajo.2014.04.017]

[52] Piñero DP, Monllor B, Camps VJ, de Fez D. Multichannel perimetric alterations in systemic lupus erythematosus treated with hydroxychloroquine. J Optom 2017; 10(2): 135-8.
[http://dx.doi.org/10.1016/j.optom.2016.04.001] [PMID: 27349992]

[53] Marmor MF. Comparison of screening procedures in hydroxychloroquine toxicity. Arch Ophthalmol 2012; 130(4): 461-9.
[http://dx.doi.org/10.1001/archophthalmol.2011.371] [PMID: 22159170]

CHAPTER 9

Branch and Central Retina Artery Occlusion and its treatment according to OCT-A Findings

Geraint J. Parfitt[1] and **Miguel A. Quiroz-Reyes, MD**[2,*]

[1] *School of Optometry & Vision Sciences, Cardiff University, Cardiff, United Kingdom*

[2] *Oftalmologia Integral ABC, Retina Department, Medical and Surgical Assistance Institution (Nonprofit Organization), Affiliated with the Postgraduate Studies Division, National Autonomous University of Mexico, Mexico City, Mexico*

Abstract: The retina requires a large blood supply to cope with the metabolic demands of the tissue, so it is vulnerable to hypoxia when the arterial blood flow is obstructed. Retinal artery occlusions are not common, but they can cause severe vision loss and may be indicative of cardiovascular disorders, such as cerebral stroke and ischemic heart disease. The central retinal artery arises from the ophthalmic artery and its branches supply blood to the inner retina via the superficial capillary plexus. Central retinal artery occlusion (CRAO) is characterized by an obstruction to the central retinal artery that often presents with severe vision loss and a poor prognosis. Branch retinal artery occlusion (BRAO) is defined by a blockage of a branch of the central retinal artery, which typically has a good prognosis if visual acuity is 20/40 or better on presentation. Optical coherence tomography-angiography (OCT-A) is a rapid, high-resolution imaging technique that can visualize the microvasculature of the retinal layers, including the superficial and deep capillary plexuses.

Therefore, it is possible to determine the microvascular changes that occur following retinal artery occlusions, and before and after potential therapies that are being actively researched. Therapies under investigation for the treatment of CRAO and BRAO include hyperbaric oxygen, fibrinolysis, and embolysis with laser therapy. In this chapter, the capabilities of OCT-A imaging to visualize and quantify retinal microvascular changes following CRAO and BRAO are assessed. Moreover, the use of OCT-A to understand the benefit of potential therapies is reviewed.

Keywords: Retinal artery occlusion, Optical coherence tomography angiography, Retinal vascular disease, Retinal ischemia.

* **Corresponding author Miguel A. Quiroz-Reyes, MD:** Oftalmologia Integral ABC, Retina Department, Medical and Surgical Assistance Institution (Nonprofit Organization), Affiliated with the Postgraduate Studies Division, National Autonomous University of Mexico, Mexico City, Mexico; Tel: +52 55 5217 2732; Fax: +52 55 1664 7180; E-mails: drquiroz@prodigy.net.mx and drquirozreyes7@gmail.com

INTRODUCTION

The central retinal artery (CRA) branches from the ophthalmic artery, which stems from the internal carotid artery, to supply blood to the inner retina layers. The inner retina is composed of the retinal nerve fiber layer, ganglion cell layer, inner plexiform layer, and inner nuclear layer, whereas the outer retina contains the photoreceptor layers, retinal pigment epithelium, and choroid. The outer retinal layers are supplied by choroidal blood vessels that form the choriocapillaris that directly underlies Bruch's membrane and the retinal pigment epithelium. The CRA travels within the dural sheath of the optic nerve and upon reaching the posterior pole, it bifurcates into two main branches (superior and inferior), which further divide into the temporal and nasal branches that supply the retinal quadrants. Embedded in the ganglion cell layer is the superficial capillary plexus (SCP), which is supplied by the CRA. The SCP is connected by anastomoses to the intermediate capillary plexus (ICP), and deep capillary plexus (DCP), which supply blood to the other inner retinal layers, including the inner nuclear layer.

Central retinal artery occlusion (CRAO) is defined as the sudden obstruction of the central retinal artery, whereas branch retinal artery occlusion (BRAO) is an occlusion of a CRA branch. Retinal artery occlusion and obstructed blood flow into the retina can cause retinal ischemia and edema that leads to tissue atrophy and vision loss. Retinal ischemia subsequently causes a loss of retinal cell viability and atrophy of photoreceptors, which results in visual defects. BRAO is restricted to the region that is supplied by the occluded vessel and the extent of vision loss correlates with the size of the area affected by the obstructed blood vessel. On the other hand, CRAO is a type of acute ischemic stroke that often causes severe vision loss of 20/400 or worse and has a poor prognosis. Both types of retinal artery occlusion are an indicator of increased risk of cerebral stroke and ischemic heart disease [1], therefore, it requires careful assessment and referral to a stroke center.

Retinal artery occlusion can be a result of embolism, thrombosis, or increased intraocular pressure and may be temporary. Damage to the affected area can occur in minutes, even when the blood flow has been restored after the initial occlusion. CRAO can result in ischemic necrosis, whitening, and opacification of the inner retina, which may last for days and cause a cherry-red spot at the fovea. Moderate retinal artery occlusions can go unnoticed when there is not a significant level of retinal opacification [2].

As outlined in Chapter 1, optical coherence tomography – angiography (OCT-A) is a non-invasive imaging approach that can generate high-resolution images of the retinal microvasculature to aid with the diagnosis and management of vascular disease, including retinal artery occlusion (Fig. **1**). OCT-A imaging can rapidly generate high-resolution cross-sections of the macula, which allows the clinical course of CRAO to be readily tracked over the long-term.

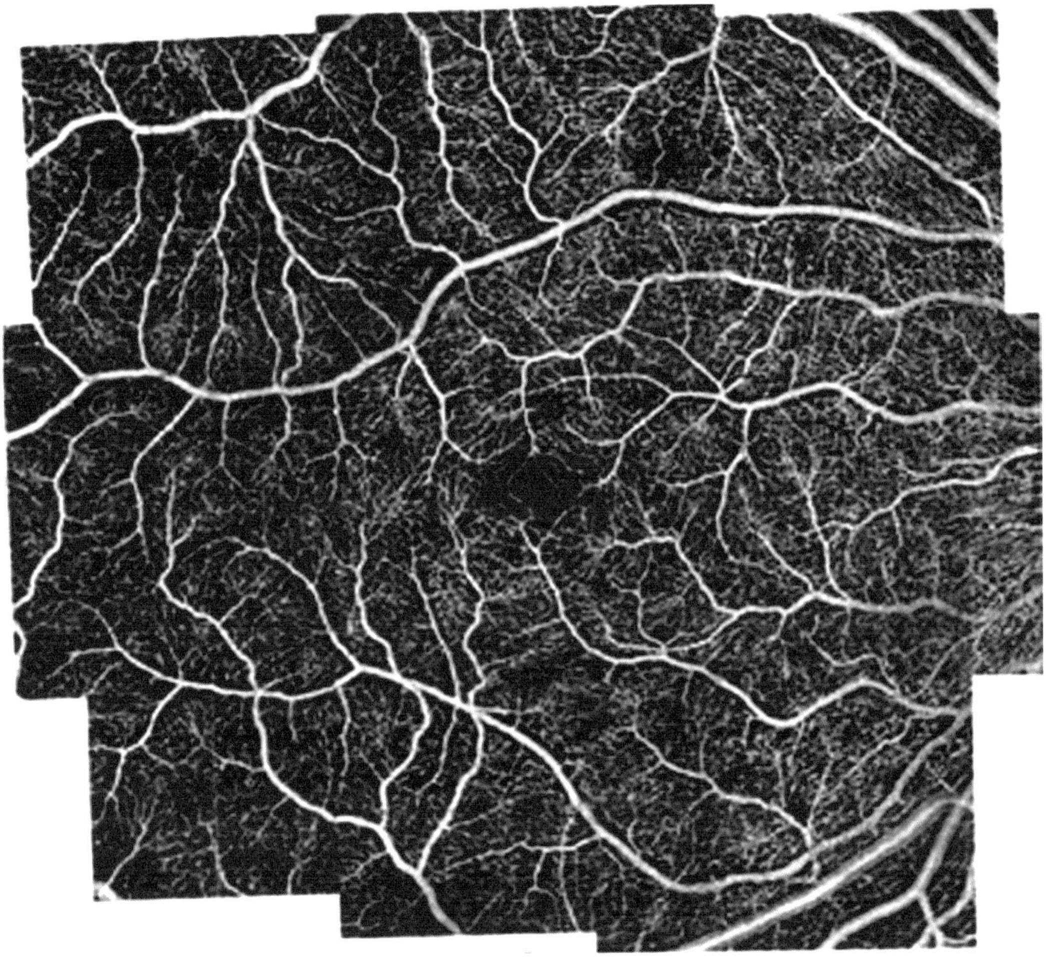

Fig. (1). OCT-A wide-field montage of vasculature in a normal retina. OCT-A images were acquired using the Angiovue software of the RTVue XR Avanti (Optovue, Inc., Fremont, CA) and montaged using Adobe Photoshop (San Jose, CA). Montage OCT-A imaging enables a large field of view like FFA with high-resolution of the retinal vasculature. Image unchanged from De Carlo, TE *et al.*,*Int J Retin Vitr* 1, 5 (2015) [4] and is used under the Creative Commons Attribution 4.0 International License (https://creativecommons.org/licenses/by/4.0/).

Fundoscopy and Fundus fluorescein angiography (FFA) are routinely used in the ophthalmology clinic as the standard of care to visualize retinal vasculature and vessel flow in retinal artery occlusion patients; however, the vascular networks cannot be depth-resolved so the separate layers of the retina cannot be quantified. For example, the ICP and DCP layers cannot be resolved using FFA imaging. However, OCT-A enables the rapid visualization of microvascular abnormalities in the retina and subsequent imaging through the clinical course of treatment without intravenous dye administration. OCT-A has revealed the variable extent of nonperfusion in the superficial and deep plexuses, which would not be possible with FFA [3]. The ability to image the retinal vasculature without intravenous dyes is important as dyes such as fluorescein and indocyanine green – angiography (ICGA) can be allergenic and cause complications with pregnancies, while intravenous injection is required for every imaging session. Importantly, OCT-A can be used for the quantification of various metrics associated with the retinal microvasculature in the superficial and deep capillary plexus, including vessel density, vessel length density, and tortuosity, while foveal avascular zone (FAZ) size and shape can also be accurately determined. In this chapter, we review the current applications of OCT-A to acute and chronic retinal artery occlusion patients and how they can be used in the management of RAO related disease.

CENTRAL RETINAL ARTERY OCCLUSION

CRAO was first described by the pioneering ophthalmologist Albrecht von Graefe in 1859. It typically presents with a sudden onset of painless, unilateral vision loss that is more common with increased age and is rarely seen in pediatric populations. CRAO related vision loss is typically severe; a study of 260 eyes with CRAO indicated that patients have significant unilateral vision loss, and up to 80% of CRAO patients exhibit a visual acuity of 20/400 or worse at presentation [5]. CRAO is often an indication of underlying atherosclerotic disease and risk of cerebral and ischemic heart disease, therefore, it is a medical emergency with a significant chance of permanent vision loss. The presence of a cilioretinal artery in up to 49.5% of patients means that some of the retina can remain perfused in the case of acute CRAO [6]. The cilioretinal artery arises from the posterior ciliary arteries and not the central retinal artery. This allows for some vision to be retained in some cases, however, 60% of eyes with a cilioretinal artery had an initial visual acuity of 6/30 or worse in one study of CRAO patients [5].

The precise location of where occlusion occurs in the central retinal artery is poorly understood. The narrowest region of the central retinal artery lumen is where it passes through the dural sheath of the optic nerve, and this is expected to be the most likely region where CRAO happens [5]. Obstruction of the central retinal artery is usually due to the presence of emboli, and carotid artery plaques formed from cholesterol (Hollenhorst plaques) are the most common origin of emboli. The most important factor in visual outcomes following CRAO is the duration of the arterial occlusion, with the retinal ganglion cells thought to be susceptible to damage within 15 minutes of CRAO [7] and retinal infarction likely after 240 minutes [8], based on animal studies. Therefore, therapeutic intervention is only likely to be effective within a golden period following CRAO, which is thought to be within 6 hours.

CRAO has been defined as four distinct clinical entities, with each classification having a different prognosis [5]:

Non-arteritic Permanent CRAO

Two-thirds of CRAO cases are caused by emboli from atherosclerotic disease and platelet fibrin thrombi, which are defined as non-arteritic permanent CRAOs. Non-arteritic permanent CRAOs have the worst prognosis and visual outcomes. Fundus imaging shows the classical cherry-red spot where the choroidal blood supply to the macula is spared, and retinal arterial changes associated with CRAO are evident, including attenuated arteries (Fig. **2**). Non-arteritic permanent CRAO risk factors include arterial hypertension, carotid artery disease, coronary artery disease, and diabetes mellitus [9].

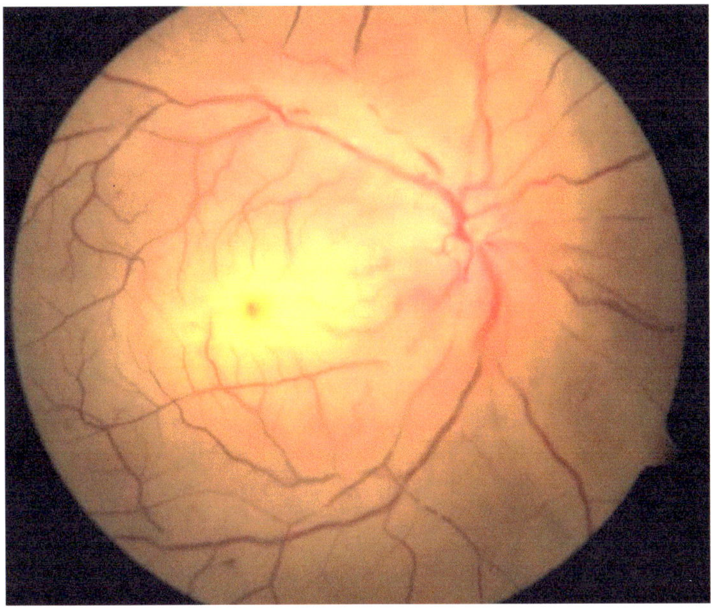

Fig. (2). Central retinal artery occlusion of the right eye shows the classical cherry-red spot at the macula. In this patient, CRAO was due to filler injections around the eyes. This image was originally published on the Retina Image Bank® website. Hyung-Woo Kwak, MD. Central Retinal Artery Occlusion. Retina Image Bank. 2022; 1683. © The American Society of Retina Specialists.

Non-arteritic CRAO with Cilioretinal Sparing

This classification of CRAO has the same clinical characterization as non-arteritic permanent CRAO, however, there is a cilioretinal artery present in these cases (Fig. **3**). Patients with a cilioretinal artery can be spared from extensive vision loss in CRAO due to the presence of an unobstructed blood supply to a portion of the inner retina, however, peripheral vision is impaired. The extent of vision that is preserved is dependent on the area of the retina that the cilioretinal artery supplies [5].

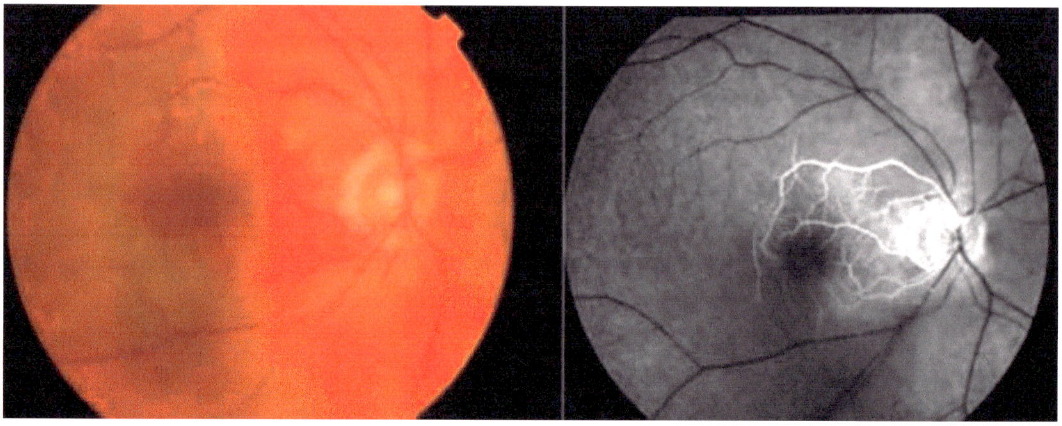

Fig. (3). Fundus photograph and fundus fluorescein angiogram of the right eye with non-arteritic CRAO with cilioretinal sparing. Image unchanged from Cugati, S. *et al.*, Curr Treat Options Neurol. 2013; 15 1: 63–77 [10] is used under the Creative Commons Attribution 4.0 International License (https://creativecommons.org/licenses/by/4.0/).

Non-arteritic Transient CRAO

Non-arteritic transient CRAO may vary in duration from minutes to hours, depending on the cause of the occlusion. Approximately 15-17% of CRAOs are of the non-arteritic transient subtype, which has the best prognosis, and visual outcome is directly dependent on the duration of transient CRAO [5]. It is analogous to a transient ischemic attack that affects the eye, where restoration of blood flow to the central retinal artery causes the symptoms to resolve.

Arteritic CRAO

Arteritic CRAO relates to a central retinal artery occlusion caused by a systemic inflammatory condition. Giant cell arteritis (GCA) is the most common cause of permanent arteritic CRAO and causes arterial inflammation, which accounts for approximately 4.5% of CRAO cases overall [5]. Fundus imaging of arteritic CRAO shows the classical findings of CRAO together with optic disk edema due to arteritic anterior ischemic optic neuropathy. GCA is thought to only affect larger vessels, so it does not affect the smaller branch vessels of the central retinal artery.

CRAO ETIOLOGY

The occurrence of an embolism is the most common reason for CRAO overall, which can be made up of either cholesterol, calcium, or platelet-fibrin. In 95% of CRAO cases, it is a result of thromboembolic disease (non-arteritic CRAO), whereas up to 5% is caused by GCA and is defined as arteritic CRAO [11]. The major cause of cholesterol and platelet-fibrin embolism that results in CRAO is carotid artery disease from atherosclerotic plaques [9], whereas calcium emboli often arise from cardiac valves [12]. Overall, 74% of emboli are found to be composed of cholesterol, while 10.5% are calcific, and 15.5% are made of fibrin [13]. Thrombosis leading to CRAO can be due to atherosclerosis, collagen-vascular disease, or hypercoagulable factors and may cause occlusion posterior to the lamina cribrosa [14].

CRAO is often associated with ipsilateral internal carotid artery stenosis, which was present in 37% of CRAO cases in one study [15] and 40% of patients in the EAGLE (European Assessment Group for Lysis in the Eye) study [1]. The risk of CRAO increases with age and is more likely in patients with a history of hypertension, hyperlipidemia, diabetes, smoking, and obesity [11]. For example, the EAGLE study found that 67% of 84 CRAO patients studied had cardiovascular risk factors as part of their medical history, with obesity (82%), hypertension (73%), smoking (49%), hypercholesterolemia (49%), and diabetes (14%) being most prevalent [16]. Iatrogenic CRAO has also been reported in the cases of injectable hyaluronic acid fillers, with CRAO being the most common arterial obstruction due to embolic hyaluronic acid filler blockage [17].

The obstruction of arterial blood flow and absence of oxygen delivery to the retina causes ischemia and subsequent vision loss. The retina is vulnerable to hypoxia, and ischemia induced in rhesus monkeys has shown that irreversible damage to the tissue only occurs after approximately 97 minutes, with 240 minutes of ischemia resulting in extensive retinal damage [8]. CRAO can result in severe, irreversible vision loss due to retinal ischemia and can occur concurrently with silent ischemic stroke, so it is a medical emergency that requires immediate attention.

Arteritic CRAO is a common cause of vision loss in giant cell arteritis (GCA), which is the most common primary vasculitis in adults [18]. Vision loss due to GCA can be prevented with early diagnosis and immediate treatment with corticosteroids that reduce inflammation and is recommended to be continued for six to twelve months. A temporal artery biopsy can be performed after steroid treatment and positive biopsy results can be found after 4 weeks after steroid treatment initiation [19].

CRAO EPIDEMIOLOGY

The incidence of CRAO is estimated at 1.9 in 100,000 people in the United States [20], 1.8 in 100,000 in South Korea [21], and 2.5 in 100,000 in Japan [22], and represents approximately 1 in 10,000 outpatient visits to an ophthalmologist [23]. After 80 years of age, the incidence of CRAO increases to 10.1 in 100,000, while men have a marginally higher incidence than women [21, 24]. The mean age of presentation has been described as early 60s [25], and less than 2% present with bilateral CRAO. CRAO patients have an estimated life expectancy of 5.5 years compared to 15.4 years for non-CRAO patients of the same age [1].

In a study of 244 patients, the mean age of non-arteritic permanent CRAO was 68 years, while non-arteritic transient CRAO was found to be 63 years of age. Non-arteritic CRAO with cilioretinal sparing mean age was 67 years, whereas arteritic CRAO mean age was 74 years of age [5].

CRAO PROGNOSIS

Typically, vision loss associated with non-arteritic permanent CRAO is severe and related to the extent and duration of retinal ischemia and edema. As mentioned above, patients typically present with severe vision loss of 20/400 or worse. When 260 eyes with CRAO were studied, 74% presented with a visual acuity of counting fingers or worse [5]. Less than 20% of patients regain functional vision in the eye affected by CRAO [26]. However, in the case of non-arteritic CRAO with cilioretinal sparing, visual acuity was observed to recover to 20/50 or better in 80% of eyes [27].

Retinal neovascularization is a known complication of CRAO, but it is not common. The prevalence of neovascularization secondary to acute CRAO has been shown to be 18.2% with an onset of 8.5 weeks post CRAO on average. Iris neovascularization has been reported in 2.5 – 31.6% of CRAO patients, with neovascular glaucoma present in 15.2% of cases [28].

OCT Imaging of CRAO

Fundoscopy of CRAO patients typically shows retina whitening as indicative of retinal ischemia, a cherry-red spot that is a result of choroidal blood supply to the fovea surrounded by ischemic retina, and slow segmental blood flow (boxcarring) in attenuated arteries [11]. OCT can supplement fundoscopy and provide new insights into microvascular changes with high-resolution, cross-section views of the macula. Moreover, it enables rapid assessment of retinal microvascular networks in the different retinal layers and is an emerging method for monitoring the progression of retinal artery occlusions [29 - 31].

Optical coherence tomography has proven to be an effective imaging approach for diagnosis, staging and prognosis of CRAO. For example, OCT can rapidly detect retinal edema in acute CRAO, whereas FFA is slower and not always necessary to confirm a CRAO diagnosis. It has been previously reported that retinal thickness is increased in the acute phase of CRAO, which decreases over time, although the level of retinal edema did not correlate with visual outcome [32]. Higher-resolution spectral domain optical coherence tomography (SD-OCT) reveals that inner retina thickness decreased in chronic CRAO, but the outer retina remained the same [33].

OCT imaging shows hyperreflectivity of the inner retina layers in the acute stages of CRAO, which is related to retinal edema following ischemia [11]. Inner and outer retinal thickening has been shown to be present at initial presentation, while the inner retina subsequently atrophies and thins out over time, which can be clearly observed in cross-section images of the macula generated by OCT [34]. Follow-up OCT shows a reduction in thickness and reflectivity of inner retinal layers, whereas the outer retina, retinal pigment epithelium and choriocapillaris increased in reflectivity after decreasing reflectivity in the acute phase. This finding suggested that there is an atrophy of the neurosensory retina in the later stages of CRAO [29]. Therefore, OCT may be a valuable tool in recognizing acute and chronic CRAO, which is important for decisions on therapeutic intervention.

OCT-A can be used for the quantification of various metrics associated with the retinal microvasculature in the superficial and deep capillary plexus, including vessel density, vessel length density, tortuosity, foveal avascular zone (FAZ) size and shape can be accurately determined. OCT-A has been used to determine reduced retinal perfusion in both the SCP and the DCP of retinal artery occlusion patients [31].

Vessel density in the SCP and DCP has been shown to be significantly reduced in retinal artery occlusion patients when compared to control eyes [30]. It has been suggested that reduced vessel density in the SCP may be a valuable predictive factor in retinal artery occlusions. There was also found to be a significant reduction in an area with a width of 300 μm surrounding the FAZ in CRAO patients when compared to control eyes. No significant alteration was found in the FAZ of either CRAO or BRAO patients and no correlation between visual acuity and FAZ was found, however, the acircularity index of the FAZ was significantly decreased in CRAO eyes (Fig. **4**). Central macular thickness was also correlated with visual acuity in CRAO patients using OCT (r = 0.626, P = 0.024) [30].

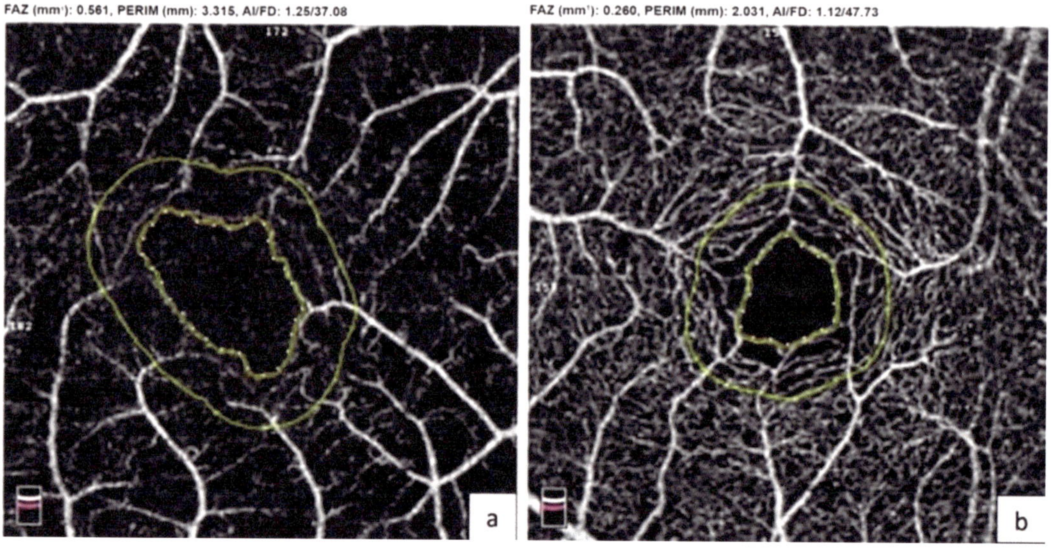

Fig. (4). Foveal avascular zone imaging of a CRAO patient using OCT-A. Yellow lines indicate the border of the FAZ and an area with a width of 300 μm surrounding the FAZ. (**A**) CRAO patient; (**B**) Fellow eye. Image unchanged from Yang, S *et al.,BMC Ophthalmology* volume 19, Article number: 147 (2019) [30] and is used under the Creative Commons Attribution 4.0 International License (https://creativecommons.org/licenses/by/4.0/).

A recent study investigated optical intensities in segment retinal layers from OCT cross-section images of CRAO patients and normal controls (Fig. **5**). They found that the optical intensities of the inner retina were increased in CRAO patients when compared to controls, with the largest increase noted in the inner nuclear layer [35]. In the outer retina, optical densities were decreased and were most prominent in the photoreceptor layers. The reduction in optical densities in the outer nuclear may be explained by a shadowing effect caused by the increased inner retina reflectivity found in CRAO patients. The optical intensity in the retinal nerve fiber layer was found to remain the same between CRAO patients and control groups, even though edema is expected to affect the superficial layer of the retina. It has been suggested that the reflectivity of the inner nuclear layers may be a diagnostic tool to establish CRAO in patients [35].

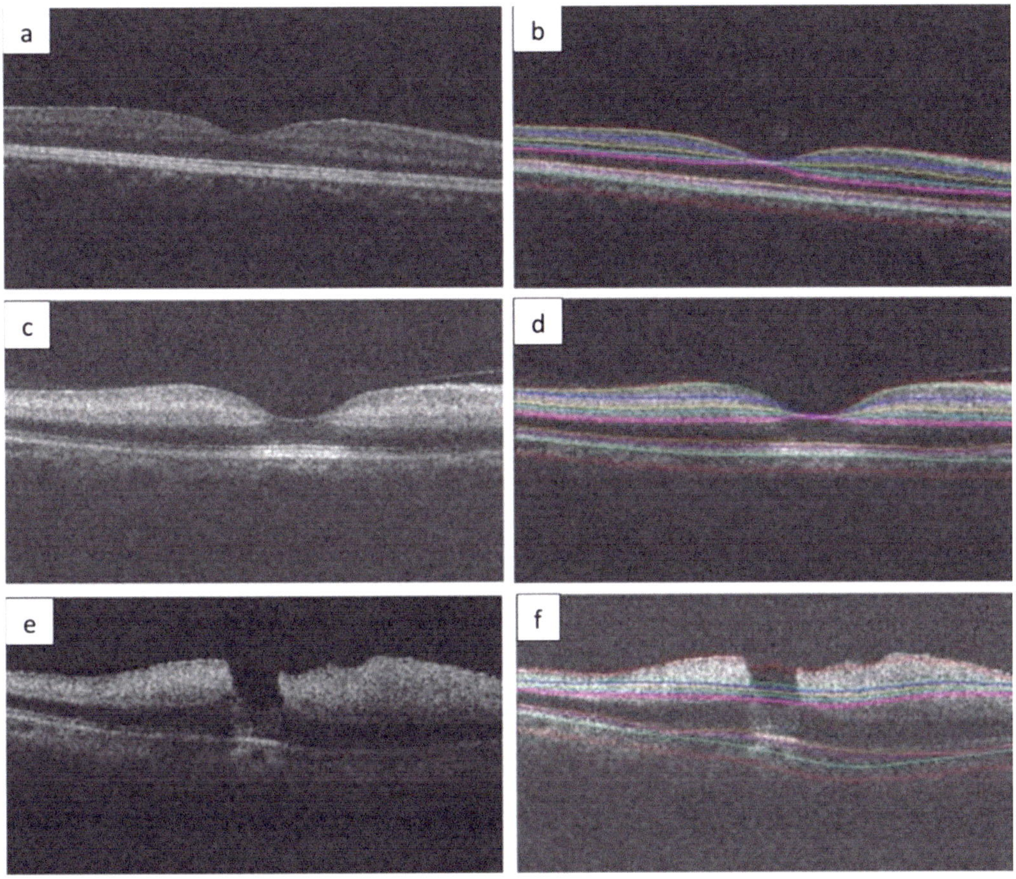

Fig. (5). Segmentation of retinal layers on macular SD-OCT images to determine optical densities in CRAO patients and normal controls. (**A** and **B**) Control eyes; (**C** and **D**) CRAO patients with segmented retinal layers; (**E** and **F**) CRAO patients with increased optical densities in the inner retina. Image unchanged from Chen, H *et al.*,*Sci Rep* 5, 9269 (2015) [35] is used under the Creative Commons Attribution 4.0 International License (https://creativecommons.org/licenses/by/4.0/).

Vessel density surrounding the optic disc and retinal nerve fiber layer thickness have also been measured in CRAO patients using OCT. In three patients with CRAO, peripapillary vessel density and retinal nerve fiber layer thickness were both reduced when compared to fellow eyes without CRAO. The vessel density inside the optic disc was also reduced in two patients with CRAO and peripapillary vessels were shown to be thinner by OCT imaging [30].

FFA and ICGA imaging are unable to confirm structural continuity between retinal arteries and the posterior ciliary arteries, which can be resolved using OCT-A. This was confirmed in a recent study that used OCT-A to understand the three-dimensional configuration of circumpapillary collaterals that developed post iatrogenic CRAO. Therefore, OCT-A is an important tool for non-invasive imaging of retinal circulatory dynamics and was used here to identify anastomosis of the retinal and posterior ciliary artery systems. Two weeks after CRAO caused by an embolization of a convexity meningioma, OCT-A showed collateral vessel development on the optic disc margin. Six months on, OCT-A was used to observe circumpapillary collaterals connecting retinal artery branches with vessels supplying the optic disc, which come from the posterior ciliary arteries [36].

Treatment of CRAO

CRAO is an emergency that requires prompt referral to a stroke center as it is indicative of potential cerebral stroke and ischemic heart disease. There should be an immediate evaluation for carotid occlusion and thromboembolic disease when CRAO is presented. This will entail a clinical workup for vasculitis or hypercoagulability in patients under 50, and a workup for embolism in patients over 50 [37]. It is understood that treatments for CRAO must be administered within 6 hours after symptoms arise for them to have a chance of being effective.

At this time, there are few options to treat CRAO that can definitively improve visual outcomes. Therapeutic options include vasodilators, hyperbaric oxygen therapy, clot-busting approaches, and fluid release; however, none have been proven to be efficacious in treating all CRAO patients. For example, pentoxifylline is a derivative of xanthine that has been used to decrease blood viscosity and increase perfusion of the retina. It has been studied for use in treating CRAO and has shown improved retinal perfusion, but visual outcomes were not improved [38]. Diet and lifestyle changes have also been advocated as important factors for the secondary prevention of CRAO and to reduce the risk factors of atherosclerosis [10].

Carbogen inhalation (95% oxygen and 5% carbon dioxide mixture) has been tested based on the idea that carbon dioxide will prevent oxygen induced vasoconstriction and improve blood flow. Carbogen is inhaled for 10 minutes every 1 – 4hrs for up to 3 days. Visual outcomes in CRAO after carbogen inhalation have been measured and were found to not reach significance [39]. Hyperbaric oxygen has also been used in the treatment of CRAO to increase the delivery of oxygen to ischemic retinas with the aim of tissue reperfusion. Hyperbaric oxygen application differs between studies, which is typically between 2 – 2.5 atm for 1.5 hrs within 8 hours of CRAO onset. Visual acuity improvements have been found when hyperbaric oxygen has combined with hemodilution [1], although no study has proven that hyperbaric oxygen is efficacious in the treatment of CRAO.

Neovascularization of the retina and anterior segment is a potential complication of vascular occlusion in the retina, so patients with retinal ischemia from CRAO require frequent follow-ups to detect neovascularization and neovascular glaucoma. Panretinal photocoagulation (PRP) with or without anti-vascular endothelial growth factor therapy (VEGF) has been recommended for CRAO patients who have developed iris or retinal neovascularization [37, 40]. PRP converts ischemic areas of the retina to anoxic regions that reduce the expression of angiogenic VEGF and platelet-derived growth factor (PDGF) and prevents the formation of new blood vessels.

Intravenous thrombolysis with tissue plasminogen activator (tPA) has been evaluated as an approach to treat CRAO and 5.8% of patients with CRAO in the United States are treated with tPA [41]. Altaplase is the most frequently used tPA agent and has been FDA approved for use in acute ischemic stroke. It has been shown that up to 50% of acute CRA patients treated with fibrinolytic drugs exhibited some clinical recovery when treated within 4.5 hours [42]. Further studies have also shown that thrombolytic treatment with intravenous low-dose recombinant tPA improves visual recovery in acute CRAO patients when administered within 6.5 hours [43]. Intra-arterial tPA is an approach to deliver tPA directly to the ophthalmic artery to reduce systemic effects, and there is a case series that suggests it can improve visual outcomes [44]. Another case study showed that endovascular surgery with an injection of tPA can significantly improve visual outcomes after CRAO. In this case, tPA (80,000 units/mL) solution was administered to the retinal artery of the optic disc for 2-3 minutes after 25-G vitrectomy. Two patients were treated within 12 hours after CRAO onset and visual acuity was improved to -0.08 and 0.1 logMAR [45]. The risk of intra-arterial tPA administration is arterial dissection, catheter-induced spasm, and distal embolization due to dislodging of atheromatous plaques in the ophthalmic circulation. Overall, fibrinolysis using tPA is a promising approach for treating CRAO that requires further investigation.

In the case of arteritic CRAO associated with GCA, immediate systemic corticosteroids are recommended to reduce inflammation [1]. Treatment for suspected GCA should begin with testing of erythrocyte sedimentation rate and C-reactive protein to confirm the diagnosis. High-dose intravenous methylprednisolone is indicated for use with arteritic CRAO associated with GCA, and a temporal artery biopsy can be performed to confirm the presence of vasculitis.

BRANCH RETINAL ARTERY OCCLUSION

BRAO is defined as an occlusion of a branch of the central retinal artery that supplies blood to the inner retina. It is estimated that BRAO accounts for 38% of all retinal artery occlusion cases [46]. Like CRAO, vision loss in BRAO is related to the extent and duration of retinal ischemia caused by the obstruction of blood flow in a branch of the central retinal artery. However, the prognosis and visual outcomes of BRAO are significantly better than CRAO. Retinal ischemia and acute edema occur alongside the occluded branch retinal artery, which is evident on fundus and OCT imaging (Fig. **6**).

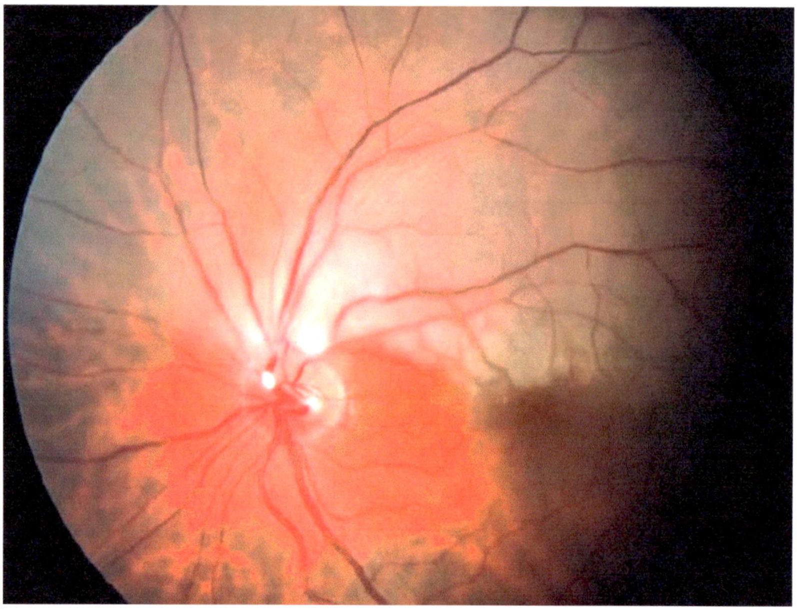

Fig. (6). Fundus photograph of half ischemic retina in BRAO with Hollenhorst plaque at the optic disc. This image was originally published on the Retina Image Bank® website. Vishal Gupta, MBBS, MS. Central Retinal Artery Occlusion. Retina Image Bank. 2022; 80937. © The American Society of Retina Specialists.

BRAO patients typically present with unilateral, partial visual loss that is painless, and occlusion of a branch retinal artery is often caused by an embolus or thrombus related to cardiovascular disease risk factors. In a study of 187 patients (201 eyes), the temporal vessels were implicated in 98% of BRAO cases and systemic hypertension was seen in 71% of cases [47].

BRAO is subdivided into permanent BRAO and transient BRAO. Permanent BRAO is associated with more severe vision loss, whereas transient BRAO is an occlusion that lasts for a shorter duration and, therefore, it generally has a better prognosis than permanent BRAO. Tissue atrophy is more likely to occur in permanent BRAO as retinal cells lose viability following hypoxia due to a lack of blood supply. Increasing severity of BRAO causes a larger area of retinal ischemia and retinal cell death. In mice, pyknotic nuclei and retinal degeneration can be observed in the inner retina at 24 hours following induced retinal artery occlusion. After 21 days, 80% of retinal ganglion cells are estimated to have nuclear loss [48].

BRAO ETIOLOGY

BRAOs are typically caused by emboli, which are from a carotid artery atheroma or myocardial thrombus. Emboli are often composed of cholesterol or fibrin, as is the case with CRAO. Emboli are less frequently derived from calcified cardiac valves, air from trauma or surgery, and talc from intravenous drug use. The embolus travels through the ophthalmic and central retinal arteries and gets lodged at the bifurcation of a branch from the central retinal artery.

BRAO risk factors are common to cardiovascular diseases and include hypertension, atherosclerosis, coronary artery disease, and hypercholesterolemia [46]. Hyperhomocysteinaemia is a cause of central and branch retinal artery occlusion in young people [49] (Fig. **7**). Smoking, diabetes, and transient ischemic attack are more likely to be a part of the medical history of BRAO patients when compared to non-BRAO cases, while increasing age is a common factor as pediatric cases are very rare [50]. BRAO is a relatively benign ophthalmic disease, however, the association with severe cardiovascular disorders requires prompt evaluation.

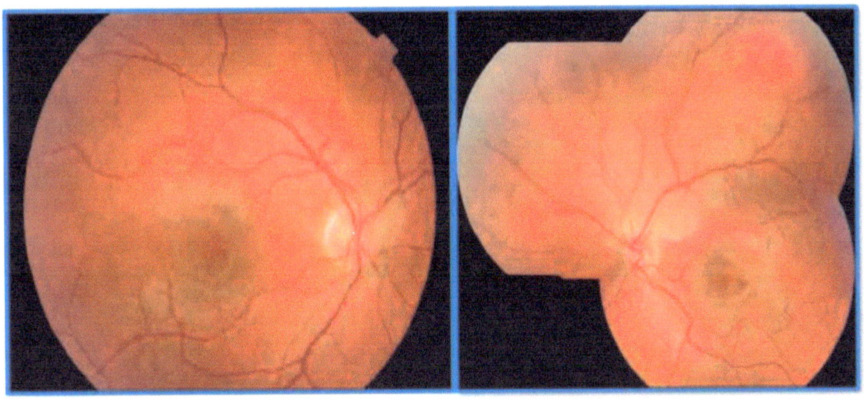

Fig. (7). Branch retinal artery occlusion in a teenager due to hyperhomocysteinaemia. (Left panel) Fundus photo of the normal right eye. (Right panel) Left eye has retinal pallor and arterial attenuation across superior retinal arcade. Image unchanged from Shute, C. *BMC Ophthalmology* volume 18, Article number: 220 (2018) [49] is used under the Creative Commons Attribution 4.0 International License (https://creativecommons.org/licenses/by/4.0/).

Non-embolic etiologies of BRAO include vasculitides, coagulopathies, and vasospasms from migraines. Susac syndrome is a rare auto-immune condition that involves antibodies targeting endothelial cells in arteries. The subsequent damage to vascular endothelial cells and thrombosis causes obstructions that result in BRAO [51]. BRAO is not caused by GCA as it only affects larger arteries such as the central retinal artery. There is also evidence that exposure to high altitudes and diabetic retinopathy are risk factors for BRAO [52].

BRAO EPIDEMIOLOGY

Occlusion of retinal arteries are rare disorders (CRAO and BRAO). The incidence of BRAO is approximately 5 people per 100,000 [53], which is higher than CRAO and accounts for 38% of all retinal artery occlusions. The cumulative 10-year incidence of emboli in asymptomatic BRAO is 2.9% in those >49 years of age [54], while the incidence of symptomatic BRAO is approximately 30% of CRAO [55]. BRAO patients are typically 70 years or older [56].

BRAO PROGNOSIS

Transient BRAO typically has a better prognosis than permanent BRAO as the duration of arterial occlusion and extent of retinal ischemia is shorter. The visual prognosis following BRAO correlates with the initial visual acuity on presentation; patients presenting with a visual acuity of 20/40 or better remained at 20/40 at least. Approximately 74% of permanent BRAO patients present with a visual acuity of 20/40 or better, and 89% of cases have a visual acuity of 20/40 or better at follow-up. On the other hand, 94% of patients with transient BRAO present with an initial visual acuity of 20/40 and 100% have a visual acuity of 20/40 or better at follow-up [26]. However, 86% of BRAO patients with a poor visual acuity of 20/100 or worse did not show a significant improvement in their visual outcome [46].

OCT-A Imaging of BRAO

Fundoscopy reveals the presence of emboli in a branch of the central retinal artery in up to 62% of patients [46]. Superficial retinal whitening is evident surrounding the obstructed branch vessel, which is indicative of retinal ischemia. Like CRAO, OCT is emerging as an imaging method to rapidly assess the changes in retinal layers of BRAO patients in the acute and chronic phases (Fig. **8**). BRAO typically has a good prognosis, with most patients presenting a visual acuity of 20/40 or better. Therefore, extensive treatment is not often carried out, but OCT can be used to track the progression of retinal ischemia and edema.

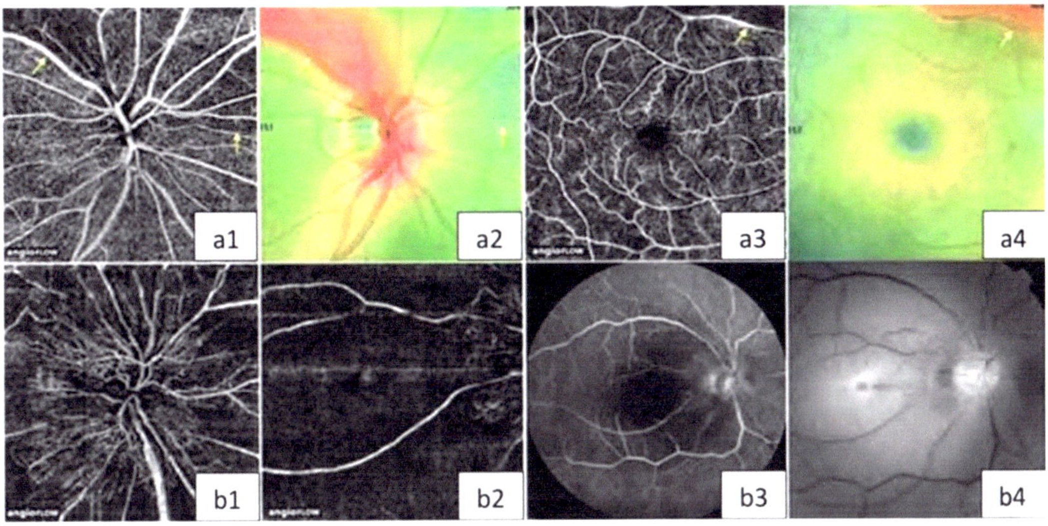

Fig. (8). OCT-A imaging of BRAO and CRAO cases. (**a**) OCT-A imaging of an acute BRAO from the right eye of a 70-year-old patients. (a1) Full thickness (4.5 x 4.5 mm) OCT-A image of the optic disc with decreased capillary perfusion supero-temporal and nasal to the optic disc (yellow arrows). (a2) En-face OCT thickness heat map shows retinal thickening (red) and thinning (blue) that highlight the decreased capillary perfusion shown in A1. (a3) Full-thickness OCT-A image shows decreased capillary perfusion supero-temporal and nasal to the optic disc (yellow arrow). (A4) En-face OCT thickness heat map shows retinal thickening (red) that relates to the area of decreased capillary perfusion shown in a3. (**b**) OCT-A imaging of a subacute CRAO in the right eye of an 81-year-old patient. (b1) Full thickness OCT-A image of the optic disc with decreased peripapillary capillary perfusion. (b2) Full thickness OCT-A image showing decreased capillary perfusion in the macula with only the large retinal and peripapillary vessels exhibiting blood flow. (b3) FFA imaging shows hypo-fluorescence in the macula and peripapillary region caused by reduced flow of blood and fluorescein dye. (b4) Red-free fundus image shows vessel attenuation in the macular and peripapillary regions. Image unchanged from De Carlo, TE *et al.,Int J Retin Vitr* 1, 5 (2015) [4] is used under the Creative Commons Attribution 4.0 International License (https://creativecommons.org/licenses/by/4.0/).

OCT studies of BRAO patients suggest that the damage in the retina is limited to the inner retina. One study of BRAO has shown that the inner plexiform layer showed the highest relative increase in optical reflectivity when compared with the inner nuclear layer and nerve fiber layer. The inner plexiform layer was increased in thickness at presentation but subsided over time. Shadowing and a subsequent decrease in the outer retina reflectivity were also observed. Interestingly, the inner plexiform layer and inner nuclear layer were unable to be differentiated in OCT images, which could point to their role in the pathophysiology of BRAO [57].

SD-OCT was also used to measure the thickness of retinal layers in the acute and chronic stages of BRAO. In acute BRAO, the thickness of retinal layers was increased in the inner layers, including the retinal nerve fiber layer, inner plexiform layer, and inner nuclear layer, and is slightly increased in the outer nuclear layer. The thickness was reduced in chronic BRAO, and the inner plexiform layer and inner nuclear layers were difficult to distinguish, which may be suggestive of tissue atrophy. However, there were no thickness changes in the photoreceptor and retinal pigment epithelium layers in both acute and chronic BRAO [57].

OCT-A imaging of a patient with BRAO revealed an occlusion in the upper temporal branch of the retinal artery. Vessel density was qualitatively assessed and the superior hemifield SCP and DCP were decreased when compared to the inferior hemifield (Fig. **9**). The vessel density was also decreased in the unaffected hemifield of the SCP and DCP of BRAO eyes when compared to the fellow eye [30]. This suggests that high-resolution OCT imaging of the deep vascular networks may help to precisely track retinal perfusion changes that occur with BRAO and over the natural clinical course after occlusion.

changes over time.

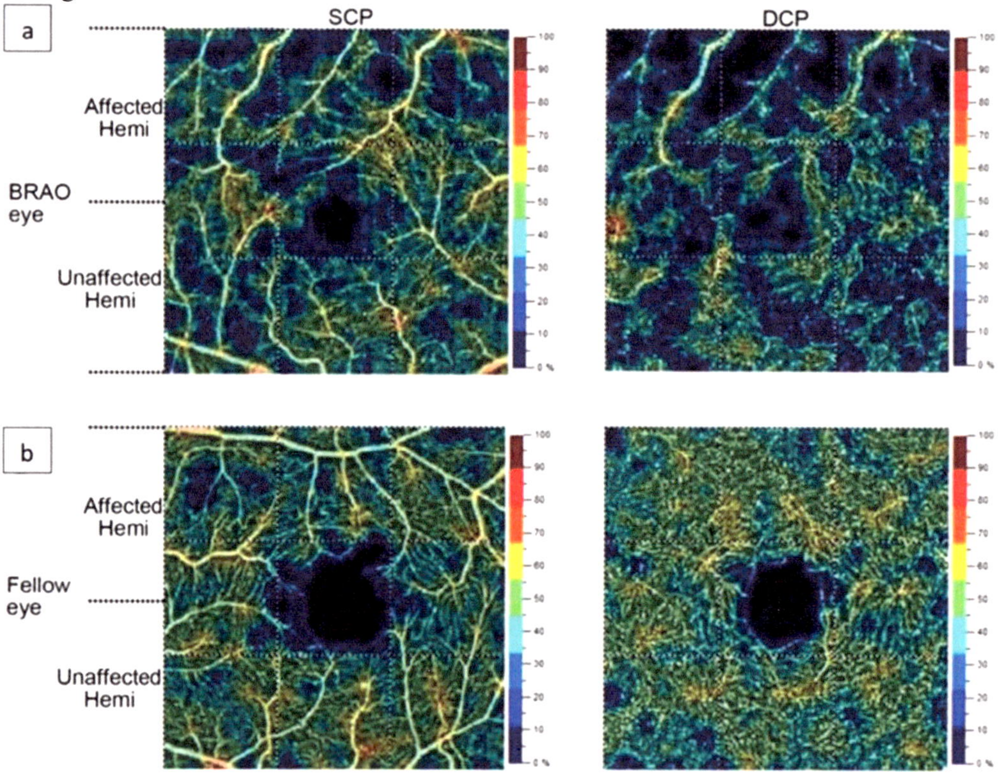

Fig. (9). OCT-A imaging of the SCP and DCP in a BRAO patient. Vessel density heat map of (**a**) BRAO eye and; (**b**) Fellow eye shows decreased vascular density in the SCP and DCP of the BRAO eye. Image unchanged from Yang, S *et al.*,*BMC Ophthalmology* volume 19, Article number: 147 (2019) [30] is used under the Creative Commons Attribution 4.0 International License (https://creativecommons.org/licenses /by/4.0/).

In one study of OCT imaging to help characterize the changes to retinal microvasculature in BRAO, 75% of acute and chronic BRAO cases had focal restoration of the DCP perfusion while the SCP was abnormal. Therefore, it is now possible to image recanalization and reorganization of the microvasculature at different vascular layers in the retina as OCT is depth-resolved [31]. One of the main advantages of OCT imaging over FFA is the ability to rapidly differentiate the superficial and deep capillary plexus layers in retinal vascular disease and their changes over time.

Treatment of BRAO

Currently, there is no single effective therapeutic intervention recommended for BRAO. It is important that the risk of stroke is assessed due to the correlation of BRAO risk factors with cardiovascular disease. Standard management of BRAO patients includes lowering intra-ocular pressure (IOP) with brimonidine administration for approximately 6 weeks, with OCT imaging used as a valuable imaging tool to monitor retinal edema [58].

Hyperbaric oxygen is a safe and inexpensive approach to try and increase the solubility of oxygen in the blood, which may improve the delivery of oxygen from the choroidal vasculature to the outer retina and further diffusion into the inner retinal layers (Fig. **10**). However, further randomized, controlled trials are required to validate the effects of hyperbaric oxygen to treat BRAO [52].

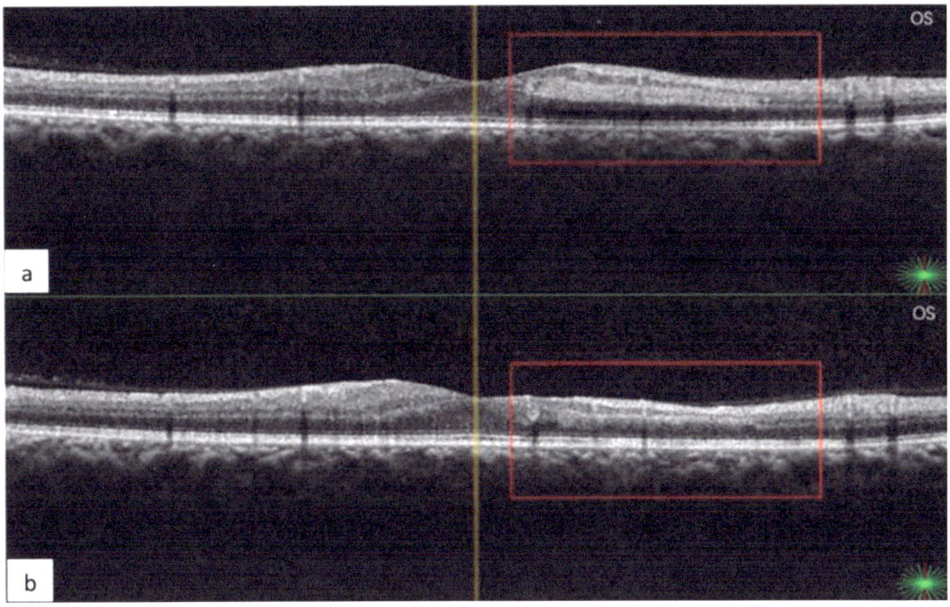

Fig. (10). SD-OCT scans of a BRAO patient before and after hyperbaric oxygen therapy. (**a**) OCT scan of the left eye with hyperreflectivity and thickening of the inner plexiform and inner nuclear layers before hyperbaric oxygen treatment. There is also a decrease in optical reflectivity in the outer retina (**b**) After hyperbaric oxygen treatment, the inner retina thinned out and optical reflectivity in the outer retina returned. Image unchanged from Feng, X *et al.,BMC Ophthalmology* volume 20, Article number: 281 (2020) [52] and is used under the Creative Commons Attribution 4.0 International License (https://creativecommons.org /licenses/by/4.0/).

Embolysis using a neodymium-doped yttrium aluminum garnet (Nd: YAG) laser has recently shown that it can restore blood flow and improve visual outcomes after BRAO. The use of Nd: YAG laser therapy has shown dramatic improvements in visual acuity and has been suggested as an effective treatment in BRAO patients with visible emboli [59]. However, there is the potential for complications such as vitreous and subretinal hemorrhage [60, 61].

Neovascularization is a rare complication of BRAO; however, it can cause sight-threatening edema through increased vascular permeability and leakage from new blood vessels. Neovascularization, as in the case with other retinal vascular disorders, can be effectively treated with anti-VEGF therapy and PRP. Neovascular glaucoma is another potential complication of retinal artery occlusions and the formation of new blood vessels in the anterior segment, so frequent follow-up for early detection of new blood vessel formation is vital for the potential treatment with anti-VEGFs and PRP.

Fibrinolysis using tissue plasminogen activators such as alteplase have been used to treat both CRAO and BRAO. Alteplase catalyses plasminogen to proteolytic plasmin which lyses fibrin and fibrinogen and disrupts fibrin-based emboli. It is currently FDA-approved to treat acute ischemic stroke. One study evaluated intravenous tPA for the treatment of CRAO/BRAO within 4.5hrs versus natural history. They found that visual outcomes were improved in CRAO/BRAO patients when treated with intravenous tPA compared to medical management after 90 days [62].

CONCLUDING REMARKS

In conclusion, CRAO and BRAO are critical conditions that demand urgent medical attention to prevent irreversible vision loss. The advent of OCT-A has revolutionized our understanding of these occlusions by providing detailed visualization of the retinal vasculature and ischemic changes that will potentially supersede FFA as the standard of care.

OCT-A is a valuable tool in clinical ophthalmology that allows for rapid and high-resolution imaging to diagnose, stage, and treat retinal artery occlusions. It generates more detailed vascular information at separate retinal layers than FFA, while it is also a non-invasive approach that can be used to track the progression of retinal vascular disease without intravenous dyes. Few treatment options exist for both CRAO and BRAO, however, OCT-A is recommended for the monitoring of retinal ischemia and edema over the clinical course. OCT-A imaging provides valuable insights into the extent of retinal ischemia and helps guide treatment decisions after retinal artery occlusion. Prompt intervention, aimed at restoring retinal perfusion and managing underlying risk factors, is crucial for maximizing visual recovery. With advances in diagnostic techniques like OCT-A, ophthalmologists have better tools to assess and manage retinal artery occlusions, ultimately improving patient outcomes.

The cardiovascular risk factors and link to acute ischemic stroke mean that retinal artery occlusions require prompt reference to an emergency department or stroke center. The visual prognosis of BRAO patients is generally good, with up to 74% of permanent BRAO patients presenting with a visual acuity of 20/40 or better, and 89% of BRAO patients having a visual acuity of 20/40 or better at follow-up. However, vision loss is severe in CRAO cases and initial presentation of visual acuity is often 20/400 or worse. The treatment of CRAO has a window of between 4 – 6 hours after onset to increase its effectiveness, due to the ischemic damage caused to retinal cells being irreversible.

Treatment options for CRAO and BRAO are not standardized, and they require further clinical trials to evaluate their efficacy in patients with retinal artery occlusions. OCT-A imaging provides detailed observation of the retinal microvasculature, at different retinal depths, to effectively track the progress of therapies to CRAO and BRAO. There is no effective treatment for all CRAO patients, but treatment approaches focus on restoring retinal perfusion and preventing further ischemic damage. Intra-arterial thrombolysis, ocular massage, hyperbaric oxygen therapy, antiplatelet therapy, and management of underlying risk factors are among the treatment options available. However, it is important to note that the success of these interventions depends on various factors, including the duration of occlusion, the extent of ischemic damage, and individual patient characteristics.

Immediate corticosteroids are recommended for arteritic CRAO as they target the inflammation of arteries caused by GCA. The standard of care for BRAO patients currently includes lowering of IOP with brimonidine and using OCT to monitor for subsequent retinal ischemia and edema. Neovascularization of the posterior and anterior segments is a potentially significant complication of retinal artery occlusions that can lead to neovascular glaucoma and macular edema, which can be treated with anti-VEGF therapeutics and PRP.

With the comprehensive assessment facilitated by OCT-A, ophthalmologists can make informed decisions regarding the most suitable treatment approach for each patient. Early intervention is critical to maximize visual recovery and prevent recurrent occlusions. Moreover, OCT-A provides a valuable tool for monitoring the response to treatment and assessing the long-term prognosis. The main findings in OCT-A of CRAO and BRAO are hyperreflectivity and increased thickness of the inner retina in the acute phase, which are subsequently decreased in the chronic stages of retinal artery occlusion. Shadowing of the outer retina by edema and increased optical density in the inner retina can cause decreased optical reflectivity that is often restored after the acute phase. Merging of the inner plexiform layer and inner nuclear layer in OCT images may point to tissue atrophy and the damage of these retinal layers following retinal artery occlusion. Importantly, OCT can be used to image the reorganization of the microvasculature at different vascular layers in the retina at high resolution. Further characterization and quantification of the SCP and DCP retinal vascular layers are needed to help define the microvasculature changes that occur with BRAO and CRAO before and after treatment.

As OCT imaging research and technology continue to advance, further refinement of OCT-A imaging and treatment strategies for retinal artery occlusions can be expected. The integration of OCT-A with other diagnostic modalities and therapeutic interventions holds the potential to enhance outcomes and improve the quality of life for patients affected by branch and central retinal artery occlusion.

In summary, OCT-A findings have revolutionized our understanding and management of branch and central retinal artery occlusion. Through its ability to visualize retinal vasculature and identify ischemic changes, OCT-A guides treatment decisions, predicts visual outcomes, and provides a foundation for ongoing research and innovation in this field. By combining early intervention with the power of OCT-A, ophthalmologists can strive to preserve and restore vision in patients affected by retinal artery occlusions.

LIST OF ABBREVIATIONS

BRAO	Branch Retinal Artery Occlusion
CRAO	Central Retinal Artery Occlusion
DCP	Deep Capillary Plexus
EAGLE	European Assessment Group for Lysis in the Eye
FAZ	Foveal Avascular Zone
FFA	Fundus Fluorescein Angiography
GCA	Giant Cell Arteritis
ICP	Intermediate Capillary Plexus

IOP Intraocular Pressure

Nd:YAG Neodymium-doped Yttrium Aluminum Garnet

OCT Optical Coherence Tomography

PDGF Platelet-derived Growth Factor

PRP Panretinal Photocoagulation

SCP Superficial Capillary Plexus

tPA Tissue Plasminogen Activator

VEGF Vascular Endothelial Growth Factor

DISCLAIMER

All the scientific comments issued in this chapter are solely the responsibility of the authors and not of the institutions with which they are affiliated.

ACKNOWLEDGMENTS

We express our deep appreciation to the technical staff of the Retina Specialists Unit at Oftalmologia Integral ABC (Nonprofit medical and Surgical Organization) affiliated with the Postgraduate Division Studies at the National Autonomous University of Mexico.

REFERENCES

[1] Shahid H, Hossain P, Amoaku WM. The management of retinal vein occlusion: Is interventional ophthalmology the way forward? Br J Ophthalmol 2006; 90(5): 627-39. Available from: www.bjophthalmol.com
[http://dx.doi.org/10.1136/bjo.2005.068668] [PMID: 16622095]

[2] Spaide RF, Fujimoto JG, Waheed NK, Sadda SR, Staurenghi G. Optical coherence tomography angiography. Prog Retin Eye Res 2018; 64: 1-55.
[http://dx.doi.org/10.1016/j.preteyeres.2017.11.003] [PMID: 29229445]

[3] Hwang CK, Kolomeyer AM, Brucker AJ. Optical coherence tomography angiography of a central retinal artery occlusion before and after anterior chamber paracentesis. Ophthalmology 2017; 124(5): 608.
[http://dx.doi.org/10.1016/j.ophtha.2016.10.030] [PMID: 28433123]

[4] de Carlo TE, Romano A, Waheed NK, Duker JS. A review of optical coherence tomography angiography (OCTA). Int J Retina Vitreous 2015; 1(1): 5. Available from: https://journal retinavitreous.biomedcentral.com/articles/10.1186/s40942-015-0005-8
[http://dx.doi.org/10.1186/s40942-015-0005-8] [PMID: 27847598]

[5] Hayreh SS, Zimmerman MB. Central retinal artery occlusion: Visual outcome. Am J Ophthalmol 2005; 140(3): 376-91. Available from: https://pubmed.ncbi.nlm.nih.gov/16138997/
[http://dx.doi.org/10.1016/j.ajo.2005.03.038]

[6] Justice J Jr, Lehmann RP. Cilioretinal arteries. Arch Ophthalmol 1976; 94(8): 1355-8. Available from: https://pubmed.ncbi.nlm.nih.gov/949278/
[http://dx.doi.org/10.1001/archopht.1976.03910040227015] [PMID: 949278]

[7] Tobalem S, Schutz JS, Chronopoulos A. Central retinal artery occlusion: Rethinking retinal survival

time. BMC Ophthalmol 2018; 18(1): 101. Available from: https://bmcophthalmol.biomedcentral.com/articles/10.1186/s12886-018-0768-4
[http://dx.doi.org/10.1186/s12886-018-0768-4] [PMID: 29301512]

[8] Hayreh SS, Zimmerman MB, Kimura A, Sanon A. Central retinal artery occlusion. Exp Eye Res 2004; 78(3): 723-36. Available from: https://pubmed.ncbi.nlm.nih.gov/15106952/
[http://dx.doi.org/10.1016/S0014-4835(03)00214-8] [PMID: 15106952]

[9] Varma DD, Cugati S, Lee AW, Chen CS. A review of central retinal artery occlusion: Clinical presentation and management. Eye 2013; 27(6): 688-97.
[http://dx.doi.org/10.1038/eye.2013.25]

[10] Cugati S, Varma DD, Chen CS, Lee AW. Treatment options for central retinal artery occlusion. Curr Treat Options Neurol 2013; 15(1): 63-77.
[http://dx.doi.org/10.1007/s11940-012-0202-9]

[11] mac Grory B, Schrag M, Biousse V, Furie KL, Gerhard-Herman M, Lavin PJ. Management of central retinal artery occlusion: A scientific statement from the American heart association. Stroke 2021; 52: E282-94. Available from: https://www.ahajournals.org/doi/abs/10.1161/STR.0000000000000366

[12] Sawant K, Ghosh A, Gupta R, Patra S. Central Retinal Artery Occlusion 2021; 5(1): 69-70. Available from: https://www.ncbi.nlm.nih.gov/books/NBK470354/

[13] Arruga J, Sanders MD. Ophthalmologic findings in 70 patients with evidence of retinal embolism. Ophthalmology 1982; 89(12): 1336-47. Available from: https://pubmed.ncbi.nlm.nih.gov/7162779/
[http://dx.doi.org/10.1016/S0161-6420(82)34626-6] [PMID: 7162779]

[14] Mangat HS. Retinal artery occlusion. Surv Ophthalmol 1995; 40(2): 145-56. Available from: https://pubmed.ncbi.nlm.nih.gov/8533103/
[http://dx.doi.org/10.1016/S0039-6257(95)80004-2] [PMID: 8533103]

[15] Chodnicki KD, Pulido JS, Hodge DO, Klaas JP, Chen JJ. Stroke risk before and after central retinal artery occlusion in a us cohort. Mayo Clin Proc 2019; 94(2): 236-41. Available from:https://pubmed.ncbi.nlm.nih.gov/30711121/
[http://dx.doi.org/10.1016/j.mayocp.2018.10.018] [PMID: 30711121]

[16] Callizo J, Feltgen N, Pantenburg S, *et al.* Cardiovascular risk factors in central retinal artery occlusion. Ophthalmology 2015; 122(9): 1881-8. Available from: https://pubmed.ncbi.nlm.nih.gov/26231133/
[http://dx.doi.org/10.1016/j.ophtha.2015.05.044] [PMID: 26231133]

[17] Kapoor KM, Kapoor P, Heydenrych I, Bertossi D. Vision loss associated with hyaluronic acid fillers: A systematic review of literature. Aesthetic Plast Surg 2020; 44(3): 929-44. Available from: https://pubmed.ncbi.nlm.nih.gov/31822960/
[http://dx.doi.org/10.1007/s00266-019-01562-8] [PMID: 31822960]

[18] Giant Cell Arteritis - NORD (National Organization for Rare Disorders). Available from: https://rarediseases.org/rare-diseases/arteritis-giant-cell/ (cited 2022 Aug 23)

[19] Davies CG, May DJ. The role of temporal artery biopsies in giant cell arteritis. Ann R Coll Surg Engl 2011; 93(1): 4.
[http://dx.doi.org/10.1308/003588411X12851639107476]

[20] Leavitt JA, Larson TA, Hodge DO, Gullerud RE. The incidence of central retinal artery occlusion in Olmsted County, Minnesota. Am J Ophthalmol 2011; 152(5): 820-823.e2. Available from: https://pubmed.ncbi.nlm.nih.gov/21794842/
[http://dx.doi.org/10.1016/j.ajo.2011.05.005] [PMID: 21794842]

[21] Park SJ, Choi NK, Seo KH, Park KH, Woo SJ. Nationwide incidence of clinically diagnosed central retinal artery occlusion in Korea, 2008 to 2011. Ophthalmology 2014; 121(10): 1933-8. Available from: https://pubmed.ncbi.nlm.nih.gov/24913283/
[http://dx.doi.org/10.1016/j.ophtha.2014.04.029] [PMID: 24913283]

[22] Kido A, Tamura H, Ikeda HO, Miyake M, Hiragi S, Tsujikawa A. Nationwide incidence of central

retinal artery occlusion in Japan: an exploratory descriptive study using the National Database of Health Insurance Claims (2011–2015). BMJ Open 2020; 10(9): e041104. Available from: https://bmjopen.bmj.com/content/10/9/e041104
[http://dx.doi.org/10.1136/bmjopen-2020-041104] [PMID: 32973068]

[23] Rumelt S, Dorenboim Y, Rehany U. Aggressive systematic treatment for central retinal artery occlusion. Am J Ophthalmol 1999; 128(6): 733-8. Available from: https://pubmed.ncbi.nlm.nih.gov/10612510/
[http://dx.doi.org/10.1016/S0002-9394(99)00359-1] [PMID: 10612510]

[24] Schumacher M, Schmidt D, Jurklies B, *et al.* Central retinal artery occlusion: Local intra-arterial fibrinolysis versus conservative treatment, a multicenter randomized trial. Ophthalmology 2010; 117(7): 1367-1375.e1. Available from: https://pubmed.ncbi.nlm.nih.gov/20609991/
[http://dx.doi.org/10.1016/j.ophtha.2010.03.061] [PMID: 20609991]

[25] Brown GC, Magargal LE. Central retinal artery obstruction and visual acuity. Ophthalmology 1982; 89(1): 14-9. Available from: https://pubmed.ncbi.nlm.nih.gov/7070767/
[http://dx.doi.org/10.1016/S0161-6420(82)34853-8] [PMID: 7070767]

[26] Hayreh SS. Ocular vascular occlusive disorders: Natural history of visual outcome. Prog Retin Eye Res 2014; 41(1): 1-25. Available from: https://pubmed.ncbi.nlm.nih.gov/24769221/
[http://dx.doi.org/10.1016/j.preteyeres.2014.04.001] [PMID: 24769221]

[27] Brown GC, Shields JA. Cilioretinal arteries and retinal arterial occlusion. Arch Ophthalmol 1979; 97(1): 84-92. Available from: https://pubmed.ncbi.nlm.nih.gov/758898/
[http://dx.doi.org/10.1001/archopht.1979.01020010024006] [PMID: 758898]

[28] Rudkin AK, Lee AW, Chen CS. Ocular neovascularization following central retinal artery occlusion: Prevalence and timing of onset. Eur J Ophthalmol 2010; 20(6): 1042-6. Available from: https://pubmed.ncbi.nlm.nih.gov/20544682/
[http://dx.doi.org/10.1177/112067211002000603] [PMID: 20544682]

[29] Falkenberry SM, Ip MS, Blodi BA, Gunther JB. Optical coherence tomography findings in central retinal artery occlusion. Ophthalmic Surg Lasers Imaging Retina 2006; 37(6): 502-5. Available from: https://pubmed.ncbi.nlm.nih.gov/17152548/
[http://dx.doi.org/10.3928/15428877-20061101-12] [PMID: 17152548]

[30] Yang S, Liu X, Li H, Xu J, Wang F. Optical coherence tomography angiography characteristics of acute retinal arterial occlusion. BMC Ophthalmol 2019; 19(1): 147. Available from: https://bmcophthalmol.biomedcentral.com/articles/10.1186/s12886-019-1152-8
[http://dx.doi.org/10.1186/s12886-019-1152-8] [PMID: 31291918]

[31] Bonini Filho MA, Adhi M, de Carlo TE, *et al.* Optical coherence tomography angiography in retinal artery occlusion. Retina 2015; 35(11): 2339-46. Available from: https://journals.lww.com/retinajournal/Fulltext/2015/11000/OPTICAL_COHERENCE_TOMOGRAPHY_ANGIOGRAPHY_IN.22.aspx
[http://dx.doi.org/10.1097/IAE.0000000000000850] [PMID: 26457398]

[32] Central retinal artery occlusion: Findings in optical coherence tomography and functional correlations. Available from: https://pubmed.ncbi.nlm.nih.gov/16820338/ (cited 2022 Aug 22)

[33] Shinoda K, Yamada K, Matsumoto CS, Kimoto K, Nakatsuka K. Changes in retinal thickness are correlated with alterations of electroretinogram in eyes with central retinal artery occlusion. Graefes Arch Clin Exp Ophthalmol 2008; 246: 949-54. Available from: https://link.springer.com/article/10.1007/s00417-008-0791-x
[http://dx.doi.org/10.1007/s00417-008-0791-x]

[34] Ahn SJ, Woo SJ, Park KH, Jung C, Hong JH, Han MK. Retinal and choroidal changes and visual outcome in central retinal artery occlusion: An optical coherence tomography study. Am J Ophthalmol 2015; 159(4): 667-676.e1. Available from: http://www.ajo.com/article/S0002939415000057/fulltext
[http://dx.doi.org/10.1016/j.ajo.2015.01.001] [PMID: 25579642]

[35] Chen H, Chen X, Qiu Z, Xiang D, Chen W, Shi F. Quantitative analysis of retinal layers' optical intensities on 3D optical coherence tomography for central retinal artery occlusion. ScientiRep 2015; 5(1): 1-6. Available from: https://www.nature.com/articles/srep09269 (cited 2022 Aug 22)

[36] Konno A, Ishibazawa A, Ro-Mase T, *et al.* Circumpapillary collateral vessel development in iatrogenic central retinal artery occlusion observed using OCT angiography. Am J Ophthalmol Case Rep 2020; 19: 100740.
[http://dx.doi.org/10.1016/j.ajoc.2020.100740] [PMID: 32490281]

[37] Flaxel CJ, Adelman MPH. Retinal and ophthalmic artery occlusions preferred practice pattern®. Ophthalmology 2019; 127(2): P259-87.
[http://dx.doi.org/10.1016/j.ophtha.2019.09.028]

[38] Fraser SG, Adams W. Interventions for acute non-arteritic central retinal artery occlusion. Cochrane Database Syst Rev 2009; 2009(1): CD001989.
[http://dx.doi.org/10.1002/14651858.CD001989.pub2]

[39] Atebara NH, Brown GC, Cater J. Efficacy of anterior chamber paracentesis and Carbogen in treating acute nonarteritic central retinal artery occlusion. Ophthalmology 1995; 102(12): 2029-35. Available from: https://pubmed.ncbi.nlm.nih.gov/9098313/
[http://dx.doi.org/10.1016/S0161-6420(95)30758-0] [PMID: 9098313]

[40] Duker JS, Brown GC. The efficacy of panretinal photocoagulation for neovascularization of the iris after central retinal artery obstruction. Ophthalmology 1989; 96(1): 92-5. Available from: https://pubmed.ncbi.nlm.nih.gov/2465523/
[http://dx.doi.org/10.1016/S0161-6420(89)32946-0] [PMID: 2465523]

[41] Schorr EM, Rossi KC, Stein LK, Park BL, Tuhrim S, Dhamoon MS. Characteristics and outcomes of retinal artery occlusion. Stroke 2020; 51(3): 800-7. Available from: https://pubmed.ncbi.nlm.nih.gov/31951154/
[http://dx.doi.org/10.1161/STROKEAHA.119.027034] [PMID: 31951154]

[42] Schrag M, Youn T, Schindler J, Kirshner H, Greer D. Intravenous fibrinolytic therapy in central retinal artery occlusion. JAMA Neurol 2015; 72(10): 1148-54. Available from: https://pubmed.ncbi.nlm.nih.gov/26258861/
[http://dx.doi.org/10.1001/jamaneurol.2015.1578] [PMID: 26258861]

[43] Hattenbach LO, Kuhli-Hattenbach C, Scharrer I, Baatz H. Intravenous thrombolysis with low-dose recombinant tissue plasminogen activator in central retinal artery occlusion. Am J Ophthalmol 2008; 146(5): 700-706.e1. Available from: https://pubmed.ncbi.nlm.nih.gov/18718570/
[http://dx.doi.org/10.1016/j.ajo.2008.06.016] [PMID: 18718570]

[44] Page PS, Khattar NK, White AC, *et al.* Intra-arterial thrombolysis for acute central retinal artery occlusion: A systematic review and meta-analysis. Front Neurol 2018; 9(FEB): 76. Available from: https://pubmed.ncbi.nlm.nih.gov/29527185/
[http://dx.doi.org/10.3389/fneur.2018.00076] [PMID: 29527185]

[45] Takata Y, Nitta Y, Miyakoshi A, Hayashi A. Retinal endovascular surgery with tissue plasminogen activator injection for central retinal artery occlusion. Case Rep Ophthalmol 2018; 9(2): 327-32. Available from: https://www.karger.com/Article/FullText/489696
[http://dx.doi.org/10.1159/000489696] [PMID: 30022948]

[46] Mason JO III, Shah AA, Vail RS, Nixon PA, Ready EL, Kimble JA. Branch retinal artery occlusion: Visual prognosis. Am J Ophthalmol 2008; 146(3): 455-7. Available from: https://pubmed.ncbi.nlm.nih.gov/18599018/
[http://dx.doi.org/10.1016/j.ajo.2008.05.009] [PMID: 18599018]

[47] Branch retinal-artery obstruction: A review of 201 eyes. Available from: https://pubmed.ncbi.nlm.nih.gov/2735694/ (cited 2022 Aug 22)

[48] Goldenberg-Cohen N, Dadon S, Avraham BCR, *et al.* Molecular and histological changes following

central retinal artery occlusion in a mouse model. Exp Eye Res 2008; 87(4): 327-33. Available from: https://pubmed.ncbi.nlm.nih.gov/18639547/
[http://dx.doi.org/10.1016/j.exer.2008.06.014] [PMID: 18639547]

[49] Shute C. A case report of branch retinal artery occlusion in a teenager due to hyperhomocysteinaemia; The interplay of genetic and nutritional defects 11 Medical and Health Sciences 1113 Ophthalmology and Optometry. BMC Ophthalmol 2018; 18(1): 1-6. Available from: https://bmcophthalmol.biomedcentral.com/articles/10.1186/s12886-018-0859-2
[PMID: 29301512]

[50] Stepanov A, Hejsek L, Jiraskova N, Feuermannova A, Rencova E, Rozsival P. Transient branch retinal artery occlusion in a 15-year-old girl and review of the literature. Biomed Pap Med Fac Univ Palacky Olomouc Czech Repub 2015; 159(3): 508-11. Available from: https://pubmed.ncbi.nlm.nih.gov/26160228/
[http://dx.doi.org/10.5507/bp.2015.031] [PMID: 26160228]

[51] Greco A, De Virgilio A, Gallo A, *et al.* Susac's syndrome : Pathogenesis, clinical variants and treatment approaches. Autoimmun Rev 2014; 13(8): 814-21. Available from: https://pubmed.ncbi.nlm.nih.gov/24727151/
[http://dx.doi.org/10.1016/j.autrev.2014.04.004] [PMID: 24727151]

[52] Feng X, Wang L, Wang H, Qi H, Zhang J, Wang Y. Branch retinal artery occlusion secondary to high-altitude exposure and diabetic retinopathy: A case report. BMC Ophthalmol 2020; 20(1): 281. Available from: https://bmcophthalmol.biomedcentral.com/articles/10.1186/s12886-020-01563-1
[http://dx.doi.org/10.1186/s12886-020-01563-1] [PMID: 32652960]

[53] Chang YS, Ho CH, Chu CC, Wang JJ, Tseng SH, Jan RL. Risk of retinal artery occlusion in patients with diabetes mellitus: A retrospective large-scale cohort study. PLoS One 2018; 13(8): e0201627. Available from: https://pubmed.ncbi.nlm.nih.gov/30091989/
[http://dx.doi.org/10.1371/journal.pone.0201627] [PMID: 30091989]

[54] Cugati S, Wang JJ, Rochtchina E, Mitchell P. Ten-year incidence of retinal emboli in an older population. Stroke 2006; 37(3): 908-10. Available from: https://www.ahajournals.org/doi/abs/10.1161/01.STR.0000204118.87477.46
[http://dx.doi.org/10.1161/01.STR.0000204118.87477.46] [PMID: 16439697]

[55] Schorr EM, Rossi KC, Stein LK, Park BL, Tuhrim S, Dhamoon MS. Characteristics and outcomes of retinal artery occlusion: Nationally representative data. Stroke 2020; 51(3): 800-7. Available from: https://www.ahajournals.org/doi/abs/10.1161/STROKEAHA.119.027034
[http://dx.doi.org/10.1161/STROKEAHA.119.027034] [PMID: 31951154]

[56] Baumal CR. Branch retinal artery occlusion.Atlas of Retinal OCT: Optical Coherence Tomography. Elsevier 2018; pp. 96-7.
[http://dx.doi.org/10.1016/B978-0-323-46121-4.00042-X]

[57] Ritter M, Sacu S, Deák GG, *et al. In vivo* identification of alteration of inner neurosensory layers in branch retinal artery occlusion. Br J Ophthalmol 2012; 96(2): 201-7. Available from: https://bjo.bmj.com/content/96/2/201
[http://dx.doi.org/10.1136/bjo.2010.198937] [PMID: 21515559]

[58] New treatment guidelines update retinal disease management. Available from: https://www.optometrytimes.com/view/new-treatment-guidelines-update-retinal-disease-management (cited 2022 Aug 22)

[59] Lim JY, Lee JY, Chung HW, Yoon YH, Kim JG. Treatment of branch retinal artery occlusion with transluminal Nd:YAg laser embolysis. Korean J Ophthalmol 2009; 23(4): 315.

[60] Mason JO III, Nixon PA, Albert MA Jr. Trans-luminal nd:YAG laser embolysis for branch retinal artery occlusion. Retina 2007; 27(5): 573-7. Available from: https://pubmed.ncbi.nlm.nih.gov/17558318/
[http://dx.doi.org/10.1097/IAE.0b013e3180546c4d] [PMID: 17558318]

[61] Opremcak M, Benner JD. Translumenal Nd:YAG laser embolysis for branch retinal artery occlusion. Retina 2002; 22(2): 213-6. Available from: https://pubmed.ncbi.nlm.nih.gov/11927856/ [http://dx.doi.org/10.1097/00006982-200204000-00013] [PMID: 11927856]

[62] Khrlobyan M, Burchette R, Modjtahedi B, Ali S, Le D, Ajani Z. Abstract P16: Alteplase within 4.5 hours *via* telemedicine and in-person for central or branch retinal artery occlusion vs medical management. Stroke 2021; 52(1): AP16.https://www.ahajournals.org/doi/abs/10.1161/str.52.suppl_1.P16

CHAPTER 10

Choroidal Neovascularization: Pathogenesis, Diagnosis, and Current Management Strategies

Sanjay Marasini[1] and **Miguel A. Quiroz-Reyes, MD**[2,*]

[1] *Department of Ophthalmology, The University of Auckland, Auckland, New Zealand*

[2] *Oftalmologia Integral ABC, Retina Department, Medical and Surgical Assistance Institution (Nonprofit Organization), Affiliated with the Postgraduate Studies Division, National Autonomous University of Mexico, Mexico City, Mexico*

Abstract: Choroidal neovascularization (CNV) is characterized by the growth of new blood vessels from the choroid to the subretinal pigment epithelium, subretinal space, or both. Newer diagnostic and treatment methods, such as, Optical Coherence Tomography Angiography and anti-vascular Endothelial Growth Factors, are becoming increasingly effective for CNV diagnosis and management, respectively. Anti-VEGF (Ranibizumab, Bevacizumab, and Aflibercept) treatment has become the first-line treatment for CNV and has replaced other methods, such as laser photocoagulation and photodynamic therapy. The current literature has established similar safety and efficacy of the three drugs (Ranibizumab, Bevacizumab, and Aflibercept) in the treatment of CNV, especially when the visual loss is mild. However, Aflibercept has been reported to result in slightly better long-term visual outcomes. Newer molecules such as Brolucizumab and Faricimab show the potential to decrease the treatment frequency and increase efficacy due to better penetration and by increasing drug concentration in the retina, addressing the limitations of the currently available drug options.

However, their investigation was in the early stages and may have taken some time before being seen in the clinic. Innovative methods for continuous drug delivery to the vitreous through the use of dedicated ocular implants filled with anti-VEGF drugs for controlled release (port delivery systems) have also shown promising results in clinical trials. The development of this technique is expected to reduce the total number of injections and maintain stable vision. Different clinical trial protocols across studies remain an issue in addressing research questions related to dosing frequency and gaps.

Keywords: Aflibercept, Anti-VEGF, Bevacizumab, Brolucizumab, Faricimab, Choroidal neovascularization (CNV), Myopic choroidal neovascularization, Age-related CNV, Idiopathic CNV, Inflammatory CNV.

* **Corresponding author Miguel A. Quiroz-Reyes, MD:** Oftalmologia Integral ABC, Retina Department, Medical and Surgical Assistance Institution (Nonprofit Organization), Affiliated with the Postgraduate Studies Division, National Autonomous University of Mexico, Mexico City, Mexico; Tel: +52 55 5217 2732; Fax: +52 55 1664 7180; E-mails: drquiroz@prodigy.net.mx and drquirozreyes7@gmail.com

Miguel A. Quiroz-Reyes and Virgilio Lima-Gomez (Eds.)

INTRODUCTION

Choroidal neovascularization (CNV) is characterized by the growth of new blood vessels from the choroid that extend into the subretinal pigment epithelium, subretinal space, or a combination of both (Fig. **1**). CNV is considered a nonspecific wound repair response to an underlying disease, the severity of which depends on the underlying condition [1]. The causes of CNV in people over 50 years of age are well characterized and include an array of retinal diseases, including age-related macular degeneration (AMD). However, this condition also occurs in young individuals. Cohen *et al.* (1996) [2] conducted a retrospective study to explore the relative incidence of various causes of CNV in people younger than 50 years of age (n = 363). They reported that CNV occurred mostly in myopic patients (62%), followed by pseudopresumed ocular histoplasmosis syndrome (12%), angioid streaks (5%), and various hereditary, traumatic, and inflammatory disorders (4%). The cause could not be identified in 17% of the cases. Visual prognosis of CNV is generally poor and may have a devastating effect on the quality of life of individuals. Yoshida *et al.* (2002) [3] studied the demographic and clinical data of patients with myopic CNV and followed them up for at least ten years after the onset of CNV. They explored the visual acuity readings during the ten years of the study period. They found that the long-term visual outcome of myopic CNV is extremely poor, dropping to 20/200 or less within 5–10 years after the onset of the disease. A good visual outcome is associated with younger age, smaller lesions, and earlier initiation of treatment.

TYPES OF CNV

Based on the proliferation pattern of new blood vessels in the retina, CNV is categorized as type 1 (subRPE), type 2 (subretinal), or type 3. In the Type 1 pattern, CNV grows between the RPE and Bruch's membrane. The vessels break through the Bruch's membrane and extend horizontally under the RPE in the natural cleavage between the basal laminar deposit and the Bruch's membrane, which has accumulated lipids (Fig. **2**). This growth pattern provides nutritional support to the RPE and outer retina [4]. Pfau *et al.* (2019) [5] evaluated the association between the presence of type 1 CNV and localized progression of atrophy in AMD. They found markedly reduced RPE atrophy progression in areas co-localized with quiescent and exudative type 1 CNV. The authors considered this to be a potential protective effect of type 1 CNV on the RPE and overlying neurosensory retina.

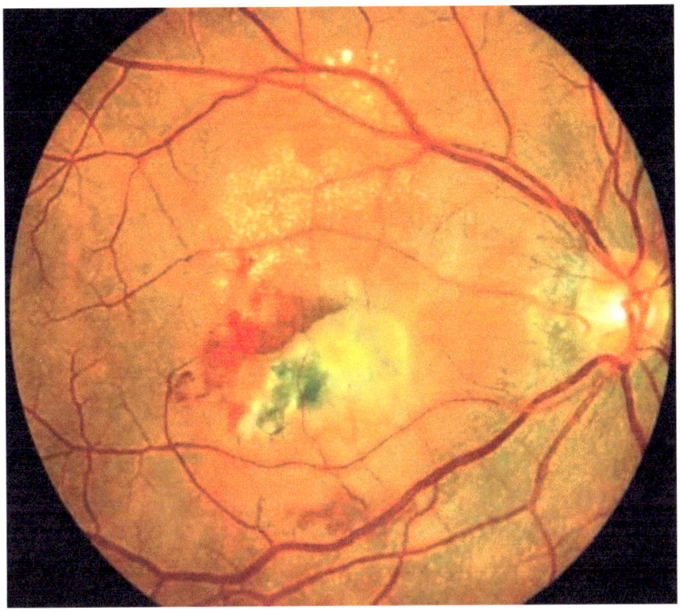

Fig. (1). CNV is characterized by the pathological growth of blood vessels involving the retinal pigment epithelium and Bruch's membrane and represents granulation tissue proliferation as seen in the wound-repair response. The growth of new vessels is known to be a final common pathway for several retinal conditions, such as AMD and idiopathic diseases.

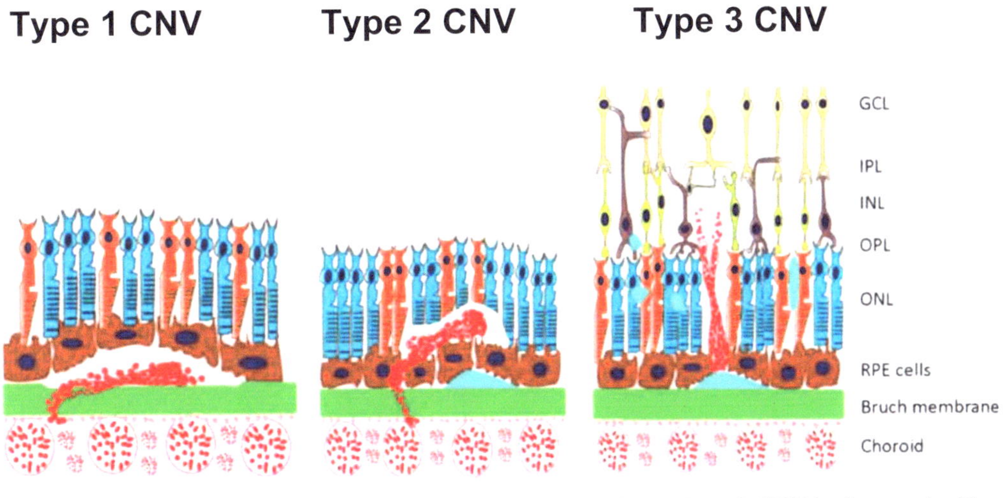

Fig. (2). Schematic diagram shows Type 1, Type 2, and Type 3 CNV. Type 1 CNV is characterized by an ingrowth of vessels originating from the choriocapillaris into the sub-RPE space; Type 2 CNV is the proliferation of new vessels arising from the choroid into the subretinal space; and Type 3 CNV is characterized by the downgrowth of vessels from the retinal vascular plexus toward the outer retina. Abbreviations: GCL, ganglion cell layer; IPL, inner plexiform layer; INL, inner nuclear layer; OPL, outer plexiform layer; ONL, outer nuclear layer; RPE, retinal pigment epithelium; MNV, macular neovascularization. The diagram was modified from the original publication by Qiang W *et al.* (2021) [7].

Type 2, or subretinal growth pattern, is most commonly observed in focal diseases and presents with single or few ingrowth sites. When there is a focal inflammatory response, a break in the Bruch membrane, and proliferation of granulation tissue, vascular leakage occurs under the RPE, which causes acute visual symptoms [6].

Type 3 CNV, also referred to as deep retinal vascular anomalous complexes (RVACs), was first reported in 1992 [8] and is characterized by unusual RPE detachments associated with retinal vessels that move down into the deep retina and form an angiomatous lesion (Fig. **2**). There have been several explanations for the origin of this disease (Fig. **3**), some suggesting an intraretinal origin [9], and others emphasizing the choroidal origin (occult chorioretinal anastomosis [10] of the intraretinal complex). However, there is now a consensus to call this type of disease a Type 3 pattern or retinal angiomatous proliferation (RAP) to emphasize the intraretinal location of the vascular complex and distinguish it from the other two well-known types of disease (Figs. **3 and 4**). However, it is important to note that growth patterns vary with diseases and individuals due to variations in individual compositions and anatomic differences of eyes, and no two CNV growth patterns appear alike [1].

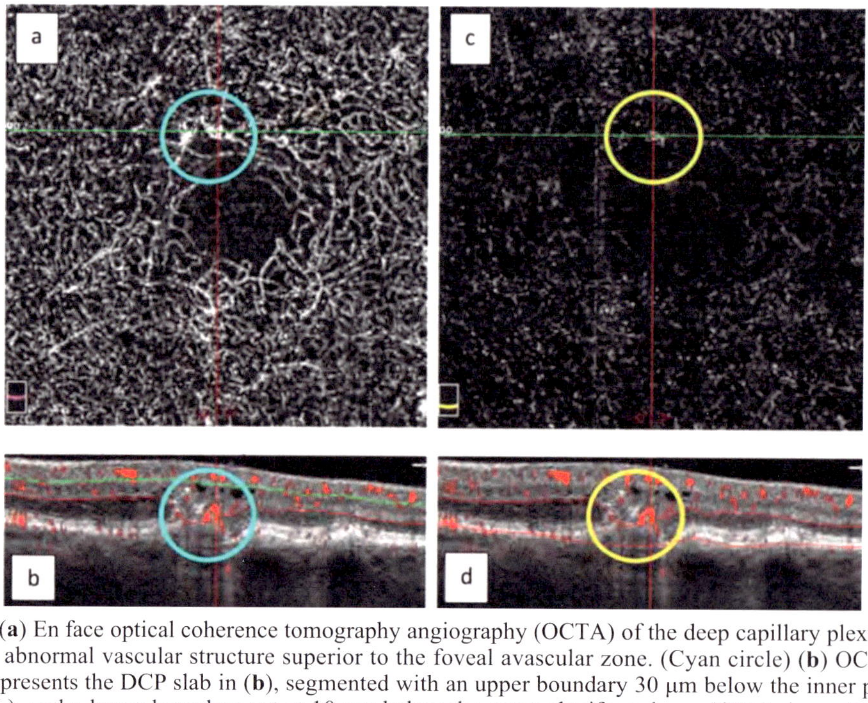

Fig. (3). (**a**) En face optical coherence tomography angiography (OCTA) of the deep capillary plexus (DCP) shows an abnormal vascular structure superior to the foveal avascular zone. (Cyan circle) (**b**) OCTA cross section represents the DCP slab in (**b**), segmented with an upper boundary 30 µm below the inner plexiform layer (IPL), and a lower boundary set at 10 µm below the outer plexiform layer (OPL) shows flow signal starting within the hyperreflective lesion arising from the DCP and traversing the outer nuclear layer (ONL) to reach the RPE. (Cyan circle) (**c**) En face OCTA of the outer avascular retina reveals a downward-growing extension of RAP from the overlying DCP. (Yellow circle) (**d**) OCTA cross section represents the outer slab in (**c**), segmented with an upper boundary set 10μm below the OPL and a lower boundary set at 10 μm above Bruch's membrane shows flow signal corresponding to the RAP lesion. (Yellow circle). This modified image from Fayed and Fawzi AA (2019) Projection resolved optical coherence tomography angiography to distinguish flow signal in retinal angiomatous proliferation from flow artifact. PloS ONE 14(5): e0217109. https://doi.org/10.1371/journal.pone.0217109 is used under the Creative Commons Attribution 4.0 International License (https://creativecommons.org/licenses/by/4.0/).

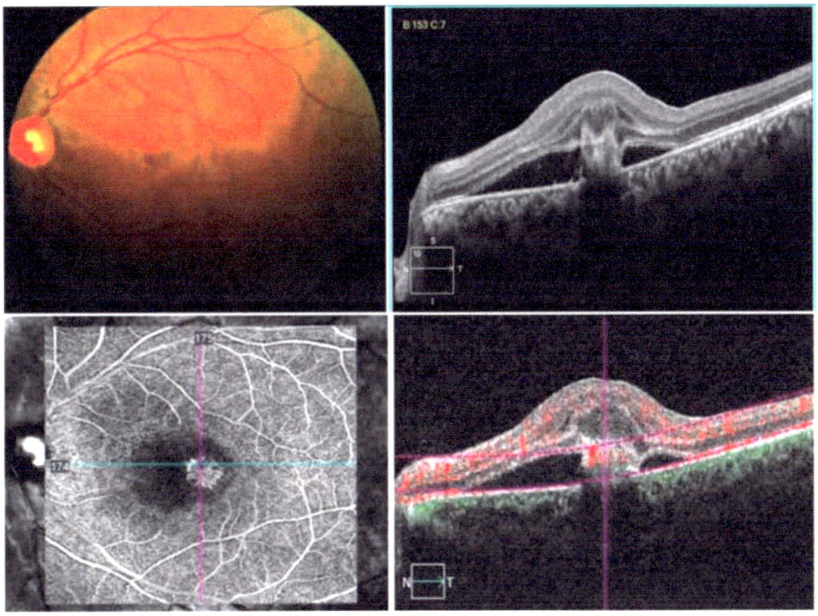

Fig. (4). Retinal angiomatous proliferation (RAP) is a distinct variant of neovascular age-related degeneration (AMD) that usually initiates at the retina and progresses posteriorly into sub-retinal space. In most recent study, it was suggested that angiogenesis may begin in the retina, choroid, or both, and introduced a new name for the process: Type 3 neovascularization. The frequency of RAP has been studied in many studies, with figures ranging from 10% to 21% of exudative AMD. Clinically, three stages were originally described as intraretinal neovascularization (IRN), subretinal neovascularization (SRN), choroidal neovascularization (CNV). RAP predominantly shows intraretinal hard exudates, and intra/pre retinal hemorrhages along with intraretinal edema, associated pigment epithelial detachment beneath it, at times retinochoroidal, retino-retinal anastomosis. Apart from conventional OCT, FFA and ICG, OCT-A has now been used primarily as a tool in the diagnosis RAP. Here we present imaging of a 30-year-old young male diagnosed as RAP stage 3 (Type 3 CNVM). Patient was started on intravitreal anti-VEGF monotherapy therapy. This image was originally published on the Retina Image Bank® website. Dhaivat Sha. Retina Image Bank. 2021; 74776. © The American Society of Retina Specialists.

CNV grows over time through the balanced activities of growth promoters and inhibitors, which is also known as the dynamic stage of angiogenesis. In the early stages, it is facilitated by the production of vascular endothelial growth factors (VEGFs) secreted by the RPE and retinal photoreceptors [11]. Macrophages migrate to the outer surface of the Bruch's membrane from the choriocapillaris and express tumor necrosis factor alpha (TNF-α), which subsequently stimulates the production of interleukin 8 (IL8) and monocyte colonization protein (MCP).

CNV then grows in size during the active inflammatory stage [12]. The vascular endothelium and macrophages produce matrix metalloproteinases (MMPs), which enable CNV to digest through the tissue planes.

PATHOPHYSIOLOGY OF CNV

The exact mechanisms underlying CNV are not fully understood. Several animal models have been developed to study CNV formation, which have helped study the pathogenesis and treatment outcomes. Despite translational limitations due to the differences in the anatomy of the animal and human retina, several pathological processes have been identified to be associated with CNV, for example, inflammatory processes [13]. However, there is consensus on the imbalance of anti-angiogenic factors in its causation, which promotes pathogenic vasculogenesis and angiogenesis. The risk factors that promote abnormal activities of pigment epithelium-derived factor (PEDF) and vascular endothelial growth factor (VEGF) have been identified, including hypoxia, high glucose, protein kinase C activation, reactive oxygen species, and abnormal cytokine production [14].

CNV pathogenesis can be classified into two groups: genetic and environmental. Recent literature supports the role of various genes related to angiogenesis and anti-angiogenesis in the causation of CNV, including VEGF [15] and FGF2 [16]. These genes have been shown to regulate CNV [17]. Other genes reported to be associated with CNV include CFI [18], RELA [19], NFKB1 [20], and RELB [19]. Cigarette smoking was the strongest environmental factor related to CNV.

Leukocytes have also been considered to play a role in AMD pathogenesis and CNV development. Sakurai *et al.* (2003) [22] investigated the role of the leukocyte adhesion molecule CD18 and intercellular adhesion molecule (ICAM)-1 in the development of CNV by inducing the disease in mice using laser photocoagulation through targeted homozygous disruption of the CD18 or ICAM-1 genes. The expression of these genes was assessed by immunostaining. They found upregulation of ICAM-1 and invasion by CD18-positive leukocytes within one day of laser injury. The authors concluded that leukocyte adhesion to the vascular endothelium plays a nonredundant role in the development of laser-induced CNV.

CNV can occur due to various ocular diseases such as AMD, high myopia, and idiopathic retinal diseases [23]. Early diagnosis and visualization of CNV are crucial for initiating and managing patients to prevent progressive and irreversible vision loss. CNV is currently diagnosed by fluorescein angiography (FA) and indocyanine green angiography using intravenous dye injection and optical coherence tomography angiography (OCTA). However, there is a large asymptomatic population with CNV, for which FFA is not considered an appropriate screening test owing to inherent potential risks related to dye injection (e.g., nausea and anaphylaxis in rare cases) [23]. OCTA has become an important non-invasive method for imaging patients with suspected CNV. In Type 1 CNV, OCT images may be used to visualize the branching CNV network below the RPE. de TE *et al.* (2015) [23] described OCT-A findings in CNV cases in an observational retrospective study. They categorized disease types based on appearance, CNV size, and the presence of subretinal fluid. They concluded that the specificity of CNV detection on OCT-A was higher than that on FA [23]. Longitudinal evaluation of subclinical CNV through OCT-A was reported by Heiferman *et al.* (2019) (Figs. **5-7**). They longitudinally evaluated OCT-A changes and their correlation with progression to exudation in AMD. They followed up 34 patients for up to 18 months and evaluated them prospectively using OCTA to detect subclinical CNV in their fellow eye. Five of the 34 fellow eyes were found to have baseline subclinical CNV, one of which was converted to exudative AMD during the follow-up period (Fig. **6**).

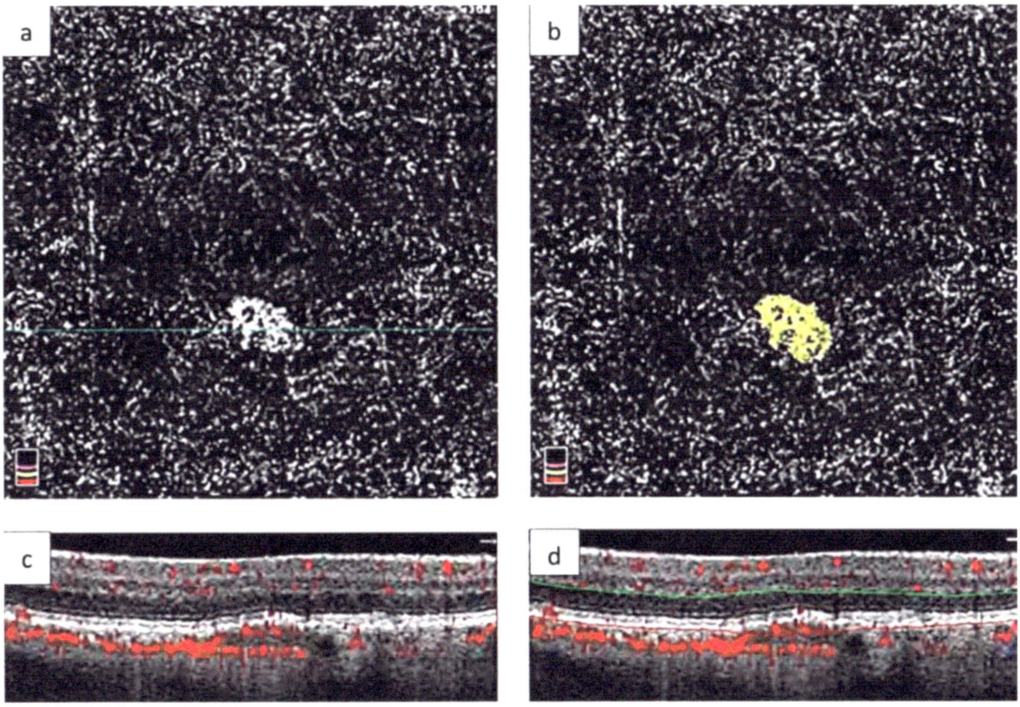

Fig. (5). (**a**) En face OCTA slab of subclinical CNV. (**b**) Flow area selection tool used in the AngioVue software. (**c**) OCTA B-scan with flow marked in red. The horizontal green line seen in Panel A marks the section of the OCTA B-scan image. (**d**) The same OCTA B-scan segmented 72 microns below (green line) the inner plexiform layer to Bruch's membrane (red line). Image courtesy of Dr. Michael J. Heiferman and Amani A. Fawzi [21].

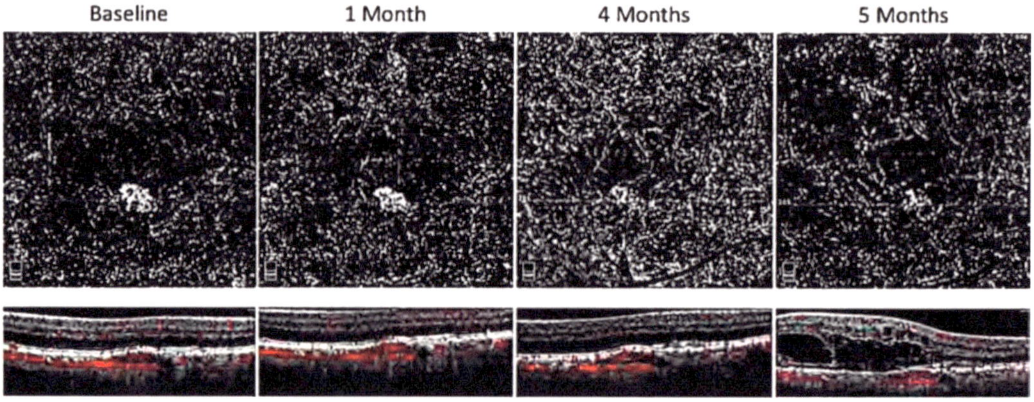

Fig. (6). Subclinical CNV can be detected with the use of OCTA. The figure shows a subclinical CNV that required anti-VEGF therapy due to the development of exudative AMD at five months of follow-up. Image courtesy of Dr. Michael J. Heiferman and Amani A. Fawzi [21].

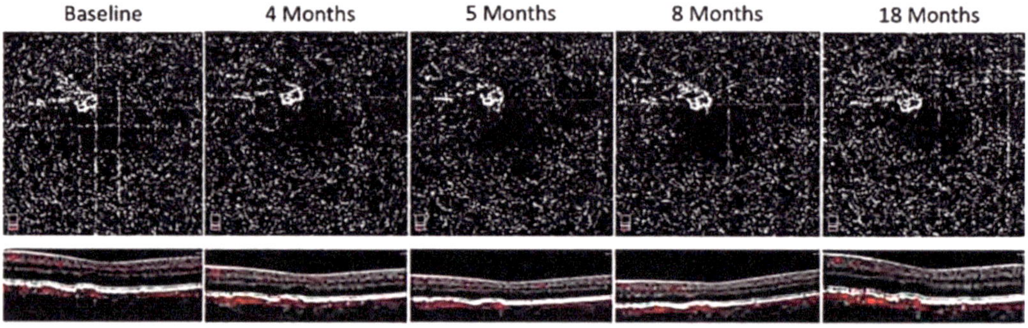

Fig. (7). Subclinical CNV that remained relatively stable in surface area and flow area during the 18-month follow-up monitored with OCTA. Image courtesy of Dr. Michael J. Heiferman and Amani A. Fawzi [21].

MYOPIC CNV

Pathological myopia (PM) is a common cause of visual impairment worldwide. PM is the most common cause of CNV in patients aged < 50 years. Pathological myopia is defined as the elongation of the globe with a refractive error of at least −6 diopters and/or an axial length greater than 26.5 mm and is associated with degenerative changes in the retina [24]. Excessive global elongation leads to mechanical stretching and thinning of the choroid and retinal pigment epithelial layers, causing various degenerative changes in the retina. These changes include posterior staphyloma, chorioretinal atrophy, retinal pigment epithelial atrophy, lacquer cracks with or without macular hemorrhage, and choroidal neovascularization. Lacquer cracks are formed by ruptures in Bruch's membrane and may predispose patients to rapid vision loss. Myopic CNV is the most dangerous complication of pathological myopia [24]. Additionally, it is estimated that 5.2%–11.3% of individuals with pathological myopia develop myopic CNV

[25]. More than 30% of patients develop CNV in the fellow eye within eight years [26]. Patients with myopic CNV generally present metamorphopsia, central or paracentral scotoma, and reduced visual acuity [27]. Patients may be asymptomatic if CNV is not central, and fundus findings vary by patient. Visual acuity depends on the location of the CNV.

Histopathological studies show that retinal degeneration is present in 11.4% of highly myopic eyes, which may coalesce and result in geographic atrophy over time. Generally, fundus examination shows a flat, small, grayish subretinal lesion near the fovea with or without macular hemorrhage (Fig. **8** (a)). The risk of developing myopic CNV increases with the severity of myopia and macular changes such as diffuse atrophy, lacquer cracks, and patchy atrophy. Leveziel *et al.* (2012) [28] investigated the potential loci related to CNV in high myopia. They assessed whether genetic factors associated with age-related macular degeneration (AMD) are related to myopic CNV. Their case-control study included myopic CNV patients and myopic controls without CNV. They also included single nucleotide polymorphisms (SNPs) from 15 genes that were reported to be related to AMD. The rs10033900 SNP located in CFI was associated with myopic CNV, and an SNP in APOE was also related to the disease. They found that the SNP (rs10033900) in the CFI gene, which encodes a protein involved in the inflammatory pathway, was significantly associated with myopic CNV.

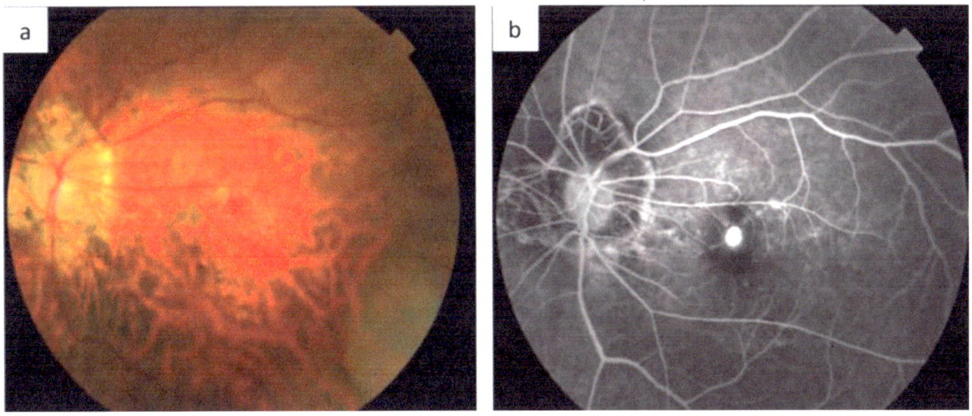

Fig. (8). A representative image of myopic CNV (**a**) and corresponding late-phase FA shows leakage due to CNV (**b**). The image was adapted from a previous publication by Timothy L and Cheung CMG (2016) [28]. Myopic CNV usually presents as a small, flat, grayish, subretinal membrane that is less than 1 disc in diameter and is located between the neurosensory retina and retinal pigment epithelium.

The clinical course of CNV in pathological myopia differs from that of CNV associated with other conditions such as AMD. Myopic CNV does not leak to the same extent as AMD but may be more pronounced in elderly patients. Therefore, these differences should be considered when managing patients with CNV caused by pathological myopia. Fundus fluorescence angiography is useful for detecting myopic CNV. On fluorescein angiography, myopic CNV may appear as a plaque-like elevation with a pigmented halo and sharply defined borders (Fig. **8** (b)). During the prearterial phase of FFA, more details of the choroidal vessels are visible owing to the thin RPE. Additionally, scleral staining was visible in the atrophic areas of the retina. Another essential tool in the assessment and management of myopic CNV is OCT. OCT showed a hyperreflective lesion with fuzzy borders at the RPE in cases of myopic CNV. Spectral-domain OCT may also reveal subretinal or intraretinal fluids.

It has been reported that using FA as the reference standard, FA and spectral-domain OCT findings agree in approximately 76% of eyes with subfoveal myopic CNV [29]. Miyata *et al.* (2016) [30] assessed whether OCTA could replace FA in detecting myopic CNV using validity and reliability analyses. They assessed whether OCTA and FA could detect CNVs in a group of 26 patients and 28 eyes. They concluded that OCTA could detect most myopic CNVs without requiring FFA, if high-quality images were available. More recently, Li *et al.* (2020) [31] evaluated OCTA findings in cases of myopic CNV and compared the data with FA results as the gold standard technique. They compared the anatomical features of CNV lesions (overall appearance, branching with tiny vessels, presence of anastomoses/loops, and dark choroidal halo) and concluded that a comprehensive diagnostic procedure combining CNV appearance, vascular branching, and anastomoses/loops using OCT-A might be a valuable strategy to evaluate neovascular activity in myopic CNV.

The management of myopic CNV has led to many discrepancies, as some authors believe that a favorable outcome can be achieved with observation alone, while others have described a poor prognosis [27]. These discrepancies are likely due to the loss of follow-up over the extended durations of the studies. However, the management of pathological myopia has come a long way over the last two decades. Laser photocoagulation has been the primary treatment; however, its use has decreased over the last decade. Patients treated with lasers show a high rate of recurrence.

Other complications, such as photothermal disruption of the RPE and Bruch's membrane and development of new lacquer cracks, retarded its application in myopic CNV. Photodynamic therapy with verteporfin increases the possibility of stabilizing or improving visual acuity in myopic CNV cases [32]. However, anti-vascular endothelial growth factor (VEGF) agents have emerged as a promising treatment for myopic CNV [25] because the visual outcome remains stable in the long term (Figs. **9** and **10**).

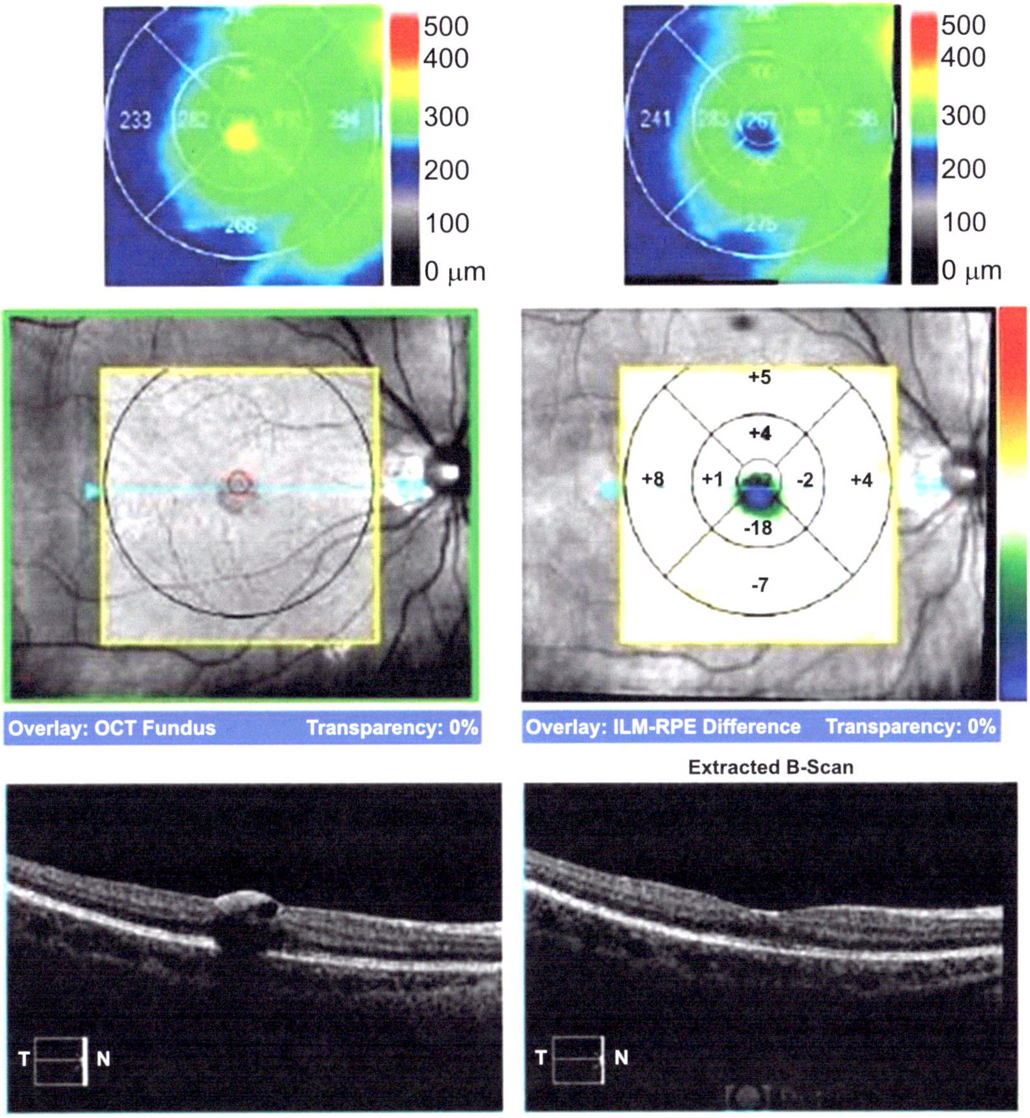

Fig. (9). Scanning laser ophthalmoscope images of myopic CNV treated with one episode of bevacizumab (Avastin) injection. The disease remained stable for nine months after the treatment. The image was adapted from the American Society of Retina Specialists.

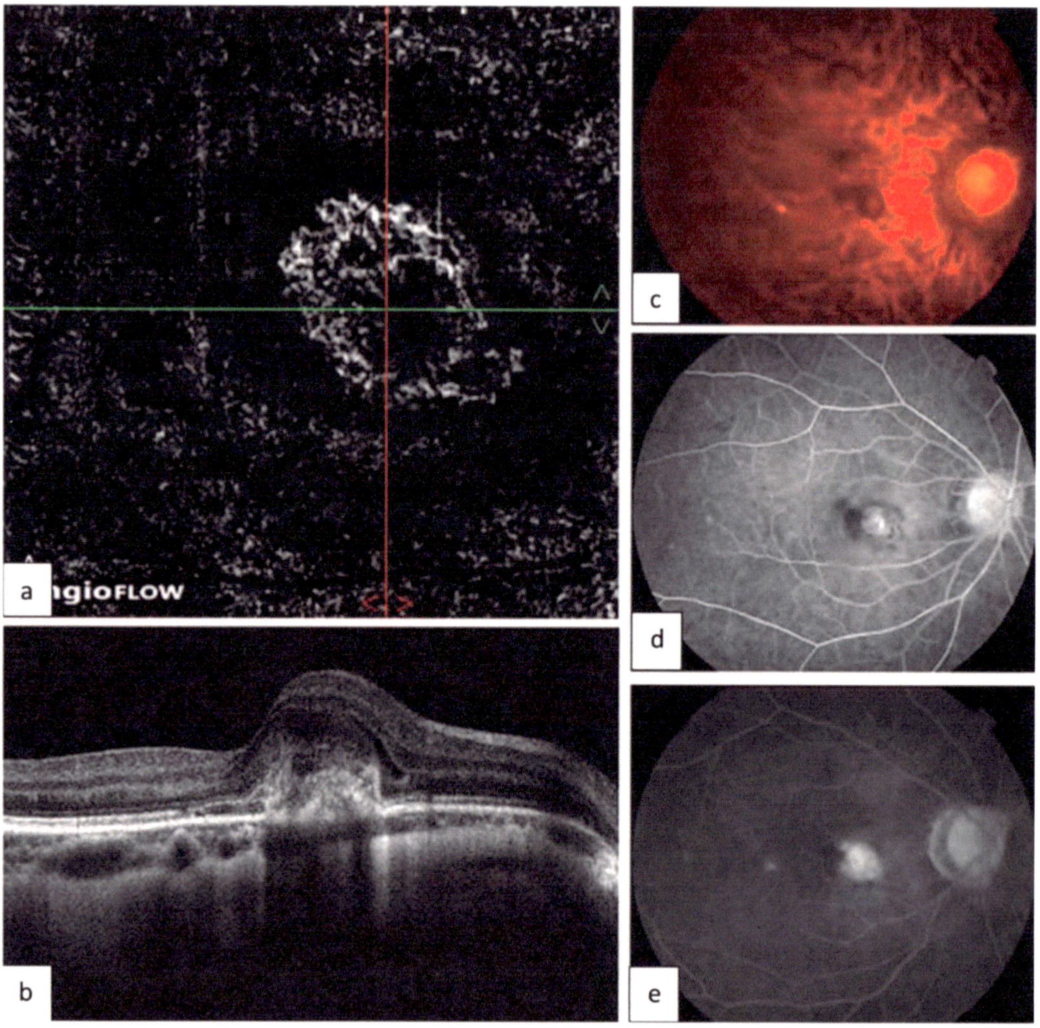

Fig. (10). CNV caused by pathological myopia. (**a**) Optical coherence tomography angiography (OCTA) of the right eye of a 52-year-old woman diagnosed with CNV caused by pathological myopia with an obvious neovascular lesion on the outer retinal layer. (**b**) Correlated OCT-B scan with intra- and subretinal hemorrhage and discontinuous retinal pigment epithelium. (**c**) Color photograph showing hemorrhage on the posterior of the ocular fundus. (**d**) Early phase of fluorescein fundus angiography shows the appearance of the hyperfluorescent lesion. (**e**) Late-phase FFA indicated persistent leakage from CNV with adjacent hemorrhage blocking the fluorescein. Image courtesy of Dr Bing Liu [33].

INFLAMMATORY CNV

After AMD and myopia, ocular inflammation is the next most frequently associated pathological condition with CNV. Inflammatory CNV can occur directly from an angiogenic stimulus mediated by local inflammation, degenerative disruption in the Bruch membrane, or both [34]. New fragile vessels progressively grow and leak, accumulating fluid in the subretinal space. CNV may occur in infectious and non-infectious uveitis, and its incidence depends on the underlying pathology.

The noninfectious causes of inflammatory CNV include choroiditis (multifocal choroiditis, punctate inner choroidopathy, acute multifocal placoid pigment epitheliopathy, etc.), stromal choroiditis (Vogt–Koyanagi–Harada syndrome and sympathetic ophthalmia), panuveitis (Behcet's disease, sarcoidosis, and multifocal choroiditis with panuveitis), and miscellaneous causes (idiopathic panuveitis and tubulointerstitial nephritis and uveitis). Similarly, infectious causes of inflammatory CNV include bacteria (*Mycobacterium tuberculosis*), protozoans (toxoplasmosis), viruses (West Nile virus and rubella retinopathy), fungi (*Candida albicans*, *Histoplasma capsulatum*, *Cryptococcus neoformans*, and *Aspergillus fumigatus*), helminths (Toxocara), and others (endophthalmitis) [35].

Wu *et al.* (2015) [36] described the demographic features and clinical and imaging characteristics of inflammatory choroidal neovascularization in a Chinese population in a retrospective case review. They observed that the proportion of patients with punctate inner choroidopathy, multifocal choroiditis, and Vogt–Koyanagi–Harada syndrome was 50.4%, 22.4%, and 8%, respectively. They also noted that inflammatory CNV tends to break through the retinal pigment epithelium and beneath the neurosensory retina.

Wijak *et al.* (2022) [37] investigated the utility of OCTA in the detection of inflammatory CNV and monitoring responses to treatment. OCTA and FFA were performed in a retrospective review of patients with uveitis associated with CNV and active exudation. They found that en face OCTA could detect CNV in 77% of patients. After CNV treatment, en face OCTA showed complete regression of CNV in 50% of eyes, partial regression in 20%, and no regression in 30%. They concluded that OCTA could be an effective tool for detailed visualization of the location, morphological structure, and flow of CNV (Figs. **11** and **12**).

Alfredo *et al.* (2007) [38] studied the effects of intravitreal bevacizumab injections as a primary treatment for inflammatory CNV. They reported that CNV resolved completely in 100% of the affected eyes. At the last examination, visual acuity improved in 88.8% of the patients, was stable in 11.2%, and worsened in 0%. They also reported that foveal thickness, as measured by OCT, decreased significantly ($P = 0.049$) after treatment. The authors concluded that intravitreal bevacizumab injection for inflammatory CNV was safe and associated with favorable visual outcomes for both subfoveal and juxtafoveal or extrafoveal inflammatory CNV.

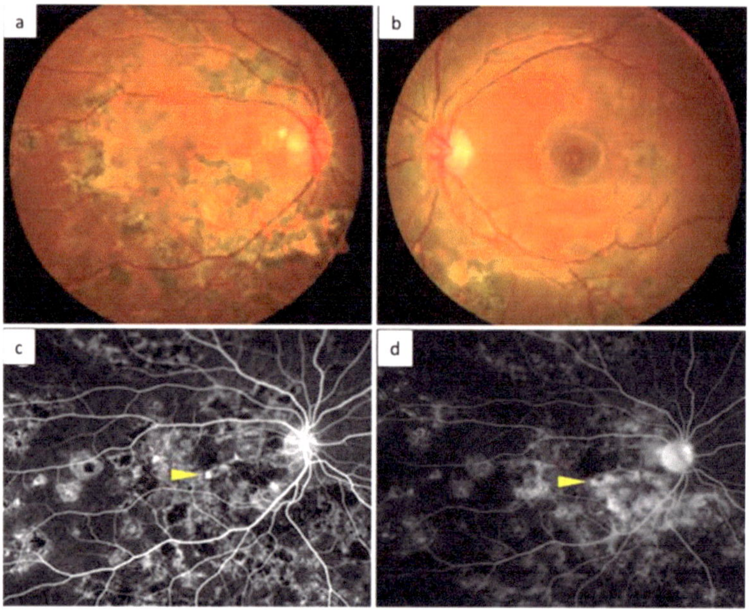

Fig. (11). (**a**) and (**b**) show healed choroiditis in the right and left eyes, respectively. (**c**) and (**d**), fluorescein angiography of the right eye shows an early hyperfluorescent lesion in the foveal region (yellow arrowhead), and the late-phase angiogram shows progressive hyperfluorescence of the foveal lesion, suggestive of CNV. The image was adapted from a publication by Agarwal *et al.* (2018) [35].

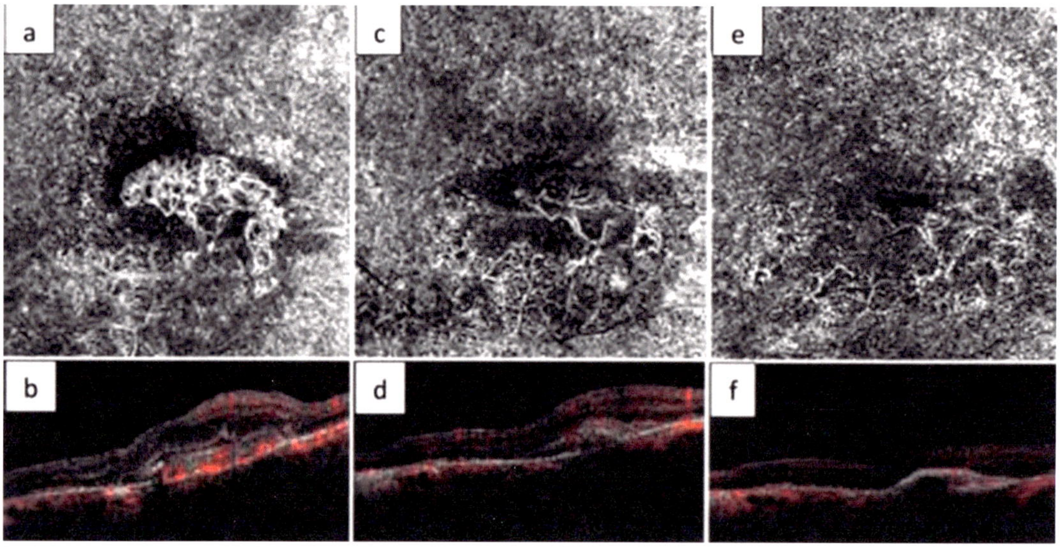

Fig. (12). OCTA images of a patient with serpiginous choroiditis and CNV. OCTA shows an en face view of the sea fan-shaped CNV in (**a**), and cross-sectional OCTA reveals neovascular flow (**b**). After anti-VEGF treatment, en face OCTA showed a reduced CNV lesion (**c**) and neovascular flow (**d**) reduction in seven days. After one month, en face OCTA showed complete regression of CNV (**e**) and no evidence of neovascular flow (**f**). The image was adapted from the publication by Wijak K *et al.* (2022) [37].

AGE-RELATED CNV

AMD is a leading cause of severe and irreversible vision loss among people aged 50 years or older in the developed world [39]. An estimated 6 million people worldwide suffer from AMD [40]. The late stages of AMD are characterized by macular CNV or atrophy of the photoreceptors, RPE, and choriocapillaris. Among AMD patients, CNV is a major cause of permanent vision loss. Neovascularization is characterized by the growth of abnormal choroidal blood vessels beneath the macula, resulting in the accumulation of serum and/or blood (Fig. **13**). Fluid accumulation causes the retinal surface to become irregular, which causes symptoms of metamorphopsia. This is often the earliest sign of AMD. With time, subretinal hemorrhage and subsequent scarring result in the death of the overlying photoreceptors, leading to permanent central scotoma. CNV associated with AMD show characteristic classic and occult fluorescein patterns. In the classic pattern, intensely bright fluorescence is seen in the early phases of the angiogram and leaks in the late phases, whereas in the occult pattern, leakage is less intense and appears in the late phases of the disease [39]. The pathological process of age-related CNV is not completely understood, but VEGF (a cytokine that promotes angiogenesis and vascular permeability) is considered to play an important role in promoting neovascularization [41].

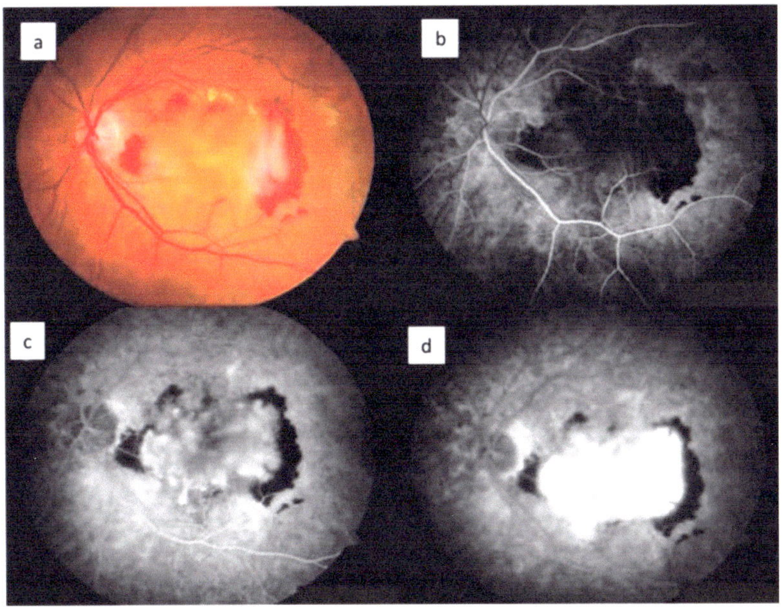

Fig. (13). (**a**) Classic CNV membrane in AMD on fluorescein angiography depicts early hyperfluorescence (**b**) and (**c**) with progressively increasing hyperfluorescence on successive images (**d**). The image was adopted from www.eyewiki.aao.org.

The FDA-approved treatment protocols for neovascular AMD include photodynamic therapy with verteporfin and intravitreal administration of pegaptanib sodium [42]. Brown *et al.* (2006) [39] compared ranibizumab, a recombinant, humanized, monoclonal antibody Fab that neutralizes all active forms of VEGF A, with photodynamic therapy with verteporfin for the treatment of predominantly classic neovascular age-related macular degeneration. The primary outcome was the proportion of patients who lost fewer than 15 letters from the baseline visual acuity at 12 months. They found that ranibizumab was superior to verteporfin as an intravitreal treatment for predominantly classic neovascular AMD, with low rates of serious ocular adverse events. Treatment improved the visual acuity by an average of one year. Rosenfild JP *et al.* (2006) [41] evaluated the treatment efficacy of ranibizumab, a recombinant humanized monoclonal antibody Fab, for neovascular age-related macular degeneration. In a randomized controlled study, they treated classic and occult CNV with intravitreal ranibizumab injections (either 0.3 mg or 0.5 mg) or sham injections for 24 months. The primary outcome measure was the proportion of patients who lost fewer than 15 letters from the baseline visual acuity at 12 months. They found that, over 24 months, the benefits of visual acuity were maintained after treatment. The authors concluded that intravitreal administration of ranibizumab for 2 years prevented vision loss and improved mean visual acuity, with low rates of serious adverse events, in patients with minimally classic or occult (with no classic lesions) CNV secondary to age-related macular degeneration.

A significant amount of research has been conducted on treatment protocols for age-related CNV. Clinical evidence suggests that ranibizumab initiation with three consecutive monthly injections is optimal, as it provides the greatest visual acuity gain. Mitchell *et al.* (2009) [43] evaluated the literature on the evidence available from prospective, multicenter studies (ANCHOR [39, 44], MARINA [41], PIER [45], SAILOR, SUSTAIN [46], and EXCITE [47]) investigating different ranibizumab treatment schedules to generate evidence-based and consensus recommendations for the treatment indication and assessment, retreatment, and monitoring of patients with neovascular AMD. They observed that ranibizumab was indicated for choroidal neovascular lesions with active disease, and the treatment was initiated with three consecutive monthly injections, followed by continued monthly injections, which provided the best visual acuity outcomes. The authors recommended continuous monitoring of patients for lesion activity if monthly injections were not feasible after initiation. This treatment protocol has been widely used worldwide. Although anti-VEGF treatment is safe and effective in delaying vision loss due to neovascular AMD, it cannot stop or halt the progression of atrophy in late-stage AMD.

IDIOPATHIC CNV

CNV in patients younger than 50 years typically appears to be associated with underlying ocular diseases such as pathological myopia or angioid streaks. However, CNV develops without any recognized ocular pathology in a distinct subset of young patients. CNV in these patients is referred to as idiopathic. Although the natural progression and visual prognosis in idiopathic CNV are more favorable than in other types of CNV, patients often suffer severe visual loss when treatment is not instituted [48]. It is estimated that 5–37% of untreated patients with idiopathic CNV may suffer from severe vision loss [49] if not treated appropriately. Liu *et al.* (2016) demonstrated that the use of OCTA could help monitor CNV changes in an idiopathic disease longitudinally (Fig. **14**) and help decide the treatment strategy [33].

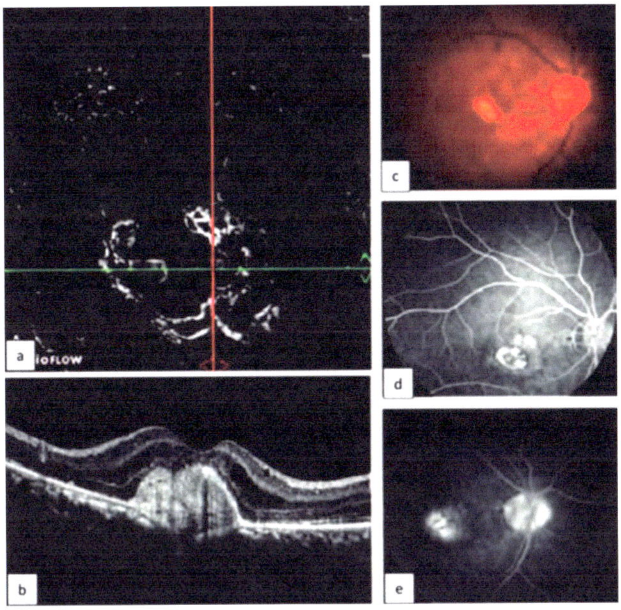

Fig. (14). Idiopathic CNV in a 47-year-old man. **A**; CNV as detected by OCTA. **B**; Stable hemorrhage and cystic macular edema on OCT-B scan. **C**; Color photograph shows the scar of the original lesion and spotted hemorrhage. **D**; Early phase of fluorescein fundus angiography shows hyperfluorescence with hemorrhage covering on the side. **E**; Late-phase of FFA demonstrating expansion or leakage. Image courtesy of Dr Bing Liu [33].

Ho *et al.* (1995) [48] studied the long-term natural history of idiopathic subfoveal CNV in young patients. In a long-term follow-up of 87 months, they observed that 95% of the patients had stable or significantly improved visual acuity, whereas only 5% had significant vision loss. Smaller lesions were associated with better visual acuity and larger lesions were associated with poor visual outcomes. Zhang *et al.* (2011) [50] evaluated the visual and anatomical outcomes of intravitreal bevacizumab in patients with subfoveal idiopathic CNV. In a prospective nonrandomized, interventional case series, they treated forty patients with a single intravitreal injection of 1.25 mg bevacizumab followed by as-needed dosing indicated by the presence and recurrence of intraretinal edema, subretinal fluid (SRF), or pigment epithelial detachment (PED) based on optical coherence tomography performed monthly. Patients were followed up for 12 months to investigate visual, clinical, angiographic, and anatomic changes. They found that intravitreal bevacizumab was well tolerated and improved visual acuity in these idiopathic CNV cases. Recent research suggests that subfoveal choroidal thickness is reduced and may be associated with the pathophysiology of idiopathic CNV, and intravitreal bevacizumab results in a significant visual and anatomical improvement in these patients [49].

Ruiz-Moreno *et al.* (2006) [51] evaluated photodynamic the efficacy of PDT in treating idiopathic and inflammatory CNV. They found that photodynamic therapy with verteporfin may be useful in stabilizing visual acuity in patients with subfoveal and juxtafoveal postinflammatory CNV and subfoveal idiopathic CNV. However, the current method involves treating macular neovascularization with anti-VEGF therapy to prevent or decrease exudation from the neovascular membranes into the surrounding retinal tissue.

TREATMENT OF CNV

Laser photocoagulation and photodynamic therapy with verteporfin are used to treat CNV; however, long-term visual outcomes tend to be similar between treated and untreated groups, showing no extended benefits of the treatments [52, 53]. Anti-VEGF agents have emerged as effective therapies for several ophthalmological diseases, including macular edema following retinal vein occlusion and diabetic macular edema. These treatments target vascular endothelial growth factor (VEGF), particularly VEGF-A, which is a key molecule involved in pathologically increased neoangiogenesis and vascular permeability. These methods have replaced photodynamic therapy and laser photocoagulation as the standard of care for treating those diseases [54].

Bevacizumab (avastin), a humanized murine monoclonal anti-VEGF-A antibody, was approved by the Food and Drug Administration (FDA) in 2004 for metastatic colorectal cancer as an intravenous chemotherapeutic agent. However, it is widely used as an intravitreal injection soon after treatment for numerous ocular indications [55]. Ranibizumab (Lucentis), a humanized murine anti-VEGF-A antibody fragment, was approved by the FDA in 2006 to treat neovascular AMD but has since been approved for other conditions, such as diabetic macular edema, diabetic retinopathy with or without diabetic macular edema, myopic CNV, and retinal vein occlusion [56]. Aflibercept (Eylea), a recombinant fusion protein of human VEGF receptors 1 and 2 binding regions to an immunoglobulin-G1 antibody Fc portion, was approved by the FDA in 2011. Aflibercept also binds and inhibits the activity of VEGF-B and placental growth factors, and has now been approved by the FDA for retinal vein occlusion, diabetic macular edema, and diabetic retinopathy with or without DME [56, 57].

Multiple studies have compared the efficacy of the three anti-VEGF treatments and reported them to be similar, mainly in patients with mild visual loss. Chan *et al.* (2007) [58] evaluated the safety and efficacy of IVB in treating idiopathic CNV and CNV secondary to central serous chorioretinopathy or punctate inner choroidopathy. They observed significant visual and anatomical improvements in the eyes after treatment. Wells *et al.* (2016) [59] compared the improvement in visual acuity after three anti-VEGF treatments in a randomized clinical trial. They observed that visual acuity outcomes were similar for eyes with better baseline VA in all three treatment groups. However, in patients with poor visual acuity at baseline, aflibercept had superior 2-year VA outcomes than bevacizumab. Wells *et al.* (2015) [60] evaluated the efficacy and safety of three treatments for diabetic macular edema in randomly assigned patients and assessed the mean change in visual acuity at one year. The drugs were administered every four weeks. They reported that the relative effect depended on baseline visual acuity, with better initial visual acuity showing no differences between the study groups. Heier JS *et al.* (2016) [61] recommended that when initiating therapy in patients with diabetic macular edema with worse visual acuity, aflibercept achieved greater visual acuity benefit than bevacizumab or ranibizumab one year later. Lim *et al.* (2015) [62] assessed whether conversion of the treatment of patients unresponsive to ranibizumab or bevacizumab to aflibercept would be beneficial in terms of mean central foveal thickness (CST) and visual acuity. They observed that eyes with DME unresponsive to multiple ranibizumab/bevacizumab injections showed better anatomical and visual improvements in conversion to aflibercept. Shah *et al.* (2016) [63] also reported improvements in CST and visual acuity after switching to aflibercept from bevacizumab or ranibizumab injections.

Although anti-VEGF treatment has shown encouraging results in halting the disease and improving vision, it may be associated with systemic adverse events and severe ocular complications. These risks may arise post-infection, such as endophthalmitis or drug class-associated adverse events. The incidence of endophthalmitis per patient has been reported to range from 0.019 to 1.6% [64]. Forooghian *et al.* (2017) [65] reported that the incidence rates of suspected endophthalmitis were 0.041%, 0.036%, and 0.06% for bevacizumab, ranibizumab, and aflibercept, respectively. For culture-positive cases, the incidence rates of bevacizumab, ranibizumab, and aflibercept were 0.017%, 0.02%, and 0.03%, respectively. Additionally, the rate of endophthalmitis did not differ when the three drugs were combined. The authors suggested that the combination of ranibizumab and aflibercept was safe in terms of the occurrence of endophthalmitis. Rayess *et al.* (2016) [66] reported that the incidence of endophthalmitis following intravitreal injections of bevacizumab, ranibizumab, and aflibercept was similar, and the visual outcomes were comparable. They suggested that treatment choice should be based on drug efficacy and patient response rather than the risk of infection.

Maloney *et al.* (2019) [67] reported that the risk of predefined systemic outcomes in patients receiving anti-VEGF therapy for retinal diseases was similar in acute myocardial infarction, acute cerebrovascular disease, major bleeding disorders, and all causes of hospitalization. They evaluated the incidence of these conditions in 87 844 patients who received anti-VEGF injections. Avery *et al.* (2017) [68] reported notable differences in systemic pharmacokinetics between the three anti-VEGF treatments. They evaluated the systemic pharmacokinetics of aflibercept, bevacizumab, and ranibizumab in patients with neovascular AMD, diabetic macular edema, and retinal vein occlusion. They treated patients ($n = 151$) with 3 monthly intravitreal injections of aflibercept 2.0 mg, bevacizumab 1.25 mg, or ranibizumab (0.5 mg for AMD/RVO, 0.3 mg for DME) and assessed the serum pharmacokinetics and plasma free-VEGF concentrations after the first and third injections. They observed that the serum concentration was highest for bevacizumab and lowest for ranibizumab, and that ranibizumab was cleared from the bloodstream more quickly than bevacizumab or aflibercept. Miao *et al.* (2012) [69] explored the relationship between the levels of inflammatory cytokines in the aqueous humor of patients with CNV with and without recent anti-VEGF therapy. They found that in the CNV groups, the aqueous levels of IL-6 and IL-8 were significantly associated with macular volume within 6 mm, whereas IL-1β, IL-10, IL-12p, and TNF-α showed no significant correlation with either the maximum macular thickness or macular volume. Additionally, they observed that in patients with exudative AMD, the level of IL-6 was significantly associated with the maximum macular thickness in patients with exudative AMD. They concluded that intraocular concentrations of IL-6 and IL-8 (particularly IL-6) were significantly associated with macular edema volume in patients with CNV. However, intravitreal injection of anti-vascular endothelial growth factor drugs did not change the intraocular levels of these inflammatory cytokines in their study cohort.

Brolucizumab, a newly developed anti-VEGF drug, is a small molecule that penetrates well into the eye and reaches high concentrations in the retina [70]. Recent evidence shows a superior reduction in retinal thickness and comparable visual acuity gains despite having the lowest injection frequency in cases of neovascular AMD [71]. More recently, faricimab has been investigated as a new drug that allows a more prolonged treatment regimen by targeting VEGF-A and the Ang-Tie/pathway. Owing to the potential of these new drugs to prolong treatment intervals, decrease treatment burden, and improve patient compliance, multiple clinical trials are underway. Innovative methods for continuous drug delivery to the vitreous humor through the use of dedicated ocular implants filled with anti-VEGF drugs for controlled release in therapeutic doses for over six months [72] have shown promising results in clinical trials (Phase 2) [73]. Ranibizumab is an ideal candidate for such a drug delivery system owing to its high stability and solubility. Multiple clinical trials are underway to test the safety and efficacy of port delivery systems, and patients have shown good tolerance to such methods. It is believed that developing this technique will reduce the total number of injections and maintain stable vision.

The treatment patterns of intravitreal anti-VEGF clinical trial protocols and routine clinical practice vary significantly. Most patients receive treatment every four weeks to three months, with the treatment protocol depending on the disease course and individual requirements. Therefore, the usability of data obtained from different clinical trials for robust decision making is very limited, and clinical practice often depends on the clinician's experience. The differences in treatment patterns are likely due to individual clinical outcomes, geographical variations, costs of care, and healthcare resource utilization. Nonetheless, the safety and efficacy of anti-VEGF treatment are well established with a low rate of ocular complications. Several attempts have been made to investigate new drugs to decrease treatment frequency and increase compliance, most of which are pending FDA approval.

CONCLUDING REMARKS

This chapter discusses the mechanisms underlying the development of different types of CNV, their diagnostic methods, and treatment options. In general, CNV is understood to be a wound repair response in the retina [1] and may be present in three basic types, type 1, type 2, and type 3, categorized based on the configuration of the angiogenesis pattern, which varies among individuals. Although multiple environmental conditions, such as smoking and other lifestyle factors, are strongly related to CNV, the genetic link has been a major research focus, with multiple genes identified in the pathogenesis related to angiogenesis and anti-angiogenesis, including VEGF [14]. FFA, the gold standard clinical method, is widely used to identify CNV cases. However, recent technologies such as OCTA have been shown to be beneficial for disease diagnosis without invasive procedures [21]. Moreover, computer-assisted diagnosis using multimodal deep learning has been found to be highly accurate for CNV diagnosis [74]. CNV may occur in pathological myopia, diabetic diseases, and retinal vascular diseases, the clinical presentation of which depends on disease severity. Disease management has changed significantly in the last two decades and has come a long way from laser photocoagulation and photodynamic therapy to anti-VEGF treatment. Anti-VEGF treatment has become the state-of-the-art treatment for these patients, although multiple ocular and systemic side effects are unavoidable. These treatments can help retain a good visual outcome in the long term and help maintain a good anatomic outcome; however, because of the difficulties related to the requirements for frequent applications (monthly to every three months), cost factors, and patient compliance, new drugs continue to be tested. Another issue with current drugs is the nonuniformity in dosing frequency, partly due to variations in clinical trial protocols. Newer treatment methods are under investigation, including liposomal sunitinib, as a potential treatment for CNV [75].

Further research is required to address this gap in the development of a universal protocol and identify the most effective drug for different pathologies. The current literature does not have much information on the ranking of commercially available drugs in terms of their safety and efficacy in treating CNV. Properly designed randomized controlled trials for a direct comparison of the available drugs for their safety, efficacy, and dosing frequency would help develop a general protocol applicable to all types of CNV.

LIST OF ABBREVIATIONS

AMD	Age-related macular degeneration
CNV	Choroidal neovascularization
FAZ	Foveal avascular zone
GA	Geographic atrophy
NV	Neovascularization
OCT	Optical coherence tomography
OCT-A	Optical coherence tomography angiography
VEGF	Vascular endothelial growth factor.

DISCLAIMER

All scientific comments issued in this chapter are solely the responsibility of the authors and not of the institutions with which they are affiliated.

ACKNOWLEDGMENTS

We express our deep appreciation to the technical staff of the Retina Specialists Unit at Oftalmologia Integral ABC (Nonprofit Medical and Surgical Organization) affiliated with the Postgraduate Division of Studies at the National Autonomous University of Mexico.

REFERENCES

[1] Grossniklaus HE, Green WR. Choroidal neovascularization. Am J Ophthalmol 2004; 137(3): 496-503. [http://dx.doi.org/10.1016/j.ajo.2003.09.042] [PMID: 15013874]

[2] Cohen SY, Laroche A, Leguen Y, Soubrane G, Coscas GJ. Etiology of choroidal neovascularization in young patients. Ophthalmology 1996; 103(8): 1241-4. [http://dx.doi.org/10.1016/S0161-6420(96)30515-0] [PMID: 8764794]

[3] Yoshida T, Ohno-Matsui K, Yasuzumi K, *et al.* Myopic choroidal neovascularization. Ophthalmology 2003; 110(7): 1297-305. [http://dx.doi.org/10.1016/S0161-6420(03)00461-5] [PMID: 12867382]

[4] Green WR, Enger C. Age-related macular degeneration histopathologic studies. The 1992 Lorenz E. Zimmerman Lecture. Ophthalmology 1993; 100(10): 1519-35. [http://dx.doi.org/10.1016/S0161-6420(93)31466-1] [PMID: 7692366]

[5] Pfau M, Möller PT, Künzel SH, *et al.* Type 1 choroidal neovascularization is associated with reduced localized progression of atrophy in age-related macular degeneration. Ophthalmol Retina 2020; 4(3): 238-48. [http://dx.doi.org/10.1016/j.oret.2019.09.016] [PMID: 31753808]

[6] Lafaut BA, Bartz-Schmidt KU, Vanden Broecke C, Aisenbrey S, De Laey JJ, Heimann K. Clinicopathological correlation in exudative age related macular degeneration: Histological differentiation between classic and occult choroidal neovascularisation. Br J Ophthalmol 2000; 84(3): 239-43. [http://dx.doi.org/10.1136/bjo.84.3.239] [PMID: 10684831]

[7] Qiang W, Wei R, Chen Y, Chen D. Clinical pathological features and current animal models of type 3 macular neovascularization (MNV3). Front Neurosci 2021; 15: 734860. [http://dx.doi.org/10.3389/fnins.2021.734860] [PMID: 34512255]

[8] Hartnett ME, Weiter JJ, Garsd A, Jalkh AE. Classification of retinal pigment epithelial detachments associated with drusen. Graefes Arch Clin Exp Ophthalmol 1992; 230(1): 11-9. [http://dx.doi.org/10.1007/BF00166756] [PMID: 1547961]

[9] Yannuzzi LA, Negrão S, Iida T, *et al.* Retinal angiomatous proliferation in age–related macular degeneration. 2001. Retina 2012; 32 (1): 416-34. [http://dx.doi.org/10.1097/IAE.0b013e31823f9b3b] [PMID: 22451953]

[10] Gass JDM, Agarwal A, Lavina AM, Tawansy KA. Focal inner retinal hemorrhages in patients with drusen: An early sign of occult choroidal neovascularization and chorioretinal anastomosis. Retina 2003; 23(6): 741-51. [http://dx.doi.org/10.1097/00006982-200312000-00001] [PMID: 14707822]

[11] Matsuoka M, Ogata N, Otsuji T, Nishimura T, Takahashi K, Matsumura M. Expression of pigment epithelium derived factor and vascular endothelial growth factor in choroidal neovascular membranes and polypoidal choroidal vasculopathy. Br J Ophthalmol 2004; 88(6): 809-15. [http://dx.doi.org/10.1136/bjo.2003.032466] [PMID: 15148217]

[12] Grossniklaus HE, Ling JX, Wallace TM, *et al.* Macrophage and retinal pigment epithelium expression of angiogenic cytokines in choroidal neovascularization. Mol Vis 2002; 8(8): 119-26.

[PMID: 11979237]

[13] Fabian-Jessing BK, Jakobsen TS, Jensen EG, *et al.* Animal models of choroidal neovascularization: A systematic review. Invest Ophthalmol Vis Sci 2022; 63(9): 11-1.
[http://dx.doi.org/10.1167/iovs.63.9.11] [PMID: 35943733]

[14] Sheng M. Identification of novel choroidal neovascularization-related genes using laplacian heat diffusion algorithm. Biomed Res Int 2021; 2021: 2295412.
[http://dx.doi.org/10.1155/2021/2295412]

[15] Zhang Y, Han Q, Ru Y, Bo Q, Wei R. Anti-VEGF treatment for myopic choroid neovascularization: From molecular characterization to update on clinical application. Drug Des Devel Ther 2015; 9: 3413-21.
[http://dx.doi.org/10.2147/DDDT.S87920] [PMID: 26170626]

[16] Kusari J, Padillo E, Zhou SX, *et al.* Effect of brimonidine on retinal and choroidal neovascularization in a mouse model of retinopathy of prematurity and laser-treated rats. Invest Ophthalmol Vis Sci 2011; 52(8): 5424-31.
[http://dx.doi.org/10.1167/iovs.10-6262] [PMID: 21482645]

[17] Nakai K, Rogers MS, Baba T, *et al.* Genetic loci that control the size of laser□induced choroidal neovascularization. FASEB J 2009; 23(7): 2235-43.
[http://dx.doi.org/10.1096/fj.08-124321] [PMID: 19237505]

[18] Fang K. Joint effect of CFH and ARMS2/HTRA1 polymorphisms on neovascular age-related macular degeneration in Chinese population. Jophthalmology 2015; 2015: 821918.

[19] Izumi-Nagai K, Nagai N, Ohgami K, *et al.* Macular pigment lutein is antiinflammatory in preventing choroidal neovascularization. Arterioscler Thromb Vasc Biol 2007; 27(12): 2555-62.
[http://dx.doi.org/10.1161/ATVBAHA.107.151431] [PMID: 17932319]

[20] Hirasawa M, Takubo K, Osada H, *et al.* Angiopoietin-like protein 2 is a multistep regulator of inflammatory neovascularization in a murine model of age-related macular degeneration. J Biol Chem 2016; 291(14): 7373-85.
[http://dx.doi.org/10.1074/jbc.M115.710186] [PMID: 26839315]

[21] Heiferman MJ, Fawzi AA. Progression of subclinical choroidal neovascularization in age-related macular degeneration. PLoS One 2019; 14(6): e0217805.
[http://dx.doi.org/10.1371/journal.pone.0217805] [PMID: 31163067]

[22] Sakurai E, Taguchi H, Anand A, *et al.* Targeted disruption of the CD18 or ICAM-1 gene inhibits choroidal neovascularization. Invest Ophthalmol Vis Sci 2003; 44(6): 2743-9.
[http://dx.doi.org/10.1167/iovs.02-1246] [PMID: 12766082]

[23] de Carlo TE, Bonini Filho MA, Chin AT, *et al.* Spectral-domain optical coherence tomography angiography of choroidal neovascularization. Ophthalmology 2015; 122(6): 1228-38.
[http://dx.doi.org/10.1016/j.ophtha.2015.01.029] [PMID: 25795476]

[24] Lai TYY, Cheung CMG. Myopic choroidal neovascularisation. Retina 2016; 36(9): 1614-21.
[http://dx.doi.org/10.1097/IAE.0000000000001227] [PMID: 27482641]

[25] Chan NSW, Teo K, Cheung CMG. Epidemiology and diagnosis of myopic choroidal neovascularization in Asia. Eye Contact Lens 2016; 42(1): 48-55.
[http://dx.doi.org/10.1097/ICL.0000000000000201] [PMID: 26448447]

[26] Ohno-Matsui K, Yoshida T, Futagami S, *et al.* Patchy atrophy and lacquer cracks predispose to the development of choroidal neovascularisation in pathological myopia. Br J Ophthalmol 2003; 87(5): 570-3.
[http://dx.doi.org/10.1136/bjo.87.5.570] [PMID: 12714395]

[27] Neelam K, Cheung CMG, Ohno-Matsui K, Lai TYY, Wong TY. Choroidal neovascularization in pathological myopia. Prog Retin Eye Res 2012; 31(5): 495-525.
[http://dx.doi.org/10.1016/j.preteyeres.2012.04.001] [PMID: 22569156]

[28] Leveziel N, Yu Y, Reynolds R, *et al.* Genetic factors for choroidal neovascularization associated with high myopia. Invest Ophthalmol Vis Sci 2012; 53(8): 5004-9. [http://dx.doi.org/10.1167/iovs.12-9538] [PMID: 22678500]

[29] Ng DSC, Lai TYY, Cheung CMG, Ohno-Matsui K. Anti-vascular endothelial growth factor therapy for myopic choroidal neovascularization. Asia Pac J Ophthalmol 2017; 6(6): 554-60. [PMID: 29057641]

[30] Miyata M, Ooto S, Hata M, *et al.* Detection of myopic choroidal neovascularization using optical coherence tomography angiography. Am J Ophthalmol 2016; 165: 108-14. [http://dx.doi.org/10.1016/j.ajo.2016.03.009] [PMID: 26973049]

[31] Li S, Sun L, Zhao X, *et al.* Assessing the activity of myopic choroidal neovascularization: Comparison between optical coherence tomography angiography and dye angiography. Retina 2020; 40(9): 1757-64. [http://dx.doi.org/10.1097/IAE.0000000000002650] [PMID: 31652198]

[32] Marticorena J, Gomez-Ulla F, Fernandez M, Pazos B, Rodriguez-Cid MJ, Sanchez-Salorio M. Combined photodynamic therapy and intravitreal triamcinolone acetonide for the treatment of myopic subfoveal choroidal neovascularization. Am J Ophthalmol 2006; 142(2): 335-7. [http://dx.doi.org/10.1016/j.ajo.2006.03.003] [PMID: 16876524]

[33] Liu B, Bao L, Zhang J. Optical coherence tomography angiography of pathological myopia sourced and idiopathic choroidal neovascularization with follow-up. Medicine 2016; 95(14): e3264. [http://dx.doi.org/10.1097/MD.0000000000003264] [PMID: 27057880]

[34] Dhingra N, Kelly S, Majid M, Bailey C, Dick A. Inflammatory choroidal neovascular membrane in posterior uveitis-pathogenesis and treatment. Indian J Ophthalmol 2010; 58(1): 3-10. [http://dx.doi.org/10.4103/0301-4738.58467] [PMID: 20029141]

[35] Agarwal A, Invernizzi A, Singh RB, *et al.* An update on inflammatory choroidal neovascularization: Epidemiology, multimodal imaging, and management. J Ophthalmic Inflamm Infect 2018; 8(1): 13. [http://dx.doi.org/10.1186/s12348-018-0155-6] [PMID: 30209691]

[36] Wu K, Zhang X, Su Y, *et al.* Clinical characteristics of inflammatory choroidal neovascularization in a Chinese population. Ocul Immunol Inflamm 2016; 24(3): 261-7. [PMID: 26171640]

[37] Kongwattananon W, Grasic D, Lin H, Oyeniran E, Sen HN, Kodati S. Role of optical coherence tomography angiography in detecting and monitroing inflammatory choroidal neovascularisation. Retina 2022; 42(6): 1047-56. [http://dx.doi.org/10.1097/IAE.0000000000003420] [PMID: 35067607]

[38] Adán A, Mateo C, Navarro R, Bitrian E, Casaroli-Marano RP. Intravitreal bevacizumab (avastin) injection as primary treatment of inflammatory choroidal neovascularization. Retina 2007; 27(9): 1180-6. [http://dx.doi.org/10.1097/IAE.0b013e31815e9834] [PMID: 18046222]

[39] Brown DM, Kaiser PK, Michels M, *et al.* Ranibizumab versus verteporfin for neovascular age-related macular degeneration. N Engl J Med 2006; 355(14): 1432-44. [http://dx.doi.org/10.1056/NEJMoa062655] [PMID: 17021319]

[40] Vos T, Allen C, Arora M, *et al.* Global, regional, and national incidence, prevalence, and years lived with disability for 310 diseases and injuries, 1990–2015: A systematic analysis for the Global Burden of Disease Study 2015. Lancet 2016; 388(10053): 1545-602. [http://dx.doi.org/10.1016/S0140-6736(16)31678-6] [PMID: 27733282]

[41] Rosenfeld PJ, Brown DM, Heier JS, *et al.* Ranibizumab for neovascular age-related macular degeneration. N Engl J Med 2006; 355(14): 1419-31. [http://dx.doi.org/10.1056/NEJMoa054481] [PMID: 17021318]

[42] Gragoudas ES, Adamis AP, Cunningham ET Jr, Feinsod M, Guyer DR. Pegaptanib for neovascular

age-related macular degeneration. N Engl J Med 2004; 351(27): 2805-16.
[http://dx.doi.org/10.1056/NEJMoa042760] [PMID: 15625332]

[43] Mitchell P, Korobelnik J-F, Lanzetta P, *et al.* Ranibizumab (Lucentis) in neovascular age-related macular degeneration: Evidence from clinical trials. Br J Ophthalmol 2010; 94(1): 2-13.
[http://dx.doi.org/10.1136/bjo.2009.159160] [PMID: 19443462]

[44] Brown DM. Ranibizumab versus verteporfin photodynamic therapy for neovascular age-related macular degeneration: Two-year results of the ANCHOR study. Ophthalmology 2009; 116(1): 57-65.e5.
[http://dx.doi.org/10.1016/j.ophtha.2008.10.018]

[45] Regillo CD. Randomized, double-masked, sham-controlled trial of ranibizumab for neovascular age-related macular degeneration: PIER Study year 1 Am J Ophthalmol 2008; 145(2): 239-48.
[http://dx.doi.org/10.1016/j.ajo.2007.10.004]

[46] Meyer C. Ranibizumab in patients with subfoveal choroidal neovascularization secondary to age-related macular degeneration. Interim results from the sustain trial. Invest Ophthalmol Vis Sci 2008; 49(13): 273-3.

[47] Bolz M, Schmidt-Erfurth U. *Ranibizumab EXCITE study: Exploring the value of optical coherence tomography for the management of ranibizumab therapy in age-related macular degeneration.* 8th EURETINA Congress.

[48] Ho AC, Yannuzzi LA, Pisicano K, DeRosa J. The natural history of idiopathic subfoveal choroidal neovascularization. Ophthalmology 1995; 102(5): 782-9.
[http://dx.doi.org/10.1016/S0161-6420(95)30968-2] [PMID: 7539905]

[49] Kim H, Lee K, Lee CS, Byeon SH, Lee SC. Subfoveal choroidal thickness in idiopathic choroidal neovascularization and treatment outcomes after intravitreal bevacizumab therapy. Retina 2015; 35(3): 481-6.
[http://dx.doi.org/10.1097/IAE.0000000000000354] [PMID: 25313710]

[50] Zhang H. Intravitreal bevacizumab for treatment of subfoveal idiopathic choroidal neovascularization: Results of a 1-year prospective trial. Am J ophthalm 2012; 153(2): 300-306. e1.

[51] Ruiz-Moreno JM, Montero JA, Arias L, *et al.* Photodynamic therapy in subfoveal and juxtafoveal idiopathic and postinflammatory choroidal neovascularization. Acta Ophthalmol Scand 2006; 84(6): 743-8.
[http://dx.doi.org/10.1111/j.1600-0420.2006.00691.x] [PMID: 17083531]

[52] Ruiz-Moreno JM, Montero JA. Long-term visual acuity after argon green laser photocoagulation of juxtafoveal choroidal neovascularization in highly myopic eyes. Eur J Ophthalmol 2002; 12(2): 117-22.
[http://dx.doi.org/10.1177/112067210201200207] [PMID: 12022283]

[53] Blinder KJ, Blumenkranz MS, Bressler NM, *et al.* Verteporfin therapy of subfoveal choroidal neovascularization in pathologic myopia. Ophthalmology 2003; 110(4): 667-73.
[http://dx.doi.org/10.1016/S0161-6420(02)01998-X] [PMID: 12689884]

[54] Stuart A, Ford JA, Duckworth S, Jones C, Pereira A. Anti-VEGF therapies in the treatment of choroidal neovascularisation secondary to non-age-related macular degeneration: A systematic review. BMJ Open 2015; 5(4): e007746.
[http://dx.doi.org/10.1136/bmjopen-2015-007746] [PMID: 25941188]

[55] Rosenfeld PJ, Moshfeghi AA, Puliafito CA. Optical coherence tomography findings after an intravitreal injection of bevacizumab (Avastin®) for neovascular age-related macular degeneration. NJ: Slack Incorporated Thorofare 2005; pp. 331-5.

[56] Maloney MH, Payne SR, Herrin J, Sangaralingham LR, Shah ND, Barkmeier AJ. Risk of systemic adverse events after intravitreal bevacizumab, ranibizumab, and aflibercept in routine clinical practice. Ophthalmology 2021; 128(3): 417-24.

[http://dx.doi.org/10.1016/j.ophtha.2020.07.062] [PMID: 32781110]

[57] Berkowitz ST, Sternberg P Jr, Feng X, Chen Q, Patel S. Analysis of anti–vascular endothelial growth factor injection claims data in US Medicare Part B beneficiaries from 2012 to 2015. JAMA Ophthalmol 2019; 137(8): 921-8.
[http://dx.doi.org/10.1001/jamaophthalmol.2019.1971] [PMID: 31219520]

[58] Chan W-M. Intravitreal bevacizumab (avastin) for choroidal neovascularization secondary to central serous chorioretinopathy, secondary to punctate inner choroidopathy, or of idiopathic origin. Am J ophthalm 2007; 143(6): 977-983. e1.

[59] Wells JA, Glassman AR, Ayala AR, *et al.* Aflibercept, bevacizumab, or ranibizumab for diabetic macular edema: Two-year results from a comparative effectiveness randomized clinical trial. Ophthalmology 2016; 123(6): 1351-9.
[http://dx.doi.org/10.1016/j.ophtha.2016.02.022] [PMID: 26935357]

[60] Wells JA, Glassman AR, Ayala AR, *et al.* Aflibercept, bevacizumab, or ranibizumab for diabetic macular edema. N Engl J Med 2015; 372(13): 1193-203.
[http://dx.doi.org/10.1056/NEJMoa1414264] [PMID: 25692915]

[61] Heier JS, Bressler NM, Avery RL, *et al.* Comparison of aflibercept, bevacizumab, and ranibizumab for treatment of diabetic macular edema: Extrapolation of data to clinical practice. JAMA Ophthalmol 2016; 134(1): 95-9.
[http://dx.doi.org/10.1001/jamaophthalmol.2015.4110] [PMID: 26512939]

[62] Lim L, Papakostas T, Kim L, *et al.* Conversion to aflibercept for diabetic macular edema unresponsive to ranibizumab or bevacizumab. Clin Ophthalmol 2015; 9: 1715-8.
[http://dx.doi.org/10.2147/OPTH.S81523] [PMID: 26396494]

[63] Shah CP, Heier JS. Aflibercept for diabetic macular edema in eyes previously treated with ranibizumab and/or bevacizumab may further improve macular thickness. Ophthal Surg Las Imag Ret 2016; 47(9): 836-9.
[http://dx.doi.org/10.3928/23258160-20160901-06] [PMID: 27631479]

[64] Mccannel CA. Meta-analysis of endophthalmitis after intravitreal injection of anti-vascular endothelial growth factor agents: causative organisms and possible prevention strategies. Retina 2011; 31(4): 654-61.
[http://dx.doi.org/10.1097/IAE.0b013e31820a67e4] [PMID: 21330939]

[65] Forooghian F, Albiani DA, Kirker AW, Merkur AB. Comparison of endophthalmitis rates following intravitreal injection of compounded bevacizumab, ranibizumab, and aflibercept. Can J Ophthalmol 2017; 52(6): 616-9.
[http://dx.doi.org/10.1016/j.jcjo.2017.04.016] [PMID: 29217032]

[66] Rayess N, Rahimy E, Storey P, *et al.* Postinjection endophthalmitis rates and characteristics following intravitreal bevacizumab, ranibizumab, and aflibercept. Am J Ophthalmol 2016; 165: 88-93.
[http://dx.doi.org/10.1016/j.ajo.2016.02.028] [PMID: 26944277]

[67] Maloney MH, Schilz SR, Herrin J, Sangaralingham LR, Shah ND, Barkmeier AJ. Risk of systemic adverse events associated with intravitreal anti–VEGF therapy for diabetic macular edema in routine clinical practice. Ophthalmology 2019; 126(7): 1007-15.
[http://dx.doi.org/10.1016/j.ophtha.2018.09.040] [PMID: 30292542]

[68] Avery RL, Castellarin AA, Steinle NC, *et al.* Systemic pharmacokinetics and pharmacodynamics of intravitreal aflibercept, bevacizumab, and ranibizumab. Retina 2017; 37(10): 1847-58.
[http://dx.doi.org/10.1097/IAE.0000000000001493] [PMID: 28106709]

[69] Miao H, Tao Y, Li XX. Inflammatory cytokines in aqueous humor of patients with choroidal neovascularization. Mol Vis 2012; 18: 574-80.
[PMID: 22419849]

[70] Tadayoni R, Sararols L, Weissgerber G, Verma R, Clemens A, Holz FG. Brolucizumab: A newly

developed anti-VEGF molecule for the treatment of neovascular age-related macular degeneration. Ophthalmologica 2021; 244(2): 93-101.
[http://dx.doi.org/10.1159/000513048] [PMID: 33197916]

[71] Finger RP, Dennis N, Freitas R, *et al.* Comparative efficacy of brolucizumab in the treatment of neovascular age-related macular degeneration: A systematic literature review and network meta-analysis. Adv Ther 2022; 39(8): 3425-48.
[http://dx.doi.org/10.1007/s12325-022-02193-3] [PMID: 35678996]

[72] Ranade SV, Wieland MR, Tam T, *et al.* The port delivery system with ranibizumab: A new paradigm for long-acting retinal drug delivery. Drug Deliv 2022; 29(1): 1326-34.
[http://dx.doi.org/10.1080/10717544.2022.2069301] [PMID: 35499315]

[73] Campochiaro PA, Marcus DM, Awh CC, *et al.* The port delivery system with ranibizumab for neovascular age-related macular degeneration: Results from the randomized phase 2 ladder clinical trial. Ophthalmology 2019; 126(8): 1141-54.
[http://dx.doi.org/10.1016/j.ophtha.2019.03.036] [PMID: 30946888]

[74] Jin K, Yan Y, Chen M, *et al.* Multimodal deep learning with feature level fusion for identification of choroidal neovascularization activity in age□related macular degeneration. Acta Ophthalmol 2022; 100(2): e512-20.
[http://dx.doi.org/10.1111/aos.14928] [PMID: 34159761]

[75] Tavakoli S, Puranen J, Bahrpeyma S, *et al.* Liposomal sunitinib for ocular drug delivery: A potential treatment for choroidal neovascularization. Int J Pharm 2022; 620: 121725.
[http://dx.doi.org/10.1016/j.ijpharm.2022.121725] [PMID: 35405282]

CHAPTER 11

Macular Perfusional Findings in Venous Obstructive Disease and Its Treatment: An OCT-A Evaluation

M. Naveed Yasin[1,2], Aftab Taiyab[2] and **Miguel A. Quiroz-Reyes, MD[3,*]**

[1] *Department of Ophthalmology, The University of Auckland, Auckland, New Zealand*

[2] *Department of Pathology and Molecular Medicine, McMaster University, Hamilton, Canada*

[3] *Oftalmologia Integral ABC, Retina Department, Medical and Surgical Assistance Institution (Nonprofit Organization), Affiliated with the Postgraduate Studies Division, National Autonomous University of Mexico, Mexico City, Mexico*

Abstract: The human retina is supplied by an extensive network of capillaries, where healthy blood flow to various parts of the retina, particularly the macula, is vital for visual functions. Any obstruction in blood flow, known as retinal vein occlusion (RVO), can reduce venous blood return. RVO can occur either at a central location (called central retinal vein occlusion [CRVO]) or a peripheral location (branch vein occlusion [BRVO]). Various techniques have been used to investigate blood flow to the retina and analyze different factors that may impact retinal blood flow. Optical coherence tomographic angiography (OCT-A) has emerged as one of the best methods, with several studies demonstrating its use to investigate changes in blood perfusion status, hemorrhage from blood vessels, and the presence of edema. Some studies have demonstrated that OCT-A is superior to other techniques.

Macular edema secondary to RVO is the most common complication that may affect visual acuity and lead to vision loss if left untreated. Several qualitative and quantitative changes caused by RVO can be detected using OCT-A, including vascular blood perfusion and vascular density. Several treatment options have been used to treat macular edema secondary to RVO and other complications. Laser photocoagulation therapy has been used extensively in the past with mixed outcomes. Glucocorticoids, especially dexamethasone (Ozurdex®), have also been used to treat macular edema secondary to RVO. Currently, anti-vascular endothelial growth factor (VEGF) agents are the gold standard for treating RVO. Ranibizumab and aflibercept are approved for the treatment of macular edema secondary to RVO, with faricimab expected to soon be approved.

* **Corresponding author Miguel A. Quiroz-Reyes, MD:** Oftalmologia Integral ABC, Retina Department, Medical and Surgical Assistance Institution (Nonprofit Organization), Affiliated with the Postgraduate Studies Division, National Autonomous University of Mexico, Mexico City, Mexico; Tel: +52 55 5217 2732; Fax: +52 55 1664 7180; E-mails: drquiroz@prodigy.net.mx and drquirozreyes7@gmail.com

Miguel A. Quiroz-Reyes and Virgilio Lima-Gomez (Eds.)

Keywords: Macular perfusion, Venous retinal illness, Blood perfusion in retinal conditions, Choroidal neovascularization, Retinal vein occlusion, Macular ischemia, Macular edema, OCT-A.

INTRODUCTION

The current understanding of blood supply to the retina, specifically the macula, was developed by exploring and understanding the blood flow in primate eyes. Primate eyes are uniquely comparable to human eyes because of the presence of a high visual acuity area in the temporal region [1]. Several studies have revealed that blood is supplied by four layers of capillary plexuses to the retina: the superficial vascular plexus (SVP), intermediate capillary plexus (ICP), deep capillary plexus (DCP), and radial peripapillary capillary plexus (RPCP) [1 - 5]. For human eyes, these capillary plexuses have been confirmed by confocal microscopic examination ex vivo [6, 7]. Further examination of human eyes via optical coherence tomography angiography (OCT) has provided three-dimensional (3D) details of the blood-supplying vasculature of the retina, including the macular region [4].

Healthy blood flow to the retina, especially in the macular region, is essential for providing nutrients and oxygen to photoreceptors, neurons, and other cells that play important roles in vision. A decrease in blood flow to the retina, especially in the macular region, is a risk factor for neovascularization (NV) and/or macular edema [8]. Systemic cardiovascular conditions, such as atherosclerosis and hypertension, have been studied as risk factors for the development of NV [9, 10]. Previous studies have also explored the role of choroidal blood flow changes as a precursor to the development of age-related macular degeneration (AMD) [9]. A hemodynamic model of pathogenesis proposed by Friedman *et al.* showed that a decrease in macular blood flow could lead to atrophic AMD, whereas an increase in macular blood flow could lead to neovascular AMD [11]. This has been further investigated in studies where a decrease in foveal blood flow was observed in atrophic AMD when compared to healthy eyes [12]. Ischemia and hypoxia associated with atrophic AMD can trigger angiogenesis, which may explain the progression of atrophic AMD to neovascular AMD [13].

A decrease in retinal venous blood return is termed retinal vein occlusion (RVO) and can be triggered by atherosclerosis, inflammation, vasospasm, or compression [14, 15]. RVO can be central (CRVO) if obstruction occurs within or posterior to the optic nerve or branch (BRVO) if obstruction occurs within a branch; BRVO is more common than CRVO [16]. Another form of RVO, hemiretinal RVO (HRVO), can occur in a major fork. RVO can lead to macular edema and ischemia, triggering neovascularization and other complications [17]. It can also cause optic neuropathy, vitreous hemorrhage, or retinal detachment [16]. Ischemic RVO is associated with poor visual acuity and requires treatment with anti-vascular endothelial growth factor (anti-VEGF) agents and corticosteroids [17, 18]. Diabetes, arterial hypertension, atherosclerosis, and thrombophilia are the common risk factors associated with RVO [16].

This chapter takes an aim explores the blood perfusion network in the retina, especially in the macular region. Retinal blood perfusion in healthy eyes was described along with optical coherence tomography angiography (OCT-A) images. After establishing the blood perfusion mechanism in healthy eyes, a detailed overview of the blood perfusion in RVO is presented with OCT-A images, presenting sequelae and macular perfusional repercussions. Treatment options for RVO and related complications are discussed in detail.

MACULAR BLOOD PERFUSION IN HEALTHY EYES

The retina is supplied by retinal and choroidal vessels, with the majority of blood supplied via the retinal artery, and almost all the blood is drained via the retinal vein [19]. The retinal and choroidal arteries form four major capillary plexuses (SVP, ICP, DCP, and RPCP) that supply optic nerves, photoreceptors, and surrounding cells. Campbell *et al.* investigated the blood supply to various regions of the retina using projection-resolved OCT-A (PR OCT-A) in healthy human eyes [4]. A significant improvement can be seen in Fig. (**1**) for studying detailed blood supply vasculature when compared to two-dimensional (2D) color fundus photographs. These findings are consistent with those of previous research carried out in primates and provide further details about the anatomy of the SVP, ICP, and DCP in the presence of an interconnecting layer (ICL) between these capillary plexuses.

Fig. (**2**) provides further exploration via OCT-A, with additional details about RPCP that seems to run along the dense nerve fiber layer (NFL), providing blood to the axons in the posterior pole around the optic nerve.

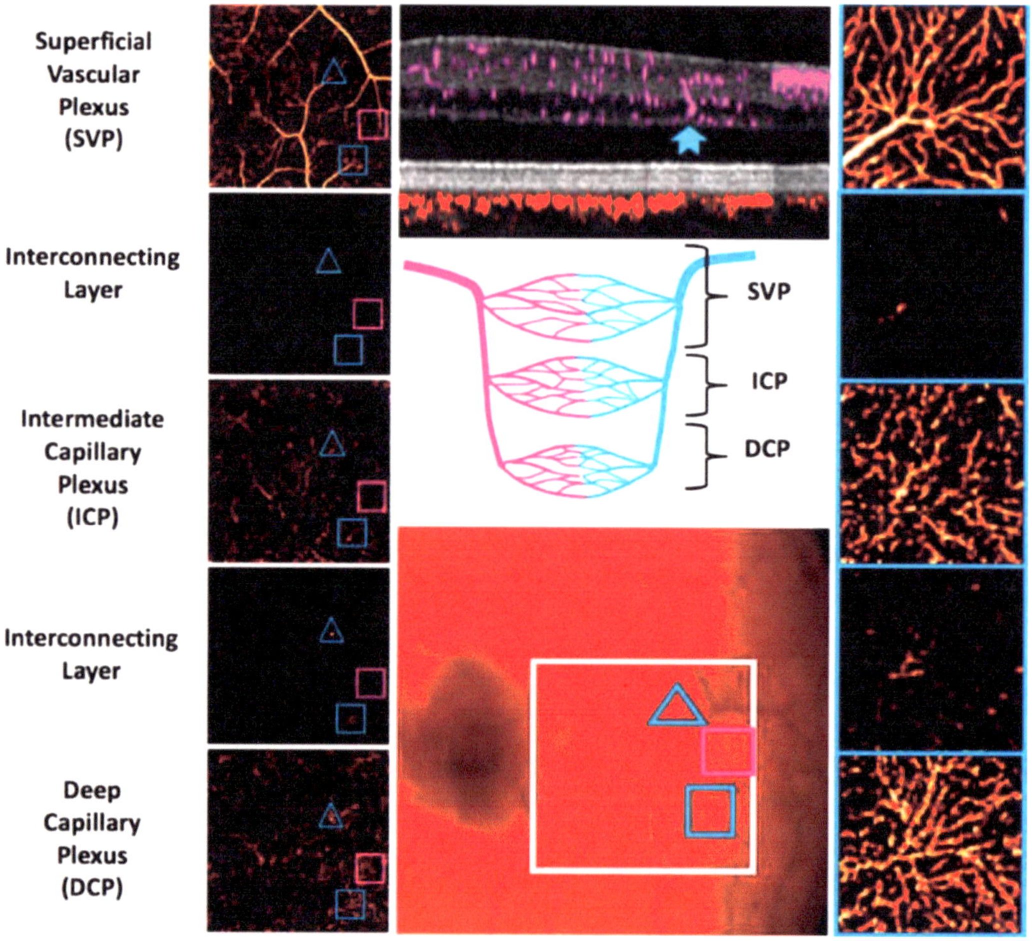

Fig. (1). ***Retinal vascular plexuses and interconnecting layers in the macula*.** Color fundus photograph (middle bottom panel) demonstrates the 2 × 2 mm region of the scan (white square). The en face PR-OCTA (left panels) are arrayed from the most superficial on top to the deepest at the bottom. The blue hollow triangles enclose a diving venule (identified on the color fundus photograph) that can be seen in the cross-sectional PR-OCT (middle top panel) traversing from the SVP to the DCP (solid blue notched arrow). The hollow pink squares enclose a diving arteriole that can be seen in the SVP, ICP, DCP, and the interconnecting layer between the ICP and the DCP. The hollow blue squares enclose a diving venule that is clearly seen in all magnified en face PR-OCTA slabs (right panels). This venule gives rise to a radiating network of capillaries in all 3 plexuses. The image (center panel) depicts the anatomical relationships between arterial and venous systems in the three vascular plexuses and the interconnecting layers (Copied from [4] with permission under CC BY 4.0 license).

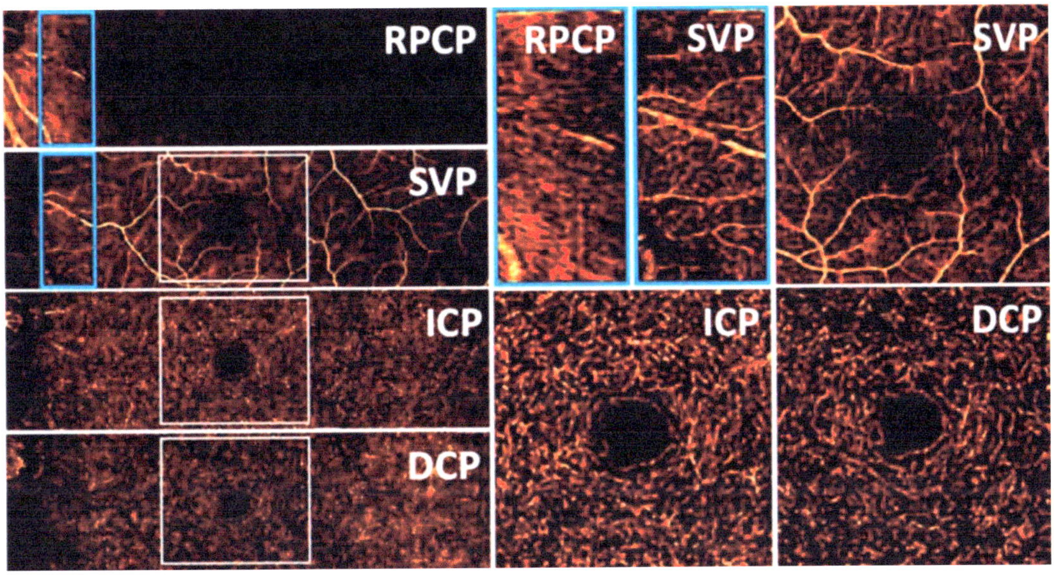

Fig. (2). En face projection-resolved optical coherence tomography angiograms of four retinal vascular plexuses in the left eye of a normal human participant. The angiograms are formed by the montage of four 2 × 2 mm scans. The radial peripapillary capillary plexus (RPCP) is found in the nerve fiber layer (NFL) slab. The superficial vascular plexus (SVP) slab was predominantly located in the ganglion cell layer (GCL), and was segmented as the inner 80% of the ganglion cell complex (GCC, defined as the NFL + GCL + inner plexiform layer [IPL]), excluding the NFL. The intermediate capillary plexus (ICP) was segmented between the outer 20% of the GCC to the inner 50% of the inner nuclear layer (INL). The deep capillary plexus was segmented between the outer 50% of the INL and the outer plexiform layer (OPL). High magnification images of the peripapillary RPCP, and parafoveal vascular networks of the SVP, ICP, and DCP are presented at the right, from corresponding sections indicated with white square (Copied from [4] with permission under CC BY 4.0 license).

The regulation of blood flow to the retina is achieved through static or dynamic autoregulation. For static blood flow regulation, local mediators are released by endothelial cells and the surrounding retinal tissue, which provide static autoregulation within the retina. Dynamic autoregulation is achieved by the intervention of the sympathetic nervous system to choroidal blood vessels, with a secondary impact on retinal blood flow [20]. Static autoregulation takes time to change blood pressure in retinal vessels; however, dynamic autoregulation provides significantly faster changes in ocular blood flow and pressure [21, 22]. Various mediators, including nitric oxide, oxygen, carbon dioxide, endothelin-1, adenosine, and angiotensin-2 [23]. In healthy eyes, autoregulation plays an important role in maintaining blood supply to the retina in response to local and external factors that may impact blood perfusion [24].

Variations in retinal blood flow among healthy eyes from one individual to another are common. Garhofer *et al.* studied blood flow variation among 64 healthy and young volunteers with normal blood pressure (BP), intraocular pressure (IOP), and reflective error of <3 diopters [25], where significant differences were observed between individual retinal blood flow. Therefore, it should be noted that the retinal blood flow measurements from clinical studies should not be used as a reference for diagnostic purposes. Ocular perfusion pressure (OPP) may differ among races; however, several other risk factors for ocular conditions also differ among individuals within a race [26]. A recent meta-analysis evaluated 72 studies to investigate the correlation between OPP and various patient characteristics to examine the risk of ocular disease. The results of a meta-analysis showed that a decrease in OPP could be a risk factor for the development of ocular diseases [27].

Macular thickness has also been extensively studied for its correlation with ocular perfusion, which may lead to ocular disease. Milani *et al.* explored the relationship between ocular conditions (i.e., ocular hypertension and/or glaucoma) and changes in macular thickness [28]. A linear correlation between the increase in macular thickness and SVP vessel density was observed in eyes with ocular hypertension/glaucoma compared to healthy eyes. Similarly, Ayhan *et al.* studied the effects of smoking on macular perfusion in healthy smokers [29]. When compared to healthy non-smoker eyes, a decrease in choriocapillary area blood flow was observed in the eyes of smokers, which could be due to the effects of nicotine and other chemical substances present in cigarettes [29]. Interestingly, yoga has been shown to significantly reduce IOP and increase the average macular thickness in healthy individuals [30]. Finally, a Turkish study found the parafoveal vascular density (VD) and foveal avascular zone (FAZ) area to be significantly higher in females when compared to males [31].

Overall, healthy blood flow to the retina is important for maintaining ocular health, visual functions, and wellbeing. The retinal artery and choroidal vessels form several capillary plexuses to provide blood to the photoreceptors, ganglion cells, neurons (including the optic nerve), and other cells. OPP is auto-regulated by static and dynamic mechanisms to maintain good blood flow in response to internal or external factors. Retinal blood flow variations can be significant between individuals; therefore, historical values should not be utilized for individual patient diagnosis. Differences in OPP, macular thickness, smoking status, and lifestyle may affect the retinal blood flow and overall ocular health.

MACULAR BLOOD PERFUSION IN RETINAL VEIN OCCLUSION

As previously described, a decrease in the venous return of retinal blood is referred to as RVO. This condition affects millions of patients globally, and BRVO is five times more prevalent than CRVO [32]. Both BRVO and CRVO can be further classified based on blood perfusion (non-ischemic) or no perfusion (ischemic) [33]. Macular edema is the most common complication of RVO and can lead to vision loss. NV is another common complication associated with RVO that can cause vision loss by vitreous hemorrhage, retinal detachment, or neovascular glaucoma [33]. Patients with RVO normally experience sudden and painless vision loss, where the extent of vision loss is normally associated with the status of macular perfusion [33].

To investigate macular perfusion in patients with RVO, OCT-A has become a popular non-invasive tool to detect changes in retinal/macular blood flow because of its ability to provide details about capillary plexuses without the need to use any dye [34]. RVO affected areas can be visualized and differentiated based on decreased vascular density and/or blood perfusion [35 - 37]. Thus, OCT-A has become an important tool to differentiate between BRVO and CRVO as well as to assess the perfusion status of the macula and other regions [38]. This is particularly important with an evolving understanding of RVO, where DCP seems to be more affected than SVP [39]. It is important to stress that OCT-A can be utilized in both CRVO and BRVO to investigate quantitative and qualitative changes [40]. Qualitative changes include nonperfusion areas (NPAs), vascular tortuosity, collateral vessel formation, disruption of perifoveal capillary plexus, dilation of capillary plexus and venous dilation, microaneurysms, cystoid spaces, intra-retinal hemorrhages, non-perfused ghost vessels, optic disc venous collaterals (OVCs) and neovascularization of disc (NVD), and neovascularization elsewhere (NVE) [35, 36, 39 - 44]. Quantitative changes include the measurement of NPAs and FAZ area [31, 40, 41, 45].

Several studies have demonstrated that OCT-A technology can be utilized for qualitative and quantitative analyses of sequelae and macular perfusional repercussions due to RVO. Koulisis *et al.* investigated the changes in the capillary plexus due to RVO using OCT-A in comparison with healthy eyes [46]. Eyes with CRVO and BRVO seemed to have significantly lower VD than healthy eyes. Additionally, eyes affected by RVO had a significantly higher vessel diameter index (VDI) than healthy eyes. Fig. (**3**) compares the OCT-A images of the healthy eye (Fig. **3** a-d) with the affected eye (Fig. **3** e-h).

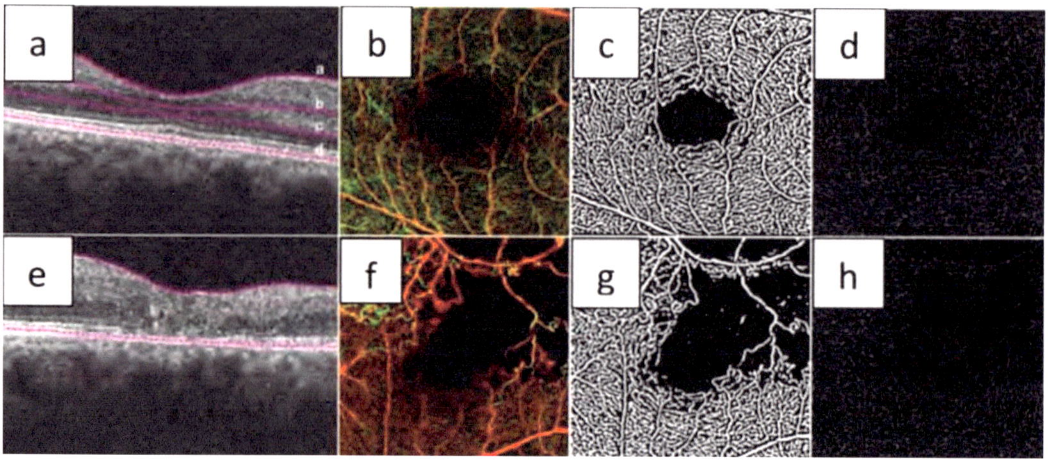

Fig. (3). (**a**) B-scan with purple dotted lines delineating the retinal vascular layers of interest in the healthy fellow eye of an RVO subject: non-segmented whole retina, NS-RL (**a-d**); Superficial retina layer, SRL (**a-b**); Deeper retina layer, DRL (**b-c**). Corresponding pseudo-colored, depth-encoded OCTA map (**B**), binarized image (**C**), and skeletonized image (**d**) of the unaffected eye. (**e-h**) Corresponding images of the RVO eye, NS-RL analysis (Copied from [46] with permission under CC BY 4.0 license).

Similarly, Mousa *et al.* performed a retrospective case series analysis of patients with ischemic RVO to optimize the grading of macular perfusion [38], which revealed that OCT-A was superior to fundus fluorescein angiography (FFA). Their analysis also revealed that the presence of SVP or DCP ischemia can lead to poor visual outcomes. Furthermore, an increase in central macular thickness (CMT), disruption of retinal outer layers (DROL), and disorganized inner retinal layers (DRIL) are sequelae and macular perfusional repercussions associated with poor visual acuity [38]. In another study of CRVO, Khodabandeh *et al.* used OCT-A to determine whether ischemia was associated with CRVO [47]. Fig. (**4**) shows foveal and parafoveal vascular density in patients with CRVO, where a significant reduction in macular blood perfusion was observed when compared to healthy eyes. This study also provides strong support for the use of OCT-A to investigate sequelae and macular perfusional repercussions due to RVO.

In addition to the previously described RVO complications, OCT-A has also been used to investigate paracentral acute middle maculopathy (PAMM) secondary to RVO [48, 49]. One case study published by Dansingani *et al.* compared the use of near-infrared (nIR) to OCT-A for the detection of lesions at the site of vein occlusion. nIR was not able to detect the lesion after one month of initial detection; however, OCT-A was able to detect the lesions, as well as changes in the retinal layer thicknesses at the occlusion site and alterations in blood perfusion to the affected area. Thinning of the ganglion cells layer (GCL), INL, and IPL and thickening of the outer nuclear layer (ONL) were observed along with a flow void in the parafoveal region [49]. Similarly, He *et al.* compared the use of FFA and OCT-A to detect improvement in retinal vasculature following pan retinal photocoagulation (PRP) treatment [50]. As displayed in Fig. (**5**), the abnormal blood vascular shape was still evident on OCT-A; however, FFA was not able to detect these details and showed no fluorescein leakage.

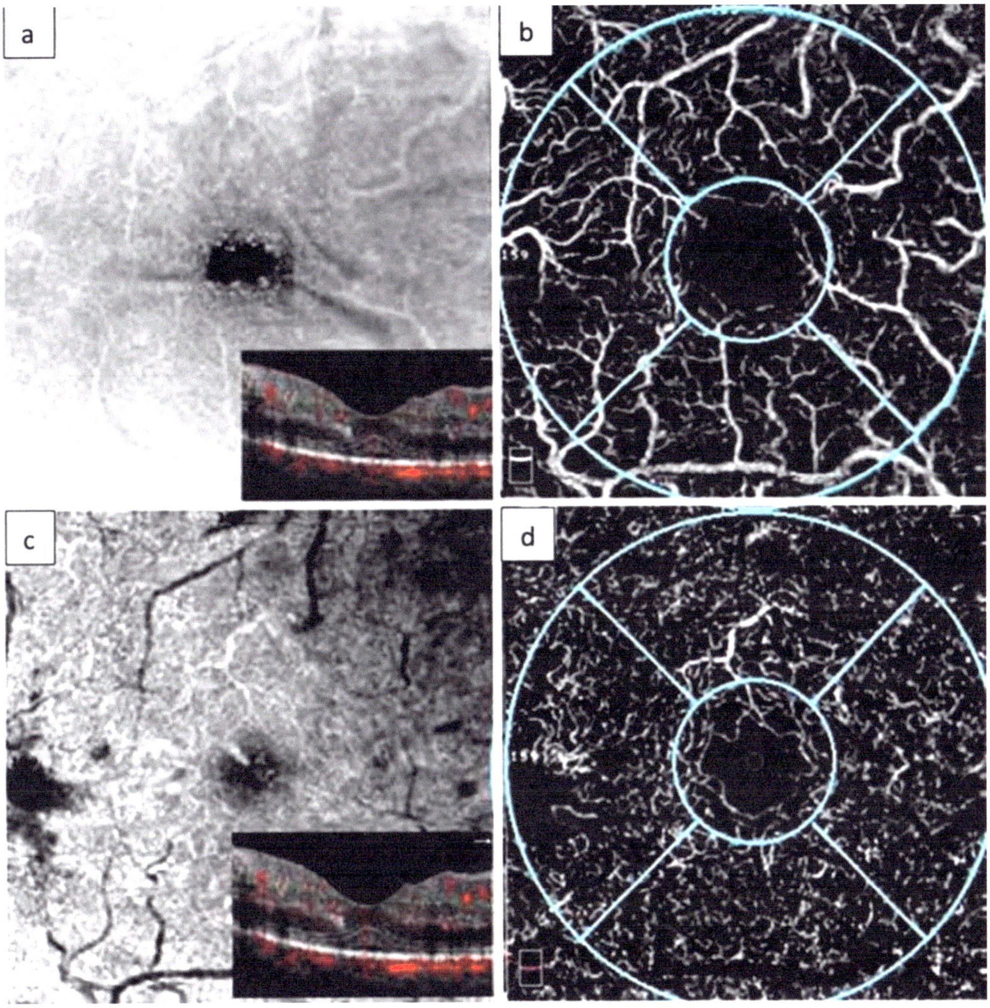

Fig. (4). ***A patient with central retinal vein occlusion.*** (**a**) En face optical coherence tomography at superficial retina layer with segmentation lines of superficial capillary layer. (**b**) Optical coherence tomography angiography (OCTA) in superficial capillary plexus, whole vascular density (larger green circle), foveal vascular density (small green circle) and parafoveal vascular density (difference between 2 circles) were calculated in superficial capillary plexuses in OCTA. (**c**) En face optical coherence tomography at deep capillary layer with segmentation lines of this plexus. d OCTA in deep capillary plexus. (Copied from [47] with permission under CC BY 4.0 license).

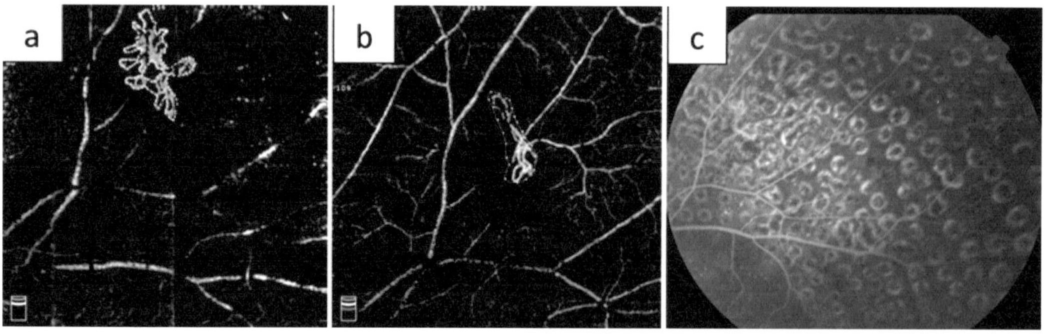

Fig. (5). (**a**) Neovascularization at baseline OCTA with an area of 0.653 mm^2 ; (**b**) OCTA still shows abnormal vascular shape at an interval of 1 year after PRP, with an area of 0.272 mm^2. (**c**) and no evidence of fluorescein leakage is seen at the FFA (right) (Copied from [50] with permission under CC BY 4.0 license).

In summary, OCT-A has become a popular and powerful tool for the evaluation of blood flow in the retina, specifically in the macular region. This provides qualitative and quantitative insights into macular perfusion. This technique has proven to be superior in investigating vascular occlusions and determining the extent of sequelae and perfusional repercussions.

TREATING SEQUELA AND MACULAR PERFUSIONAL REPERCUSSIONS IN RETINAL VEIN OCCLUSION

Herein, we discuss the options available for treating sequelae and macular perfusional repercussions due to RVO. Macular edema secondary to RVO is the 2nd most frequent macular disease after diabetic retinopathy [32]. Depending on the complications of RVO, the extent of ischemia, and the presence of macular edema, the following treatment options are utilized most frequently:

Laser Treatment

Laser treatment is one of the most popular methods for treating RVO complications, including macular edema. It must be noted that this treatment option is only effective for BRVO and does not improve CRVO. In the Central Vein Occlusion Study Report, 155 eyes were treated with laser photocoagulation therapy and followed up for up to 3 years. This study showed that laser treatment did not significantly improve visual acuity in these patients. However, a significant reduction in macular edema was observed on fluorescein angiography (FA) [51]. In contrast, The Branch Vein Occlusion Study Group treated 139 eyes with laser photocoagulation therapy and followed up for up to 3.1 years. This study showed a significant visual acuity gain in eyes treated with a laser when compared to untreated eyes [52]. The same clinical trial (Branch Vein Occlusion Study Group) also explored the use of laser photocoagulation therapy to reduce neovascularization and retinal hemorrhage in patients with BRVO. A total of 319 eyes were treated with laser to evaluate the effectiveness of laser treatment in reducing neovascularization. The study showed a significant reduction in neovascularization in treated eyes compared to untreated eyes. Similarly, a significant reduction in the development of vitreous hemorrhage was observed in eyes treated with laser therapy compared to untreated eyes [53].

Overall, laser photocoagulation therapy may provide benefits for BRVO patients; however, this treatment option is not commonly used because of the availability of other superior treatment options.

Glucocorticoids

The intravitreal use of glucocorticoids has been explored to reduce macular edema and improve visual acuity in patients with RVO. Among glucocorticoids, triamcinolone acetonide and dexamethasone have been widely studied for the treatment of BRVO and CRVO, respectively. Triamcinolone intravitreal injections were compared with laser therapy to improve visual acuity in patients with BRVO in the SCORE study [54]. A total of 411 patients were randomly assigned to receive either a triamcinolone intravitreal injection (1 mg or 4 mg) or standard treatment (laser therapy). The study results revealed no significant differences between the laser therapy and triamcinolone intravitreal injection treatment groups 12 months after baseline. Overall, an increased risk of high intraocular pressure (IOP) was observed in patients receiving higher doses of triamcinolone [54]. Similarly, the SCORE study in patients with CRVO compared observation (no treatment) to intravitreal triamcinolone injections (1 or 4 mg) in 271 patients [55]. Results from this investigation showed a significant improvement in visual acuity in patients treated with triamcinolone 12 months after the baseline. There was no significant difference in efficacy between 1 mg and 4 mg triamcinolone; however, 1 mg injection provided a superior safety profile [55].

Dexamethasone has recently gained popularity for the treatment of macular edema secondary to RVO owing to the approval of an intravitreal implant (Ozurdex®, 0.7 mg dexamethasone). This implant is used in the treatment and management of macular edema in both CRVO and BRVO [56]. In two landmark studies, Haller *et al.* investigated the use of dexamethasone implants in 1267 patients with vision loss due to RVO (CRVO or BRVO). These patients were randomized to receive either a 0.7 mg dexamethasone implant, or a 0.35 mg dexamethasone implant, or a sham. The number of patients with ≥15 letters of improvement from baseline in best-corrected visual acuity (BCVA) was significantly higher in the dexamethasone-treated group than in the sham group. At the end of 180 days of evaluation, no significant changes in IOP were detected in dexamethasone-treated patients when compared to sham [56]. These findings provide concrete evidence for the efficacy and safety of Ozurdex in treating macular edema secondary to RVO. Mastropasqua *et al.* investigated changes in the macular region as well as the resolution of edema in RVO patients after dexamethasone implant injection [42]. Fig. (**6**) shows that the vascular density decreased after treatment with Ozurdex, with an improvement in vessel perfusion after the resolution of macular edema.

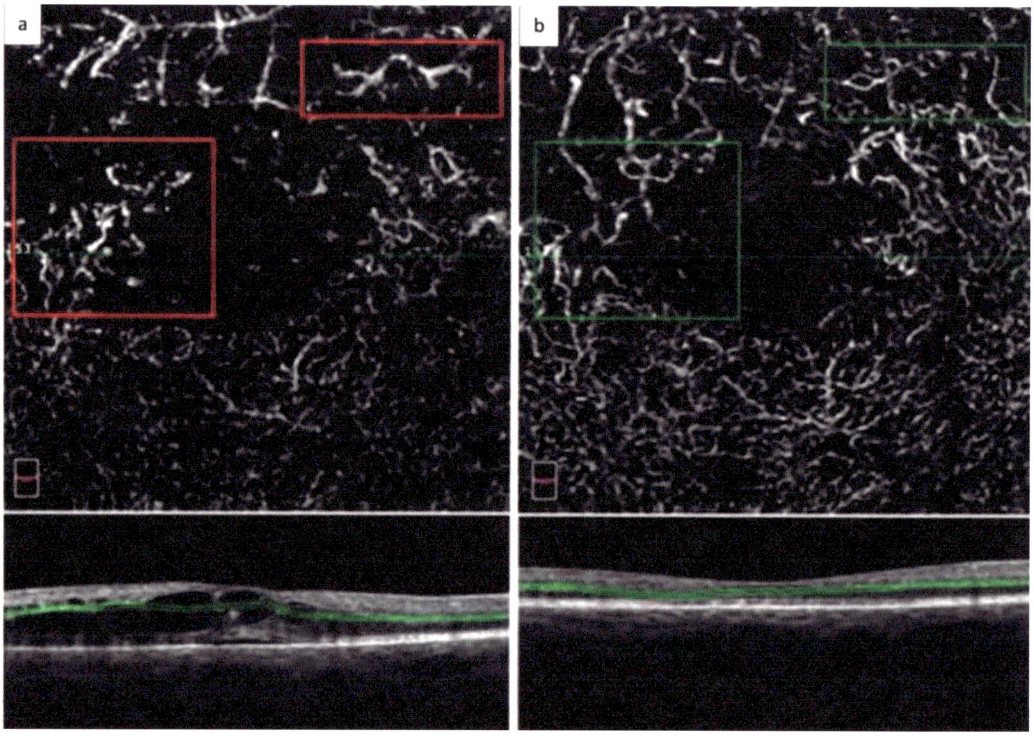

Fig. (6). Optical coherence tomography (OCT) angiography images of a patient with supero-temporal branch retinal vein occlusion: deep retinal plexus before dexamethasone implant (panel a) showing areas of telangiectatic vessels (red squares) and after dexamethasone implant (panel b), showing vessel caliber reduction (green squares) (Copied from [42] with permission under CC BY 4.0 license).

Anti-VEGF Agents

Anti-VEGF agents have become the first-line therapy or gold standard for treating macular edema and other complications related to RVO. A recent meta-analysis by Qian *et al.* provided solid support for their use in improving visual acuity and other complications in patients [57]. Anti-VEGF therapy seems superior in improving BCVA and reducing CMT compared to corticosteroids or laser therapy. Additionally, anti-VEGF agents are deemed safer because they are less likely to increase IOP. The same meta-analysis also concluded that anti-VEGF agents are more effective in treating BRVO than CRVO [57]. Previous research has investigated an increase in VEGF concentration following RVO, which could compromise the vascular integrity of blood vessels in the macular region and cause neovascularization, leading to macular edema [58, 59].

Ranibizumab (Lucentis®) was the first anti-VEGF agent approved for the treatment of macular edema secondary to RVO. Two landmark studies, BRAVO and CRUISE, investigated the use of intravitreal ranibizumab for the treatment of BRVO and CRVO, respectively [60, 61]. BRAVO included 397 patients with macular edema secondary to BRVO, whereas CRUISE included 392 patients with macular edema secondary to CRVO. Patients in both studies were randomized to receive 0.3 mg ranibizumab (0.5 mg), or sham. Ranibizumab (specifically 0.5 mg dose) significantly improved BCVA and reduced central foveal thickness (CFT) in patients within 6 months from baseline [60, 61]. The 12-months follow up established the long-term safety and efficacy of ranibizumab in patients with BRVO and CRVO [62, 63]. A follow-up study beyond BRAVO and CRUISE, called HORIZON, provided further support and guidance for the use of ranibizumab in treating RVO. This study further strengthened the use of ranibizumab in treating BRVO and CRVO, with a recommendation to individualize dosing regimens for patients with CRVO after 12 months of treatment [64]. Recently, Lida-Miwa *et al.* investigated improvements in macular edema secondary to BRVO in patients treated with ranibizumab using FA and OCT-A. Fig. (**7**) provides details about the reduction in NPA with ranibizumab treatment; interestingly, neovascularization was also seen as a complication following BRVO [65].

Bevacizumab (Avastin®) has also been used off-label for the treatment of macular edema and other complications related to BRVO and CRVO. A prospective 18-months long clinical study by Zhang *et al.* demonstrated that bevacizumab could improve visual acuity by improving BCVA and reducing CMT when compared to sham [66]. Choi *et al.* investigated improvements in macular edema among patients with BRVO following bevacizumab treatment. Fig. (**8**) provides details of the affected area in a 69-year-old patient who improved after bevacizumab injection, with no recurrence of macular edema [67].

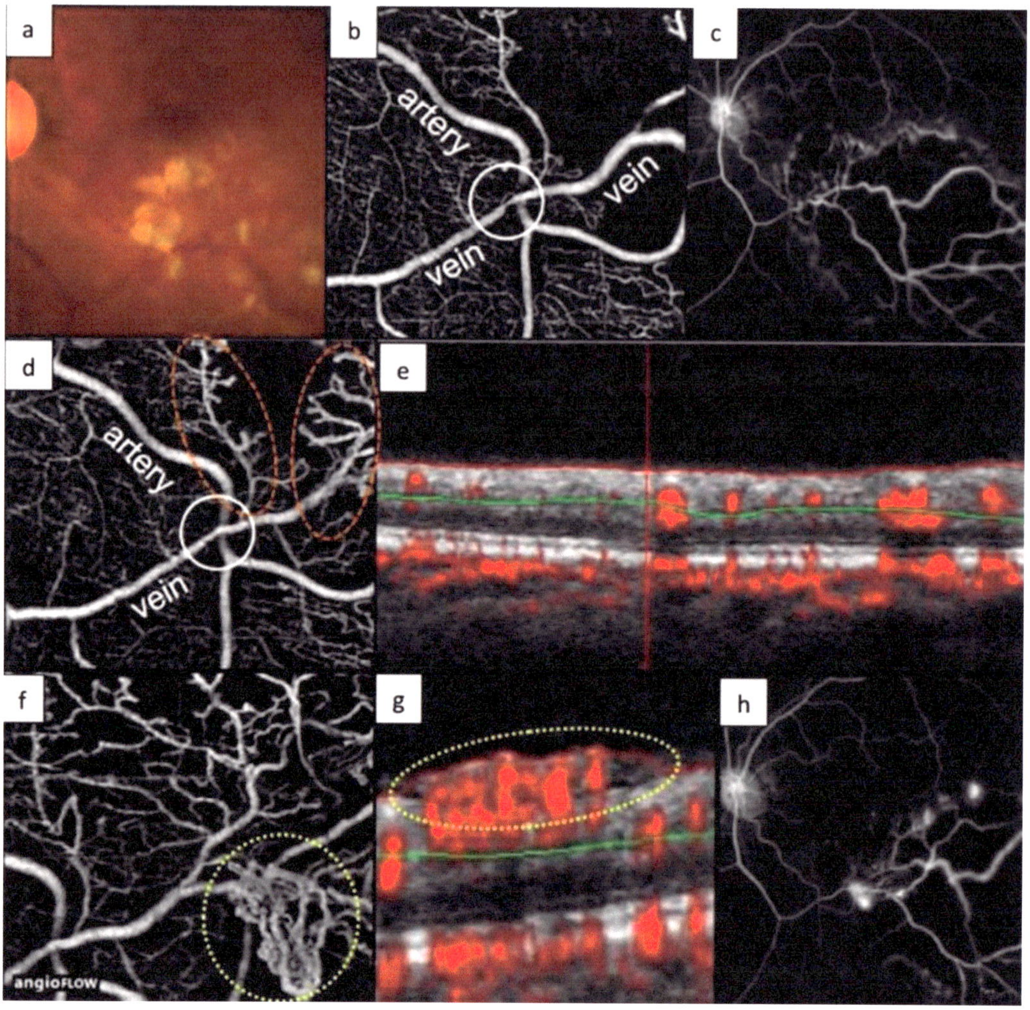

Fig. (7). ***Retinal neovascularization in an eye with major branch retinal vein occlusion (BRVO) and affected venous overcrossing***. At baseline (**a–c**), a color fundus photograph (**a**), an optical coherence tomography (OCT) angiograph (**b**), and an ultra-wide field fluorescein angiography image (**c**) show marked retinal whitening, affected venous overcrossing, and a large retinal nonperfusion area (NPA) without any neovascularization, respectively. The initial Snellen visual acuity was 20/67. At month 9 (**d**,**e**), an OCT angiography image shows the resolution of the narrowing of the affected vein (white circle) and an improvement in the circulation of the venules and capillaries around the affected crossing site (orange circles, **d**). An OCT-B scan of the retinal area showing improved retinal circulation does not show any retinal neovascularization at the vitreoretinal interface (**e**). At month 12 (**f-h**), an OCT angiography image clearly shows retinal neovascularization at the periphery of the crossing site (yellow circle, **f**) and the vitreoretinal interface (yellow circle, **g**). An ultra-wide field fluorescein angiography image shows active dye leakage, consistent with retinal neovascularization (**h**). The patient received three ranibizumab injections (no pro re nata injections were necessary) for macular edema. The time between neovascularization and the last ranibizumab injection was approximately 10 months (Copied from [65] with permission under CC BY 4.0 license).

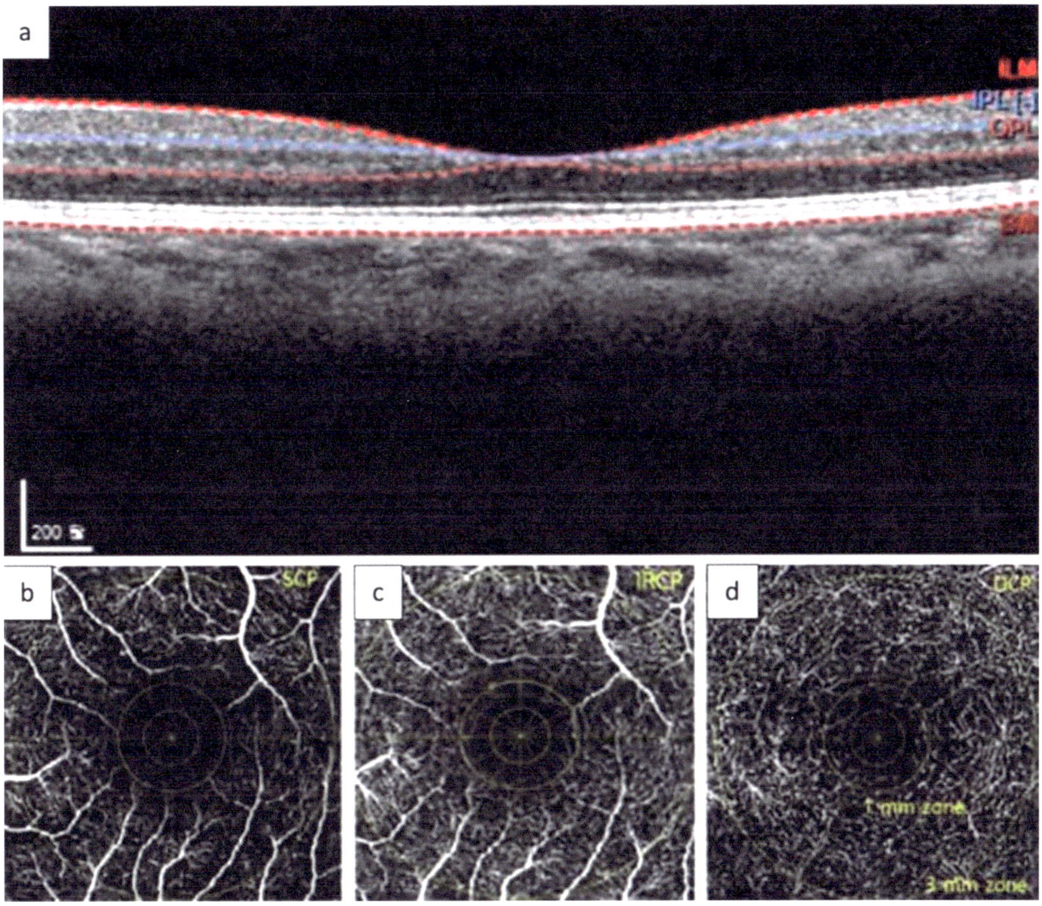

Fig. (8). (**a**) OCT image and (**b–d**) OCTA images of the fellow eye in a 69-year-old male patient from the nonrecurrence group. OCTA image of (**d**) the DCP showing a more prominent FAZ than in (**b**) the SVP. Single-layered capillaries are shown to be adherent to the FAZ within (**c**) the inner retinal capillary plexus layer (IRCP) and (**d**) the DCP but not (**b**) the SVP (Copied from [67] with permission under CC BY 4.0 license).

Aflibercept (Eylea®), another anti-VEGF agent, was approved for the treatment of macular edema and other RVO complications in 2014. In a landmark study to investigate the safety and efficacy of aflibercept in CRVO (COPERNICUS), 189 patients were randomized to receive either aflibercept 2 mg intravitreally or sham during the first 6 months. The results revealed that the aflibercept treatment group experienced significant improvement in visual acuity at the end of the initial 6-months treatment period when compared to the sham group. This study also confirmed that aflibercept is generally safe and well-tolerated [68]. The VIBRANT study is another landmark study that investigated the use of aflibercept in treating macular edema secondary to BRVO. This study recruited treatment-naïve patients who were randomized to receive either aflibercept 2 mg intravitreal or laser photocoagulation therapy. The results confirmed that aflibercept was significantly superior to laser photocoagulation therapy in improving visual acuity and decreasing CMT [69]. Ghashut *et al.* recently investigated changes in the macular region in patients with macular edema secondary to CRVO via OCT-A. Aflibercept treatment reversed changes in the macular region and improved visual acuity in patients with a relatively small NPA and no foveal photoreceptor damage. However, for patients with a relatively large NPA and mild foveal photoreceptor damage, aflibercept significantly reduces macular edema, but improvement in visual acuity is limited [70]. Similarly, Amer *et al.* investigated the improvement in macular edema secondary to CRVO following aflibercept treatment, and a significant reduction was observed in the central subfield thickness (CST), as shown in Fig. (**9**) [71].

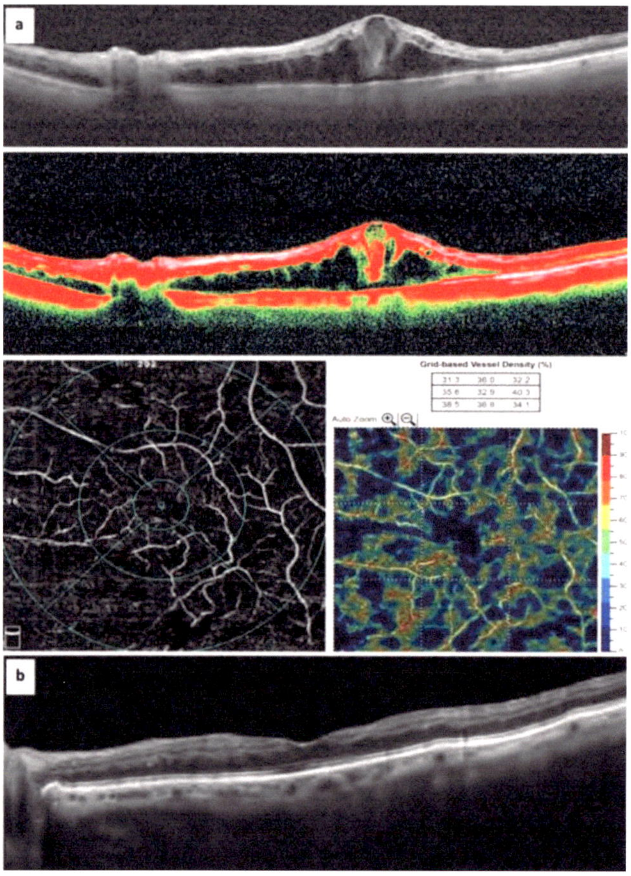

Fig. (9). (**a**) CST shows a significant reduction over time (at baseline [570.7 ± 59 Um], 6 months [388.5 ± 80 Um], and (**b**) 12 months [328.2 ± 72 Um], $p < 0.001$) (Copied from [71] with permission under CC BY 4.0 license).

Faricimab (Vabysmo®) is the most recently approved anti-VEGF and anti-angiopoietin-2 (anti-Ang2) agent that is being investigated in two Phase 3 clinical trials, BALATON and COMINO, for the treatment of macular edema secondary to BRVO and CRVO, respectively [72, 73]. A recent literature review by Heier *et al.* analyzed the angiopoietin-tie pathway and potential application of faricimab to treat RVO, where Ang-2 seems to be elevated in the retina of patients with RVO [74]. Therefore, it is expected that faricimab could significantly improve RVO treatment as a dual anti-VEGF/anti-Ang-2 agent.

Finally, the Port Delivery System (PDS, commercially available as Susvimo®), a novel device capable of delivering anti-VEGF agents to the retina for a prolonged duration (6 months or beyond), was recently approved by the US FDA [75, 76]. It is a first-of-its-kind drug delivery system that has been approved for treating neovascular AMD, and it has the potential to be used in treating macular edema and other complications of RVO by providing sustained delivery of anti-VEGF agents. The previous approval and use of Ozurdex have been highlighted in a recent literature review, hinting at the potential use of PDS to treat RVO by providing sustained delivery of anti-VEGF agents [76]. PDS is also being investigated for sustained delivery of faricimab, which could provide significant advantages by targeting both VEGF and Ang-2 pathways, as well as delivering drugs in a sustained manner [77].

CONCLUDING REMARKS

Healthy blood flow to the retina, particularly in the macular region, is essential for good ocular health. Several techniques, including nIR, FFA, and OCT-A, have been utilized to understand the normal retinal blood flow mechanisms and assess any changes. OCT-A has been used to understand retinal blood vasculature and to investigate any differences based on race, age, sex, or lifestyle. The use of OCT-A in the diagnosis of diseases in which retinal blood flow is affected (*e.g.*, RVO: CRVO and BRVO) is advantageous because of its ability to provide a detailed picture of retinal blood vessels and perfusion without the use of any dye in a noninvasive way. A few studies have shown that OCT-A can provide a better understanding of sequelae and blood perfusional repercussions secondary to RVO than other imaging and visualization techniques such as nIR or FFA. This is because of the high resolution and depth achievable only by OCT-A. In this book chapter, we explored a few studies in which the retinal blood vasculature details captured by OCT-A were missed by other techniques. Additionally, nIR can damage vision by causing cataracts; however, this is not the case with OCT-A. Similarly, FFA requires the use of fluorescein dye, which is not required for OCT-A. The use of OCT-A has significantly improved our understanding of RVO mechanisms by mapping and tracking the retinal vascular network and blood flow. Several qualitative and quantitative changes in retinal blood flow can be visualized and investigated using OCT-A. In addition to diagnosis, it can also be useful in determining treatment effects by investigating and quantifying any improvements in retinal blood flow. To date, several therapeutics, including glucocorticoids and anti-VEGF agents, have been approved for RVO treatment. Among glucocorticoids, dexamethasone implants (Ozurdex) are frequently used to treat RVO complications and improve visual acuity. However, anti-VEGF agents are considered the gold standard for the treatment of RVO. Currently, ranibizumab and aflibercept are widely used as first-line treatment options for RVO and its related complications. Bevacizumab is also used (off-label) to treat RVO and related complications. New treatment options, such as the approval of a novel dual acting agent (faricimab), may provide further advantages in RVO treatment when compared to current options. Additionally, the potential application of sustained drug delivery devices, such as PDS, to treat RVO may provide superior therapeutic outcomes and enhance patient compliance. Overall, improvements in understanding and treating RVO may significantly improve visual acuity and prevent blindness among patients.

LIST OF ABBREVIATIONS

2D	Two dimensional
3D	Three dimensional
AMD	Age related macular degeneration
Ang2	Angiopoietin-2
BCVA	Best corrected visual acuity
BP	Blood pressure
BRVO	Branch retinal vein occlusion
CMT	Central macular thickness
CRVO	Central retinal vein occlusion
CST	Central subfield thickness
DCP	Deep capillary plexus
DRIL	Disorganized Inner retinal layers
DROL	Disruption of retinal outer layers
FAZ	Foveal avascular zone
FA	Fluorescein Angiography
FFA	Fundus fluorescein angiography
GCC	Ganglion cell complex
GCL	Ganglion cell layer
HRVO	Hemiretinal vein occlusion

ICL	Inner connecting layer
ICP	Inner capillary plexus
INL	Inner nuclear layer
IOP	Intraocular pressure
IPL	Inner plexiform layer
NFL	Nerve fiber layer
NPAs	Non-perfusion areas
NV	neovascularization
NVD	Neovascularization of the disc
NVE	Neovascularization elsewhere
OCT-A	Optical coherence tomography angiography
ONL	Outer nuclear layer
OVCs	Optic disc venous collateral
PAMM	Paracentral acute middle maculopathy
PRP	Pan-retinal photocoagulation
PDS	Port delivery system
RPCP	Radial peripapillary plexus
SVP	Superficial vascular plexus
VD	Vascular density
VDI	Vessel diameter index
VEGF	Vascular endothelial growth factor

DISCLAIMER

All scientific comments issued in this chapter are solely the responsibility of the authors and not of the institutions with which they are affiliated.

ACKNOWLEDGMENTS

We express our deep appreciation to the technical staff of the Retina Specialists Unit at Oftalmologia Integral ABC (Nonprofit Medical and Surgical Organization) affiliated with The Postgraduate Division Studies at the National Autonomous University of Mexico.

REFERENCES

[1] Provis J. Development of the primate retinal vasculature. Prog Retin Eye Res 2001; 20(6): 799-821. [http://dx.doi.org/10.1016/S1350-9462(01)00012-X] [PMID: 11587918]

[2] Alterman M, Henkind P. Radial peripapillary capillaries of the retina. II. Possible role in Bjerrum scotoma. Br J Ophthalmol 1968; 52(1): 26-31.

[http://dx.doi.org/10.1136/bjo.52.1.26] [PMID: 5635900]

[3] Henkind P. Radial peripapillary capillaries of the retina. I. Anatomy: Human and comparative. Br J Ophthalmol 1967; 51(2): 115-23.
[http://dx.doi.org/10.1136/bjo.51.2.115] [PMID: 4959937]

[4] Campbell JP, Zhang M, Hwang TS, *et al.* Detailed vascular anatomy of the human retina by projection-resolved optical coherence tomography angiography. Sci Rep 2017; 7(1): 42201.
[http://dx.doi.org/10.1038/srep42201] [PMID: 28186181]

[5] Snodderly DM, Weinhaus RS, Choi JC. Neural-vascular relationships in central retina of macaque monkeys (Macaca fascicularis). J Neurosci 1992; 12(4): 1169-93.
[http://dx.doi.org/10.1523/JNEUROSCI.12-04-01169.1992] [PMID: 1556592]

[6] Chan G, Balaratnasingam C, Yu PK, *et al.* Quantitative morphometry of perifoveal capillary networks in the human retina. Invest Ophthalmol Vis Sci 2012; 53(9): 5502-14.
[http://dx.doi.org/10.1167/iovs.12-10265] [PMID: 22815351]

[7] Tan PEZ, Yu PK, Balaratnasingam C, *et al.* Quantitative confocal imaging of the retinal microvasculature in the human retina. Invest Ophthalmol Vis Sci 2012; 53(9): 5728-36.
[http://dx.doi.org/10.1167/iovs.12-10017] [PMID: 22836777]

[8] Boltz A, Luksch A, Wimpissinger B, *et al.* Choroidal blood flow and progression of age-related macular degeneration in the fellow eye in patients with unilateral choroidal neovascularization. Invest Ophthalmol Vis Sci 2010; 51(8): 4220-5.
[http://dx.doi.org/10.1167/iovs.09-4968] [PMID: 20484590]

[9] Vingerling JR, Dielemans I, Bots ML, Hofman A, Grobbee DE, de Jong PTVM. Age-related macular degeneration is associated with atherosclerosis. The Rotterdam Study. Am J Epidemiol 1995; 142(4): 404-9.
[http://dx.doi.org/10.1093/oxfordjournals.aje.a117648] [PMID: 7625405]

[10] Hyman L, Schachat AP, He Q, Leske MC. Hypertension, cardiovascular disease, and age-related macular degeneration. Arch Ophthalmol 2000; 118(3): 351-8.
[http://dx.doi.org/10.1001/archopht.118.3.351] [PMID: 10721957]

[11] Friedman E. A hemodynamic model of the pathogenesis of age-related macular degeneration. Am J Ophthalmol 1997; 124(5): 677-82.
[http://dx.doi.org/10.1016/S0002-9394(14)70906-7] [PMID: 9372722]

[12] Grunwald JE, Hariprasad SM, DuPont J, *et al.* Foveolar choroidal blood flow in age-related macular degeneration. Invest Ophthalmol Vis Sci 1998; 39(2): 385-90.
[PMID: 9477998]

[13] Grunwald JE, Metelitsina TI, DuPont JC, Ying GS, Maguire MG. Reduced foveolar choroidal blood flow in eyes with increasing AMD severity. Invest Ophthalmol Vis Sci 2005; 46(3): 1033-8.
[http://dx.doi.org/10.1167/iovs.04-1050] [PMID: 15728562]

[14] Yen YC, Weng SF, Chen HA, Lin YS. Risk of retinal vein occlusion in patients with systemic lupus erythematosus: A population-based cohort study. Br J Ophthalmol 2013; 97(9): 1192-6.
[http://dx.doi.org/10.1136/bjophthalmol-2013-303265] [PMID: 23832964]

[15] O'Mahoney PRA, Wong DT, Ray JG. Retinal vein occlusion and traditional risk factors for atherosclerosis. Arch Ophthalmol 2008; 126(5): 692-9.
[http://dx.doi.org/10.1001/archopht.126.5.692] [PMID: 18474782]

[16] Ip M, Hendrick A. Retinal vein occlusion review. Asia Pac J Ophthalmol 2018; 7(1): 40-5.
[PMID: 29280368]

[17] Sivaprasad S, Amoaku WM, Hykin P. The royal college of ophthalmologists guidelines on retinal vein occlusions: Executive summary. Eye 2015; 29(12): 1633-8.
[http://dx.doi.org/10.1038/eye.2015.164] [PMID: 26315705]

[18] Singer M, Cohen S, Groth S, Porbandarwalla S. Comparing bevacizumab and ranibizumab for initial reduction of central macular thickness in patients with retinal vein occlusions. Clin Ophthalmol 2013; 7(Jul): 1377-83.
[http://dx.doi.org/10.2147/OPTH.S46235] [PMID: 23874079]

[19] Onda E, Cioffi GA, Bacon DR, van BUSKIRK M. Microvasculature of the human optic nerve. Am J Ophthalmol 1995; 120(1): 92-102.
[http://dx.doi.org/10.1016/S0002-9394(14)73763-8] [PMID: 7611333]

[20] Delaey C, van de Voorde J. Regulatory mechanisms in the retinal and choroidal circulation. Ophthalmic Res 2000; 32(6): 249-56.
[http://dx.doi.org/10.1159/000055622] [PMID: 11015035]

[21] Iester M, Torre PG, Bricola G, Bagnis A, Calabria G. Retinal blood flow autoregulation after dynamic exercise in healthy young subjects. Ophthalmologica 2007; 221(3): 180-5.
[http://dx.doi.org/10.1159/000099298] [PMID: 17440280]

[22] Liang Y, Fortune B, Cull G, Cioffi GA, Wang L. Quantification of dynamic blood flow autoregulation in optic nerve head of rhesus monkeys. Exp Eye Res 2010; 90(2): 203-9.
[http://dx.doi.org/10.1016/j.exer.2009.10.009] [PMID: 19853603]

[23] Lesk MR, Wajszilber M, Deschenes MC. The effects of systemic medications on ocular blood flow. Can J Ophthalmol 2008; 43(3): 351-5.
[http://dx.doi.org/10.3129/i08-057] [PMID: 18493276]

[24] Pournaras C. Autoregulation of ocular blood flow.Ocular Blood Flow: Glaucoma Meeting 1995. Basel, Switzerland: Karger Basel Publications 1996; pp. 40-50.

[25] Garhofer G, Werkmeister R, Dragostinoff N, Schmetterer L. Retinal blood flow in healthy young subjects. Invest Ophthalmol Vis Sci 2012; 53(2): 698-703.
[http://dx.doi.org/10.1167/iovs.11-8624] [PMID: 22247463]

[26] Siesky B, Harris A, Verticchio Vercellin AC, Guidoboni G, Tsai JC. Ocular blood flow as it relates to race and disease on glaucoma. Adv Ophthalmol Optom 2021; 6: 245-62.
[http://dx.doi.org/10.1016/j.yaoo.2021.04.016] [PMID: 35252630]

[27] Kim KE, Oh S, Baek SU, Ahn SJ, Park KH, Jeoung JW. Ocular perfusion pressure and the risk of open-angle glaucoma: Systematic review and meta-analysis. Sci Rep 2020; 10(1): 10056.
[http://dx.doi.org/10.1038/s41598-020-66914-w] [PMID: 32572072]

[28] Milani P, Bochicchio S, Urbini LE, *et al.* Diurnal measurements of macular thickness and vessel density on oct angiography in healthy eyes and those with ocular hypertension and glaucoma. J Glaucoma 2020; 29(10): 918-25.
[http://dx.doi.org/10.1097/IJG.0000000000001580] [PMID: 32555061]

[29] Ayhan Z, Kaya M, Ozturk T, Karti O, Hakan Oner F. Evaluation of macular perfusion in healthy smokers by using optical coherence tomography angiography. Ophthalmic Surg Lasers Imaging Retina 2017; 48(8): 617-22.
[http://dx.doi.org/10.3928/23258160-20170802-03] [PMID: 28810036]

[30] Galina D, Etsuo C, Takuhei S, *et al.* Immediate effect of Yoga exercises for eyes on the macular thickness. Int J Yoga 2020; 13(3): 223-6.
[http://dx.doi.org/10.4103/ijoy.IJOY_28_20] [PMID: 33343152]

[31] Kaya M, Ayhan Z, Ozturk AT, Kocak N, Arikan G, Kaynak S. Evaluation of the macular and choroidal perfusion in healthy turkish population using optical coherence tomography angiography. Korean J Ophthalmol 2021; 35(5): 360-7.
[http://dx.doi.org/10.3341/kjo.2020.0122] [PMID: 34344137]

[32] Rogers S, McIntosh RL, Cheung N, *et al.* The prevalence of retinal vein occlusion: Pooled data from population studies from the United States, Europe, Asia, and Australia. Ophthalmology 2010; 117(2): 313-319.e1.

[http://dx.doi.org/10.1016/j.ophtha.2009.07.017] [PMID: 20022117]

[33] Wong TY, Scott IU. Retinal-vein occlusion. N Engl J Med 2010; 363(22): 2135-44. [http://dx.doi.org/10.1056/NEJMcp1003934] [PMID: 21105795]

[34] Bonini Filho MA, Adhi M, de Carlo TE, *et al.* Optical coherence tomography angiography in retinal artery occlusion. Retina 2015; 35(11): 2339-46. [http://dx.doi.org/10.1097/IAE.0000000000000850] [PMID: 26457398]

[35] Glacet-Bernard A, Sellam A, Coscas F, Coscas G, Souied EH. Optical coherence tomography angiography in retinal vein occlusion treated with dexamethasone implant: A new test for follow-up evaluation. Eur J Ophthalmol 2016; 26(5): 460-8. [http://dx.doi.org/10.5301/ejo.5000829] [PMID: 27405288]

[36] Adhi M, Filho MAB, Louzada RN, *et al.* Retinal capillary network and foveal avascular zone in eyes with vein occlusion and fellow eyes analyzed with optical coherence tomography angiography. Invest Ophthalmol Vis Sci 2016; 57(9): OCT486-94. [http://dx.doi.org/10.1167/iovs.15-18907] [PMID: 27442342]

[37] Suzuki N, Hirano Y, Yoshida M, *et al.* Microvascular abnormalities on optical coherence tomography angiography in macular edema associated with branch retinal vein occlusion. Am J Ophthalmol 2016; 161: 126-132.e1. [http://dx.doi.org/10.1016/j.ajo.2015.09.038] [PMID: 26454243]

[38] Moussa M, Leila M, Bessa AS, *et al.* Grading of macular perfusion in retinal vein occlusion using en-face swept-source optical coherence tomography angiography: A retrospective observational case series. BMC Ophthalmol 2019; 19(1): 127. [http://dx.doi.org/10.1186/s12886-019-1134-x] [PMID: 31182069]

[39] Coscas F, Glacet-Bernard A, Miere A, *et al.* Optical coherence tomography angiography in retinal vein occlusion: Evaluation of superficial and deep capillary plexa. Am J Ophthalmol 2016; 161: 160-171.e2, 2. [http://dx.doi.org/10.1016/j.ajo.2015.10.008] [PMID: 26476211]

[40] Singh RP, Tsai G, Banaee T, Conti FF. Optical coherence tomography angiography in eyes with retinal vein occlusion. J Ophthalmic Vis Res 2018; 13(3): 315-32. [http://dx.doi.org/10.4103/jovr.jovr_264_17] [PMID: 30090189]

[41] Rispoli M, Savastano MC, Lumbroso B. Capillary network anomalies in branch retinal vein occlusion on optical coherence tomography angiography. Retina 2015; 35(11): 2332-8. [http://dx.doi.org/10.1097/IAE.0000000000000845] [PMID: 26502008]

[42] Mastropasqua R, Toto L, Di Antonio L, *et al.* Optical coherence tomography angiography microvascular findings in macular edema due to central and branch retinal vein occlusions. Sci Rep 2017; 7(1): 40763. [http://dx.doi.org/10.1038/srep40763] [PMID: 28098203]

[43] Kashani AH, Lee SY, Moshfeghi A, Durbin MK, Puliafito CA. Optical coherence tomography angiography of retinal venous occlusion. Retina 2015; 35(11): 2323-31. [http://dx.doi.org/10.1097/IAE.0000000000000811] [PMID: 26457395]

[44] Sogawa K, Nagaoka T, Ishibazawa A, Takahashi A, Tani T, Yoshida A. En-face optical coherence tomography angiography of neovascularization elsewhere in hemicentral retinal vein occlusion. Int Med Case Rep J 2015; 8(Oct): 263-6. [http://dx.doi.org/10.2147/IMCRJ.S93702] [PMID: 26604832]

[45] Kadomoto S, Muraoka Y, Ooto S, *et al.* Evaluation of macular ischemia in eyes with branch retinal vein occlusion. Retina 2018; 38(2): 272-82. [http://dx.doi.org/10.1097/IAE.0000000000001541] [PMID: 28221256]

[46] Koulisis N, Kim AY, Chu Z, *et al.* Quantitative microvascular analysis of retinal venous occlusions by spectral domain optical coherence tomography angiography. PLoS One 2017; 12(4): e0176404.

[http://dx.doi.org/10.1371/journal.pone.0176404] [PMID: 28437483]

[47] Khodabandeh A, Shahraki K, Roohipoor R, *et al.* Quantitative measurement of vascular density and flow using optical coherence tomography angiography (OCTA) in patients with central retinal vein occlusion: Can OCTA help in distinguishing ischemic from non-ischemic type? Int J Retina Vitreous 2018; 4(1): 47. [http://dx.doi.org/10.1186/s40942-018-0152-9] [PMID: 30607260]

[48] Casalino G, Williams M, McAvoy C, Bandello F, Chakravarthy U. Optical coherence tomography angiography in paracentral acute middle maculopathy secondary to central retinal vein occlusion. Eye 2016; 30(6): 888-93. [http://dx.doi.org/10.1038/eye.2016.57] [PMID: 27034199]

[49] Dansingani KK, Inoue M, Engelbert M, Freund KB. Optical coherence tomographic angiography shows reduced deep capillary flow in paracentral acute middle maculopathy. Eye 2015; 29(12): 1620-4. [http://dx.doi.org/10.1038/eye.2015.180] [PMID: 26381094]

[50] He F, Yu W. Longitudinal neovascular changes on optical coherence tomography angiography in proliferative diabetic retinopathy treated with panretinal photocoagulation alone versus with intravitreal conbercept plus panretinal photocoagulation: A pilot study. Eye 2020; 34(8): 1413-8. [http://dx.doi.org/10.1038/s41433-019-0628-3] [PMID: 31719675]

[51] Clarkson JG, Chuang E, Gass D, *et al.* Evaluation of grid pattern photocoagulation for macular edema in central vein occlusion. The Central Vein Occlusion Study Group M report. Ophthalmology 1995; 102(10): 1425-33. [http://dx.doi.org/10.1016/S0161-6420(95)30849-4] [PMID: 9097788]

[52] The Branch Vein Occlusion Study Group. Argon laser photocoagulation for macular edema in branch vein occlusion. Am J Ophthalmol 1984; 98(3): 271-82. [http://dx.doi.org/10.1016/0002-9394(84)90316-7] [PMID: 6383055]

[53] Branch Vein Occlusion Study Group. Argon laser scatter photocoagulation for prevention of neovascularization and vitreous hemorrhage in branch vein occlusion. A randomized clinical trial. Arch Ophthalmol 1986; 104(1): 34-41. [http://dx.doi.org/10.1001/archopht.1986.01050130044017] [PMID: 2417579]

[54] Scott IU, Ip MS, VanVeldhuisen PC, *et al.* A randomized trial comparing the efficacy and safety of intravitreal triamcinolone with standard care to treat vision loss associated with macular Edema secondary to branch retinal vein occlusion: The Standard Care vs Corticosteroid for Retinal Vein Occlusion (SCORE) study report 6. Arch Ophthalmol 2009; 127(9): 1115-28. [http://dx.doi.org/10.1001/archophthalmol.2009.233] [PMID: 19752420]

[55] Ip MS, Scott IU, VanVeldhuisen PC, *et al.* A randomized trial comparing the efficacy and safety of intravitreal triamcinolone with observation to treat vision loss associated with macular edema secondary to central retinal vein occlusion: The Standard Care vs Corticosteroid for Retinal Vein Occlusion (SCORE) study report 5. Arch Ophthalmol 2009; 127(9): 1101-14. [http://dx.doi.org/10.1001/archophthalmol.2009.234] [PMID: 19752419]

[56] Haller JA, Bandello F, Belfort R Jr, *et al.* Randomized, sham-controlled trial of dexamethasone intravitreal implant in patients with macular edema due to retinal vein occlusion. Ophthalmology 2010; 117(6): 1134-1146.e3. [http://dx.doi.org/10.1016/j.ophtha.2010.03.032] [PMID: 20417567]

[57] Qian T, Zhao M, Xu X. Comparison between anti-VEGF therapy and corticosteroid or laser therapy for macular oedema secondary to retinal vein occlusion: A meta-analysis. J Clin Pharm Ther 2017; 42(5): 519-29. [http://dx.doi.org/10.1111/jcpt.12551] [PMID: 28639290]

[58] Campochiaro PA, Akhlaq A. Sustained suppression of VEGF for treatment of retinal/choroidal vascular diseases. Prog Retin Eye Res 2021; 83: 100921.

[http://dx.doi.org/10.1016/j.preteyeres.2020.100921] [PMID: 33248215]

[59] Stahl A, Buchwald A, Martin G, *et al.* Vitreal levels of erythropoietin are increased in patients with retinal vein occlusion and correlate with vitreal VEGF and the extent of macular edema. Retina 2010; 30(9): 1524-9.
[http://dx.doi.org/10.1097/IAE.0b013e3181d37539] [PMID: 20664492]

[60] Brown DM, Campochiaro PA, Singh RP, *et al.* Ranibizumab for macular edema following central retinal vein occlusion: six-month primary end point results of a phase III study. Ophthalmology 2010; 117(6): 1124-1133.e1.
[http://dx.doi.org/10.1016/j.ophtha.2010.02.022] [PMID: 20381871]

[61] Campochiaro PA, Heier JS, Feiner L, *et al.* Ranibizumab for macular edema following branch retinal vein occlusion: Six-month primary end point results of a phase III study. Ophthalmology 2010; 117(6): 1102-1112.e1.
[http://dx.doi.org/10.1016/j.ophtha.2010.02.021] [PMID: 20398941]

[62] Brown DM, Campochiaro PA, Bhisitkul RB, *et al.* Sustained benefits from ranibizumab for macular edema following branch retinal vein occlusion: 12-month outcomes of a phase III study. Ophthalmology 2011; 118(8): 1594-602.
[http://dx.doi.org/10.1016/j.ophtha.2011.02.022] [PMID: 21684606]

[63] Campochiaro PA, Brown DM, Awh CC, *et al.* Sustained benefits from ranibizumab for macular edema following central retinal vein occlusion: Twelve-month outcomes of a phase III study. Ophthalmology 2011; 118(10): 2041-9.
[http://dx.doi.org/10.1016/j.ophtha.2011.02.038] [PMID: 21715011]

[64] Heier JS, Campochiaro PA, Yau L, *et al.* Ranibizumab for macular edema due to retinal vein occlusions: Long-term follow-up in the HORIZON trial. Ophthalmology 2012; 119(4): 802-9.
[http://dx.doi.org/10.1016/j.ophtha.2011.12.005] [PMID: 22301066]

[65] Iida-Miwa Y, Muraoka Y, Iida Y, *et al.* Branch retinal vein occlusion: Treatment outcomes according to the retinal nonperfusion area, clinical subtype, and crossing pattern. Sci Rep 2019; 9(1): 6569.
[http://dx.doi.org/10.1038/s41598-019-42982-5] [PMID: 31024035]

[66] Zhang H, Liu ZL, Sun P, Gu F. Intravitreal bevacizumab for treatment of macular edema secondary to central retinal vein occlusion: Eighteen-month results of a prospective trial. J Ocul Pharmacol Ther 2011; 27(6): 615-21.
[http://dx.doi.org/10.1089/jop.2011.0050] [PMID: 21823986]

[67] Choi KE, Yun C, Cha J, Kim SW. OCT angiography features associated with macular edema recurrence after intravitreal bevacizumab treatment in branch retinal vein occlusion. Sci Rep 2019; 9(1): 14153.
[http://dx.doi.org/10.1038/s41598-019-50637-8] [PMID: 31578437]

[68] Brown DM, Heier JS, Clark WL, *et al.* Intravitreal aflibercept injection for macular edema secondary to central retinal vein occlusion: 1-year results from the phase 3 copernicus study. Am J Ophthalmol 2013; 155(3): 429-437.e7.
[http://dx.doi.org/10.1016/j.ajo.2012.09.026] [PMID: 23218699]

[69] Campochiaro PA, Clark WL, Boyer DS, *et al.* Intravitreal aflibercept for macular edema following branch retinal vein occlusion: The 24-week results of the VIBRANT study. Ophthalmology 2015; 122(3): 538-44.
[http://dx.doi.org/10.1016/j.ophtha.2014.08.031] [PMID: 25315663]

[70] Ghashut R, Muraoka Y, Ooto S, *et al.* Evaluation of macular ischemia in eyes with central retinal vein occlusion. Retina 2018; 38(8): 1571-80.
[http://dx.doi.org/10.1097/IAE.0000000000001749] [PMID: 28671896]

[71] Amer AA, Aldghaimy AH, Abdellah MM. Ranibizumab versus aflibercept for macular edema secondary to nonischemic central retinal vein occlusion in young adult patients. Res Sq 2022.
[http://dx.doi.org/10.21203/rs.3.rs-1490565/v1]

[72] A study to evaluate the efficacy and safety of faricimab in participants with macular edema secondary to branch retinal vein occlusion (BALATON). Available from: https://clinicaltrials.gov/ct2/show/NCT04740905

[73] A study to evaluate the efficacy and safety of faricimab in participants with macular edema secondary to central retinal or hemiretinal vein occlusion (COMINO). Available from:https://clinicaltrials.gov/ct2/show/NCT04740931

[74] Heier JS, Singh RP, Wykoff CC, *et al.* The angiopoietin/tie pathway in retinal vascular diseases. Retina 2021; 41(1): 1-19.
[http://dx.doi.org/10.1097/IAE.0000000000003003] [PMID: 33136975]

[75] FDA Approves genentech's susvimo, a first-of-its-kind therapeutic approach for wet age-related macular degeneration (AMD). Available from: https://www.gene.com/media/press-releases/14935/2021-10-22/fda-approves-genentechs-susvimo-a-first-

[76] Ranade S v, Wieland MR, Tam T, Rea JC, Horvath J, Hieb AR. The port delivery system with ranibizumab: A new paradigm for long-acting retinal drug delivery. Drug Delivery 2022; 29(1): 1326-234.

[77] Ghanchi F, Bourne R, Downes SM, *et al.* An update on long-acting therapies in chronic sight-threatening eye diseases of the posterior segment: AMD, DMO, RVO, uveitis and glaucoma. Eye 2022; 36(6): 1154-67.
[http://dx.doi.org/10.1038/s41433-021-01766-w] [PMID: 34974541]

Supplementary Material

Table S1. Shapiro-Wilk normality test results in the Buckled group.

S. No.	Object	W	p value
1	Age	0.954	**0.001**
2	Preoperative BCVA (logMAR)	0.930	**0.001**
3	Postoperative BCVA (logMAR)	0.790	**0.001**
4	ERM Detection (weeks)	0.961	0.319
5	BCVA after ERM surgery (logMAR)	0.951	0.211
6	CSFT (microns)	0.888	**0.001**
7	Follow-up period (months)	0.959	**0.001**

The variables that do not follow a normal distribution are in bold writing ($p<0.05$).
W (Shapiro-Wilk normality test): BCVA: best corrected visual acuity; CSFT: central subfoveal thickness.

Table S2. Descriptive statistics for the numeric variables in the Buckle group.

S. No.	Object	Mean	Min	Max	Standard Deviation	Length of Sample (n=125)
1	Age (years)	44.34	18.00	76.00	15.94	125
2	Preoperative macula-off (weeks)	3.60	1.00	12.00	2.47	125
3	Preoperative BCVA (logMAR)	1.03	0.48	1.60	0.28	125
4	Postoperative BCVA (logMAR)	0.40	0.10	1.30	0.33	125
5	ERM detection (weeks)	11.93	5.00	22.00	4.59	125
6	BCVA after ERM surgery(logMAR)	0.43	0.18	0.70	0.14	125
7	CSFT (microns)	243.57	32.00	402.00	41.95	125
8	Follow-up period (months)	26.11	2.00	73.00	13.42	125

Non-parametric Mann-Whitney U-test. min: minimum; max: maximum; BCVA: best corrected visual acuity; ERM: epiretinal membrane; CSFT: central subfoveal thickness.

Table S3. Summarized statistics for the categorical variables in the Buckle group.

Variable	Value	n	Freq
Sex	Female	75	0.6
	Male	50	0.4

Miguel A. Quiroz-Reyes and Virgilio Lima-Gomez (Eds.)

(Table S3) cont.....

Eye	Left	59	0.472
	Right	66	0.528
Preop Lens Status	Phakic	98	0.784
	Pseudophakic	27	0.216
Preop BCVA	20/100	26	0.208
	20/160	14	0.112
	20/200	35	0.28
	20/300	12	0.096
	20/400	21	0.168
	20/60	1	0.008
	20/70	3	0.024
	20/80	2	0.016
	20/800	11	0.088
Postop BCVA	20/100	11	0.088
	20/120	1	0.008
	20/160	1	0.008
	20/200	4	0.032
	20/25	16	0.128
	20/30	35	0.28
	20/300	3	0.024
	20/40	31	0.248
	20/400	6	0.048
	20/50	4	0.032
	20/60	8	0.064
	20/70	1	0.008
	20/80	4	0.032
Redetachment	No	114	0.912
	Yes	11	0.088

(Table S3) cont.....

Additional Surgery		114	0.912
	BUCKLE REVISION	4	0.032
	PHAKO-VITRECTOMY	3	0.024
	PHAKO-VITRECTOMY-ERM PEELING	1	0.008
	VITRECTOMY	2	0.016
	VITRECTOMY-ERM PEELING	1	0.008
Postop ERM proliferations	No	96	0.768
	Yes	29	0.232
ERM Surgery	No	98	0.784
	Yes	27	0.216
BCVA after ERM surgery		97	0.776
	20/100	2	0.016
	20/30	2	0.016
	20/40	7	0.056
	20/50	6	0.048
	20/60	4	0.032
	20/70	4	0.032
	20/80	3	0.024
Retinal perforation	No	118	0.944
	Yes	7	0.056
Submacular blood	No	120	0.96
	Yes	5	0.04
Through and through scleral drainage complication phenomenon	No	117	0.936
	Yes	8	0.064
Retinal entrapment	No	122	0.976
	Yes	3	0.024
Foveal contour OCT alterations	Normal	14	0.112
	Abnormal	19	0.152
	Normal	92	0.736
Ellipsoid band OCT alterations		14	0.112
	Disrupted	25	0.2
	Normal	86	0.688

(Table S3) cont.....

DONFL OCT defects		14	0.112
	Not Present	80	0.64
	Present	31	0.248
ELM line OCT alterations		15	0.12
	Abnormal	24	0.192
	Normal	86	0.688
mfERG registration		26	0.208
	Abnormal	54	0.432
	Normal	45	0.36
Microperimetry results		18	0.144
	Abnormal	51	0.408
	Normal	56	0.448

Fisher's exact test. freq: frequency; preop: preoperative: postop: postoperative: BCVA: best corrected visual acuity; CSFT: central subfoveal thickness; ERM: epiretinal membrane; DONFL: diffuse optic nerve fiber layer; ELM: external limiting membrane: mfERG: multifocal electroretinography.

Table S4. Correlations among the numeric variables in the Buckle group (sample size N=125 eyes).

	Age	Preoperative macula-off (weeks)	Preoperative BCVA (logMAR)	Postoperative BCVA (logMAR)	ERM Detection (weeks)	BCVA After ERM Surgery (logMAR)	CSFT (microns)	Follow-up Period (months)
Age	1 (p=NA)							
Preoperative macula-off (weeks)	0.12 (p=0.17)	1 (p=NA)						
Preoperative BCVA (logMAR)	0.01 (p=0.88)	0.04 (p=0.63)	1 (p=NA)					
Postoperative BCVA (logMAR)	-0.06 (p=0.48)	-0.02 (p=0.78)	0.02 (p=0.85)	1 (p=NA)				
ERM detection (weeks)	-0.27 (p=0.15)	-0.19 (p=0.31)	-0.19 (p=0.31)	0.06 (p=0.74)	1 (p=NA)			

(Table S4) cont.....

BCVA after ERM surgery (logMAR)	0.05 (p=0.79)	-0.21 (p=0.28)	0.26 (p=0.17)	**0.57 (p=0.00)**	0.04 (p=0.82)	1 (p=NA)		
CSFT (microns)	0.01 (p=0.9)	0.01 (p=0.93)	0.09 (p=0.37)	0.13 (p=0.17)	0.04 (p=0.85)	-0.06 (p=0.78)	1 (p=NA)	
Follow-up period (months)	-0.17 (p=0.06)	-0.17 (p=0.06)	0.03 (p=0.71)	**-0.2 (p=0.03)**	0.08 (p=0.68)	-0.05 (p=0.79)	0.12 (p=0.2)	1 (p=NA)

Spearman's rank correlation coefficient test. The significant correlations are in bold text. BCVA: best corrected visual acuity; ERM: epiretinal membrane; CSFT: central subfoveal thickness; NA: not applicable.

Table S5. Mann-Whitney U tests results in the Buckle group (N=125 eyes). (a) Preoperative best-corrected visual acuity (BCVA). (b) Postoperative BCVA. (c) BCVA after epiretinal membrane surgery.

(a) preoperative BCVA (logMAR) Mann-Whitney U tests results	-	-
Object	U	**p value**
Age	7875	**0.001**
Preoperative macula-off (weeks)	7140	**0.001**
Postoperative BCVA (logMAR)	201.5	**0.001**
ERM detection (weeks)	465	**0.001**
BCVA after ERM surgery (logMAR)	0	**0.001**
CSFT (microns)	6105	**0.001**
Follow-up period (months)	7875	**0.001**
(b) postoperative BCVA (logMAR) Mann-Whitney U tests results		
Object	U	**p value**
Age	7875	**0.001**
Preoperative macula-off (weeks)	7866	**0.001**
Preoperative BCVA (logMAR)	7301.5	**0.001**
ERM detection (weeks)	465	**0.001**
BCVA after ERM surgery (logMAR)	0	**0.001**
CSFT (microns)	6105	**0.001**
Follow-up period (months)	7875	**0.001**
(c) BCVA after ERM surgery (logMAR) Mann–Whitney U tests results		
Object	U	**p value**
Age	406	**0.001**

(Table S5) cont.....

Preoperative macula-off (weeks)	406	**0.001**
Preoperative BCVA (logMAR)	378	**0.001**
Postoperative BCVA (logMAR)	406	**0.001**
ERM detection (weeks)	406	**0.001**
CSFT (microns)	406	**0.001**
Follow-up period (months)	406	**0.001**

Mann-Whitney U tests. The statistically significant variables ($p < 0.05$) are in bold text. U test BCVA: best corrected visual acuity; ERM: epiretinal membrane; CSFT: central subfoveal thickness.

Table S6. Kruskal-Wallis test results in the Buckle group.

(a) Kruskal-Wallis test results of the preoperative best-corrected visual acuity (BCVA) with the categorical variables.

S. No.	**Object**	**Kruskal-Wallis x^2.**	**df**	**p value**	**Number of eyes**	**No of NAs**
1	Male	3.117	1	0.077	125	0
2	Eye	2.132	1	0.144	125	0
3	Preoperative Lens Status	0.130	1	0.718	125	0
4	**Preoperative BCVA**	**124.000**	**8**	**0.000**	**125**	**0**
5	Postoperative BCVA	5.342	12	0.946	125	0
6	Re-Detachment	1.018	1	0.313	125	0
7	Additional surgery	1.238	4	0.872	125	114
8	Postoperative ERM proliferations	0.035	1	0.851	125	0
9	ERM surgery	0.090	1	0.764	125	0
10	BCVA after ERM surgery	4.763	6	0.575	125	97
11	Retinal perforation	0.222	1	0.638	125	0
12	Submacular blood	1.057	1	0.304	125	0
13	Through and through	2.829	1	0.093	125	0
14	Retinal entrapment	0.001	1	0.980	125	0
15	Foveal contour	0.006	1	0.936	125	14
16	Ellipsoid	0.236	1	0.627	125	14
17	DONFL	1.581	1	0.209	125	14
18	ELM	0.384	1	0.535	125	15
19	mfERG	0.242	1	0.623	125	26
20	Microperimetry	0.653	1	0.419	125	18

(Table S6) cont.....

(b) Kruskal-Wallis test results of the postoperative BCVA with the categorical variables.

S. No.	Object	Kruskal-Wallis x^2.	df	p value	Number of eyes	No of NAs
1	Male	0.026	1	0.871	125	0
2	Eye	0.047	1	0.828	125	0
3	Preoperative Lens Status	0.234	1	0.629	125	0
4	Preoperative BCVA	3.950	8	0.862	125	0
5	**Postoperative BCVA**	**124.000**	**12**	**0.000**	**125**	**0**
6	**Re-Detachment**	**7.484**	**1**	**0.006**	**125**	**0**
7	Additional surgery	5.331	4	0.255	125	114
8	**Postoperative ERM proliferations**	**68.187**	**1**	**0.000**	**125**	**0**
9	**ERM surgery**	**63.098**	**1**	**0.000**	**125**	**0**
10	**BCVA after ERM surgery**	**13.048**	**6**	**0.042**	**125**	**97**
11	Retinal perforation	1.214	1	0.271	125	0
12	**Submacular blood**	**9.449**	**1**	**0.002**	**125**	**0**
13	Through and Through	0.357	1	0.550	125	0
14	Retinal Entrapment	0.612	1	0.434	125	0
15	**Foveal contour**	**15.821**	**1**	**0.000**	**125**	**14**
16	Ellipsoid	3.479	1	0.062	125	14
17	**DONFL**	**18.677**	**1**	**0.000**	**125**	**14**
18	ELM	0.303	1	0.582	125	15
19	**mfERG**	**20.558**	**1**	**0.000**	**125**	**26**
20	**Microperimetry**	**11.826**	**1**	**0.001**	**125**	**18**

(c) Kruskal-Wallis tests results of the BCVA after epiretinal membrane surgery with the categorical variables.

S. No.	Object	Kruskal-Wallis x^2.	df	p value	Number of eyes	No of NAs
1	Male	0.499	1	0.480	125	0
2	Eye	0.967	1	0.325	125	0
3	Preoperative Lens Status	1.070	1	0.301	125	0
4	Preoperative BCVA	6.587	7	0.473	125	0
5	Postoperative BCVA	11.572	6	0.072	125	0
6	Re-Detachment	0.428	1	0.513	125	0
7	Additional surgery	1.716	3	0.633	125	114

(Table S6) cont.....

8	Postoperative ERM proliferations	0.063	1	0.801	125	0
9	ERM surgery	0.063	1	0.801	125	0
10	BCVA after ERM surgery	27.000	6	**0.000**	125	97
11	Retinal perforation	1.847	1	0.174	125	0
12	Submacular blood	2.783	1	0.095	125	0
13	Through and Through	1.144	1	0.285	125	0
14	Retinal entrapment	0.776	1	0.378	125	0
15	Foveal contour	0.178	1	0.673	125	14
16	Ellipsoid	1.235	1	0.266	125	14
17	DONFL	1.230	1	0.267	125	14
18	ELM	0.138	1	0.710	125	15
19	mfERG	0.115	1	0.734	125	26
20	Microperimetry	1.033	1	0.310	125	18

The statistically significant variables ($p < 0.05$) are in bold text. df: difference no: number; NA: not applicable; BCVA: best corrected visual acuity; ERM: epiretinal membrane; DONFL: diffuse optic nerve fiber layer; ELM: external limiting membrane: mfERG: multifocal electroretinography.

Table S7. Generalized linear model results of the preoperative best-corrected visual acuity (BCVA), postoperative BCVA, and BCVA after epiretinal membrane surgery in the Buckle group (n=125 eyes).

Preoperative BVCA	**Estimate**	**Std. Error**	**t value**	**Pr(>|t|)**	
(Intercept)	0.972	0.033	29.046	**<2e-16**	***
Sex Male	0.106	0.051	2.07	**0.040**	*
Through and Through scleral drainage complication phenomenon	0.164	0.102	1.605	**0.111**	
Generalized	-	-	-	-	-
Postoperative BCVA	**Estimate**	**Std. Error**	**t value**	**Pr(>|t|)**	
(Intercept)	0.218	0.056	3.854	**0.001**	***
Postop ERM proliferations	0.676	0.035	19.055	**< 2e-16**	***
Retinal entrapment	-0.206	0.097	-2.112	**0.036**	*
Preop BCVA logMAR	0.029	0.052	0.567	0.572	
BCVA after ERM surgery	**Estimate**	**Std. Error**	**t value**	**Pr(>|t|)**	
(Intercept)	-0.170	0.130	-1.303	0.206	
Post BCVA logMAR	0.323	0.080	4.003	**0.001**	***

(Table S7) cont.....

Preop BCVA logMAR	0.194	0.072	2.694	**0.013**	*
Retinal perforation	0.151	0.067	2.251	**0.034**	*
Age	0.002	0.001	1.712	0.100	
Sex Male	-0.021	0.043	-0.498	0.623	

The statistically significant variables ($p < 0.05$) are in bold text and marked with *.
Pr: Probabilities using the t distribution, gives the p-value for that t-test; BCVA: best corrected visual acuity; Postop: postoperative; Preop: preoperative: ERM: epiretinal membrane.

Table S8. Shapiro-Wilk normality test results in the Vitrectomy group (n=105 eyes).

Object	**W**	**P value**
Age (years)	0.974	**0.039**
Macula-off (weeks)	0.924	**0.001**
Preoperative BCVA (logMAR)	0.923	**0.001**
Follow-up period (days)	0.971	**0.023**
BCVA before ERM-ILM removal (logMAR)	0.888	**0.001**
Final postoperative BCVA (logMAR)	0.924	**0.001**
CSFT (microns)	0.939	**0.008**
Follow-up period (months)	0.970	**0.023**

The variables that do not follow a normal distribution are in bold text ($p < 0.05$). BCVA: best corrected visual acuity; ERM: epiretinal membrane; ILM: internal limiting membrane; CSFT: central subfoveal thickness.

Table S9. Descriptive statistics for the numeric variables in the Vitrectomy group.

Object	**Mean**	**Min**	**Max**	**Standard Deviation**
Age (years)	47.92	18.00	76.00	14.60
Macula-off (weeks)	4.42	1.00	12.00	2.56
Preoperative BCVA (logMAR)	1.06	0.54	1.60	0.27
Follow-up period (months)	24.2	1.0	58.66	13.02
BCVA before ERM-ILM removal (logMAR)	0.52	0.10	1.30	0.36
ERM detection (weeks)	13.75	5.00	30.00	5.33
Final postoperative BCVA (logMAR)	0.37	0.10	1.00	0.20
CSFT (microns)	256.55	198.00	320.00	35.16
Follow-up period (months)	23.42	1.00	57.00	12.98

Wilcoxon rank sum test. Min: minimum; Max: maximum; BCVA: best corrected visual acuity; ERM: epiretinal membrane; ILM: internal limiting membrane; CSFT: central subfoveal thickness.

Table S10. Summarized statistics for the categorical variables in the vitrectomy group (peeling and nonpeeling groups).

Variable	Group	n	freq	% freq
Additional Surgery	BUCKLE REVISION	3	0.03	2.9%
	No	92	0.88	87.6%
	PHAKO VITRECTOMY ERM PEELING	1	0.01	1.0%
	VITRECTOMY	2	0.02	1.9%
	VITRECTOMY REVISION	7	0.07	6.7%
DONFL	Absent	34	0.32	32.4%
	Present	60	0.57	57.1%
	NA	11	0.10	10.5%
Ellipsoid	Disrupted	29	0.28	27.6%
	Normal	76	0.72	72.4%
ELM	Disrupted	27	0.26	25.7%
	Normal	74	0.70	70.5%
	NA	4	0.04	3.8%
ERM 2nd Surgery	VIT and MACULA REVISION	1	0.01	1.0%
	VIT REVISION ERM-ILM REMOVAL	45	0.43	42.9%
	VIT REVISION ERM-ILM REMOVAL	5	0.05	4.8%
	VIT REVISION ERM-ILM REMOVAL	1	0.01	1.0%
	NA	53	0.50	50.5%
Eye	Left	50	0.48	47.6%
	Right	55	0.52	52.4%
First Surgery	BUCKLE	27	0.26	25.7%
	ONLY VITRECTOMY	68	0.65	64.8%
	VIT ERM-ILM REMOVAL	10	0.10	9.5%
Foveal contour	Abnormal	24	0.23	22.9%
	Normal	77	0.73	73.3%
	NA	4	0.04	3.8%
Sex	Female	37	0.35	35.2%
	Male	68	0.65	64.8%

(Table S10) cont.....

mfERG	Abnormal	43	0.41	41.0%
	Normal	30	0.29	28.6%
	NA	32	0.30	30.5%
Microperimetry	Abnormal	35	0.33	33.3%
	Normal	42	0.40	40.0%
	NA	28	0.27	26.7%
Postoperative ERM proliferations	No	54	0.51	51.4%
	Yes	51	0.49	48.6%
Preoperative ERM proliferations	No	55	0.52	52.4%
	Yes	50	0.48	47.6%
Preop Lens Status	Phakic	68	0.65	64.8%
	Pseudophakic	37	0.35	35.2%
Recurrent RRD	No	92	0.88	87.6%
	Yes	13	0.12	12.4%

Fisher's exact test. freq: frequency; ERM: epiretinal membrane; DONFL: diffuse optic nerve fiber layer; ELM: external limiting membrane; VIT: vitrectomy; ILM: internal limiting membrane; mfERG: multifocal electroretinography; RRD: rhegmatogenous retinal detachment.

Table S11. Descriptive statistics with respect to the Vitrectomy (preoperative ERM proliferations) group (nonpeeling and peeling).

Vitrectomy groups	**Nonpeeling**	**Peeling**	**p**	-
	(N=55)	(N=50)	-	-
	-	-	-	-
Age	50.455 ± 13.52	45.140 ±15.36	0.054	-
	-	-	-	-
Sex	-	-	1	-
- Female	19 (34.545%)	18 (36.0%)	-	-
- Male	36 (65.455%)	32 (64.0%)	-	-
	-	-	-	-
Eye	-	-	0.698	-
- Left	25 (45.455%)	25 (50.0%)	-	-
- Right	30 (54.545%)	25 (50.0%)	-	-
	-	-	-	-

(Table S11) cont.....

Preoperative Lens Status	-	-	0.068	-
- Phakic	31 (56.364%)	37 (74.0%)	-	-
- Pseudophakic	24 (43.636%)	13 (26.0%)	-	-
	-	-	-	-
Macula-off (weeks)	4.527 ±2.403	4.300 ±2.750	0.425	-
	-	-	-	-
Preoperative BCVA (logMAR)	1.036 ±0.258	1.077 ±0.277	0.386	-
	-	-	-	-
Follow-up period (days)	768.6 ±373.01	679.90 ±407.98	0.131	-
	-	-	-	-
First Surgery	-	-	**0**	***
- BUCKLE	0 (0.0%)	27 (54.0%)	-	-
- ONLY VITRECTOMY	55 (100.000%)	13 (26.0%)	-	-
- VIT ERM and ILM REMOVAL	0 (0.0%)	10 (20.0%)	-	-
BCVA Before ERM-ILM removal (logMAR)	**0.297 ±0.23**	**0.756 ±0.319**	**0.001**	***
Recurrent RRD			**0.001**	***
- No	54 (98.182%)	38 (76.0%)		
- YES	1 (1.818%)	12 (24.0%)		
Additional Surgery			**0.004**	***
- BUCKLE REVISION	0 (0.0%)	3 (6.0%)		
- No	54 (98.182%)	38 (76.0%)		
- PHAKO VITRECTOMY ERM PEELING	0 (0.0%)	1 (2.0%)		
- VITRECTOMY	0 (0.0%)	2 (4.0%)		
- VITRECTOMY REVISION	1 (1.818%)	6 (12.0%)		
ERM Detection (weeks)	**18.00 ±6.45**	**12.575 ±4.385**	**0.009**	***
ERM 2nd Surgery			**0**	***
- VIT and MACULA REVISION	0 (0.0%)	1 (2.439%)		
- VIT REVISION ERM and ILM	5 (45.455%)	40 (97.561%)		
- VIT REVISION ERM and ILM REMOVAL	5 (45.455%)	0 (0.0%)		
- VIT REVISION ERM.ILM REMOVAL	1 (9.091%)	0 (0.0%)		
Final Postoperative BCVA (logMAR)	**0.280 ±0.192**	**0.477 ±0.161**	**0.001**	***

(Table S11) cont.....

CSFT (microns)	266.71 ±32.75	253.073 ±35.66	0.173	
Foveal Contour			**0.002**	***
- Abnormal	6 (11.321%)	18 (37.5%)		
- Normal	47 (88.679%)	30 (62.5%)		
Ellipsoid integrity			0.828	
- Disrupted	16 (29.091%)	13 (26.0%)		
- Normal	39 (70.909%)	37 (74.0%)		
DONFL defects			**0**	***
- Absent	39 (88.63%)	21 (42.0%)		
- Present	5 (11.36%)	29 (58.0%)		
ELM line appearance			0.654	
- Disrupted	16 (29.091%)	11 (23.913%)		
- Normal	39 (70.909%)	35 (76.087%)		
mfERG result			**0**	***
- Abnormal	13 (33.333%)	30 (88.235%)		
- Normal	26 (66.667%)	4 (11.765%)		
Microperimetry evaluation			**0**	***
- Abnormal	11 (25.581%)	24 (70.588%)		
- Normal	32 (74.419%)	10 (29.412%)		
Follow-up period (months)	24.80 ±12.34	21.880 ±13.324	0.133	

The p-values (p) are the results from the Wilcoxon rank sum test for the numerical variables and Fisher's Exact test for the categorical variables. The variables that showed a statistically significant difference ($p < 0.05$) among the groups of the peeling (preoperative ERM proliferation) are in bold text and marked with *. sig: significance ; BCVA: best corrected visual acuity; VIT: vitrectomy; ERM: epiretinal membrane; ILM: internal limiting membrane; RRD: rhegmatogenous retinal detachment; CSFT: central subfoveal thickness; DONFL: diffuse optic nerve fiber layer; ELM: external limiting membrane: mfERG: multifocal electroretinography.

Table S12. Correlations among the numeric variables in the Vitrectomy group (peeling and nonpeeling groups).

	Age	**Preoperative Macula-Off (weeks)**	**Preoperative BCVA (logMAR)**	**BCVA Before ERM and ILM removal (logMAR)**	**ERM Detection (Weeks)**	**Final Postoperative BCVA (logMAR)**	**CSFT (microns)**	**Follow-up period (months)**
Age	1							
Preoperative Macula-off (weeks)	0.03 (p=0.78)	1						
Preoperative BCVA (logMAR)	-0.07 (p=0.47)	0.04 (p=0.68)	1					
BCVA Before ERM and ILM removal (logMAR)	-0.18 (p=0.07)	-0.16 (p=0.1)	-0.10 (p=0.33)	1				
ERM Detection (weeks)	-0.18 (p=0.21)	0.03 (p=0.83)	**-0.29 (p=0.04)**	-0.16 (p=0.26)	1			
Final Postoperative BCVA (logMAR)	-0.04 (p=0.72)	-0.05 (p=0.62)	0.10 (p=0.3)	**0.78 (p=0)**	0.04 (p=0.76)	1		
CSFT (microns)	0.15 (p=0.28)	**0.32 (p=0.02)**	0.02 (p=0.89)	-0.14 (p=0.32)	0.02 (p=0.89)	0.02 (p=0.88)	1	
Follow-up period (months)	-0.14 (p=0.18)	-0.08 (p=0.42)	0.09 (p=0.36)	-0.2 (p=0.05)	0.12 (p=0.42)	-0.05 (p=0.61)	-0.08 (p=0.6)	1

Wilcoxon rank sum test. The p-values in parenthesis (p); significant correlations ($p < 0.05$) are in bold text. BCVA: best corrected visual acuity; ERM: epiretinal membrane; ILM: internal limiting membrane; CSFT: central subfoveal thickness. Spearman Rank Test nonpeeling sample=55 eyes. Peeling sample=50 eyes.

Table S13. Mann-Whitney U tests results in the Vitrectomy group (peeling and nonpeeling groups). (a) Preoperative best-corrected visual acuity (BCVA). (b) Postoperative BCVA. (c) Final BCVA.

(a) preoperative BCVA (logMAR) Mann-Whitney U tests results		
Object	U	**p-value**
Age	5565	**0.001**
Macula-off (weeks)	5341	**0.001**

(Table S13) cont.....

Follow-up period (days)	5565	**0.001**
BCVA before ERM-ILM removal (logMAR)	238	**0.001**
ERM detection (weeks)	1326	**0.001**
Final postoperative BCVA (logMAR)	0	**0.001**
CSFT (microns)	1540	**0.001**
Follow-up period (months)	4950	**0.001**
(b) postoperative BCVA (logMAR) Mann-Whitney U tests results		
Object	U	**p-value**
Age	5565	**0.001**
Macula-off (weeks)	5556	**0.001**
Preoperative BCVA (logMAR)	4712	**0.001**
Follow-up period (days)	5565	**0.001**
ERM detection (weeks)	1326	**0.001**
Final postoperative BCVA (logMAR)	101.5	**0.001**
CSFT (microns)	1540	**0.001**
Follow-up period (months)	5049	**0.001**
(c) final BCVA after ERM proliferation removal (logMAR)		
Object	U	**p-value**
Age	5565	**0.001**
Macula-off (weeks)	5565	**0.001**
Preoperative BCVA (logMAR)	5460	**0.001**
Follow-up period (days)	5565	**0.001**
BCVA before ERM-ILM removal (logMAR)	1074.5	**0.001**
ERM detection (weeks)	1326	**0.001**
CSFT (microns)	1540	**0.001**
Follow-up period (months)	5050	**0.001**

The statistically significant variables ($p < 0.05$) are in bold text. BCVA: best corrected visual acuity; ERM: epiretinal membrane; ILM: internal limiting membrane; CSFT: central subfoveal thickness.

Table S14. Kruskal-Wallis test results in the Vitrectomy group (peeling and nonpeeling groups). (a) Preoperative best-corrected visual acuity (BCVA). (b) Postoperative BCVA. (c) Final BCVA.

(a) preoperative BCVA (logMAR) Kruskal-Wallis tests results			
Object	**Kruskal-Wallis x^2.**	**df**	**p-value**
Male	0.458	1	0.499
Eye	1.878	1	0.171
Preoperative Lens Status	1.640	1	0.200
Preoperative ERM proliferations	0.760	1	0.383
First Surgery	1.055	2	0.590
BCVA Before ERM-ILM removal	9.412	12	0.667
Recurrent RRD	0.208	1	0.649
Additional surgery	1.360	4	0.851
Postoperative ERMs	0.038	1	0.846
ERM 2nd surgery	3.135	3	0.371
Final Postoperative BCVA	11.718	10	0.304
Foveal contour abnormalities	0.385	1	0.535
Ellipsoid disruption	4.175	1	**0.041**
DONFL defects	1.402	1	0.236
ELM line alterations	0.144	1	0.704
mfERG alterations	0.109	1	0.741
Microperimetry alterations	1.623	1	0.203
(b) postoperative BCVA (logMAR) Kruskal-Wallis tests results			
Object	**Kruskal-Wallis x^2.**	**df**	**p-value**
Male	0.355	1	0.552
Eye	0.001	1	0.979
Preoperative Lens Status	6.083	1	**0.014**
Preoperative BCVA	12.845	8	0.117
Preoperative ERM proliferations	50.177	1	**0.001**
First surgery	47.013	2	**0.000**
Recurrent RRD	11.364	1	**0.001**
Additional surgery	12.324	4	**0.015**
Postoperative ERM proliferations	68.366	1	**0.001**

(Table S14) cont.....

ERM 2nd surgery	5.469	3	0.141
Foveal Contour abnormalities	10.021	1	**0.002**
Ellipsoid disruption	1.091	1	0.296
DONFL defect	19.206	1	**0.001**
ELM line alterations	0.746	1	0.388
mfERG alterations	31.253	1	**0.001**
Microperimetry alterations	19.749	1	**0.001**
(c) final BCVA after ERM proliferation removal (logMAR)			
Object	**Kruskal-Wallis x^2.**	**df**	**p-value**
Male	1.561	1	0.211
Eye	0.121	1	0.728
Preoperative Lens Status	1.855	1	0.173
Preoperative ERM proliferations	33.337	1	**0.001**
First surgery	13.877	2	**0.001**
Recurrent RRD	9.223	1	**0.002**
Additional surgery	10.697	4	**0.030**
Postoperative ERM proliferations	38.068	1	**0.001**
ERM 2nd surgery	1.113	3	0.774
Foveal contour abnormalities	6.168	1	**0.013**
Ellipsoid disruption	0.894	1	0.344
DONFL defect	16.777	1	**0.001**
ELM line alterations	0.375	1	0.540
mfERG alterations	16.522	1	**0.001**
Microperimetry alterations	13.150	1	**0.001**

The statistically significant variables ($p < 0.05$) are in bold text. df: degrees of freedom: BCVA: best corrected visual acuity; ERM: epiretinal membrane; ILM: internal limiting membrane; RRD: rhegmatogenous retinal detachment; DONFL: diffuse optic nerve fiber layer; ELM: external limiting membrane: mfERG: multifocal electroretinography.

Table S15. Generalized linear model results in the Vitrectomy group (peeling and nonpeeling groups). (a) Preoperative best-corrected visual acuity (BCVA). (b) Postoperative BCVA. (c) Final BCVA.

(a) preoperative BCVA (logMAR) GLM results				
	Estimate	**SE**	**t value**	**p**
(Intercept)	1.055	0.026	40.60	**0.001**
(b) postoperative BCVA (logMAR) GLM results				
	Estimate	**SE**	**t value**	**p**
(Intercept)	0.515	0.067	7.72	**0.001**
Postoperative ERM proliferations	0.448	0.050	8.97	**0.001**
First surgery - ONLY VITRECTOMY	-0.235	0.055	-4.30	**0.001**
First surgery - VIT ERM and ILM REMOVAL	0.034	0.090	0.38	0.704
Macula-off (weeks)	-0.019	0.008	-2.50	**0.014**
Recurrent RRD	0.118	0.061	1.94	0.055
(c) final BCVA after ERM proliferation removal (logMAR) GLM results				
	Estimate	**SE**	**t value**	**p**
(Intercept)	-0.213	0.070	-3.05	**0.003**
BCVA Before ERM-ILM removal (logMAR)	0.552	0.046	11.98	**0.001**
First Surgery - ONLY VITRECTOMY	0.201	0.038	5.22	**0.001**
First Surgery - VIT ERM and ILM REMOVAL	0.275	0.051	5.42	**0.001**
Preoperative BCVA (logMAR)	0.106	0.046	2.29	**0.024**
Gender - Male	0.052	0.026	2.03	**0.045**

The statistically significant variables ($p < 0.05$) are in bold text. BCVA: best corrected visual acuity; GLM: generalized linear models; SE: standard error; ERM: epiretinal membrane; VIT: vitrectomy; ILM: internal limiting membrane; mfERG: multifocal electroretinography; RRD: rhegmatogenous retinal detachment.

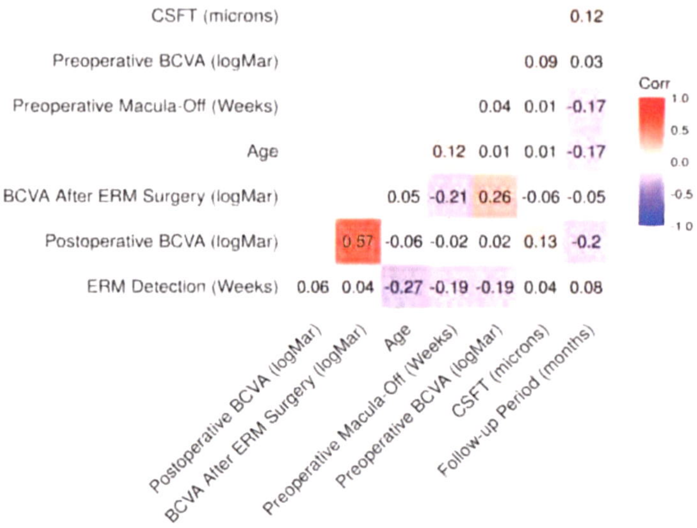

Additional Fig. S1. The Spearman's rank correlation coefficient test showed that there was a moderate to strong positive correlation (rho= 0.57, p<0.01) of the postoperative BCVA in logMAR units with the BCVA after ERM surgery. In addition, there was a weak negative correlation (rho = -0.2, p<0.05) between postoperative BCVA in logMAR units and follow-up period in months.

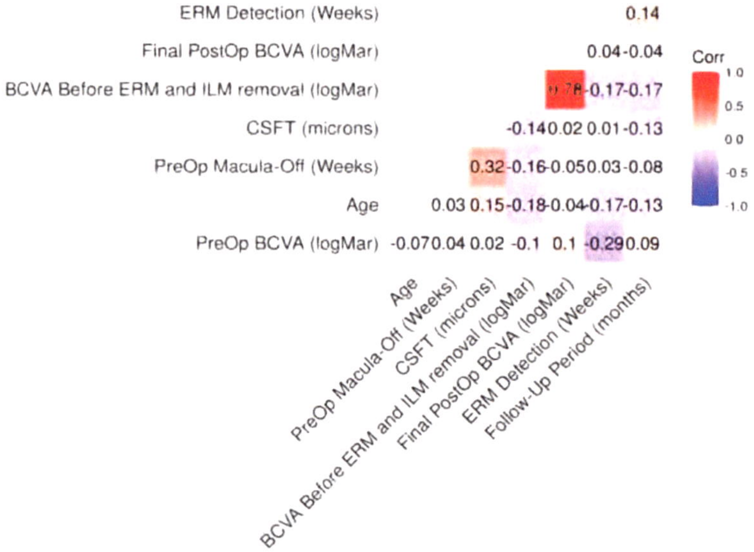

Additional Fig. S2. The Spearman's rank correlation coefficient test showed a weak positive correlation (rho= 0.32, p<0.05) between the preoperative period with the macula-off in weeks and the CSFT findings in microns; it also showed a weak negative correlation (rho= -0.29, p<0.05) between the preoperative BCVA in logMAR units and ERM detection in weeks.

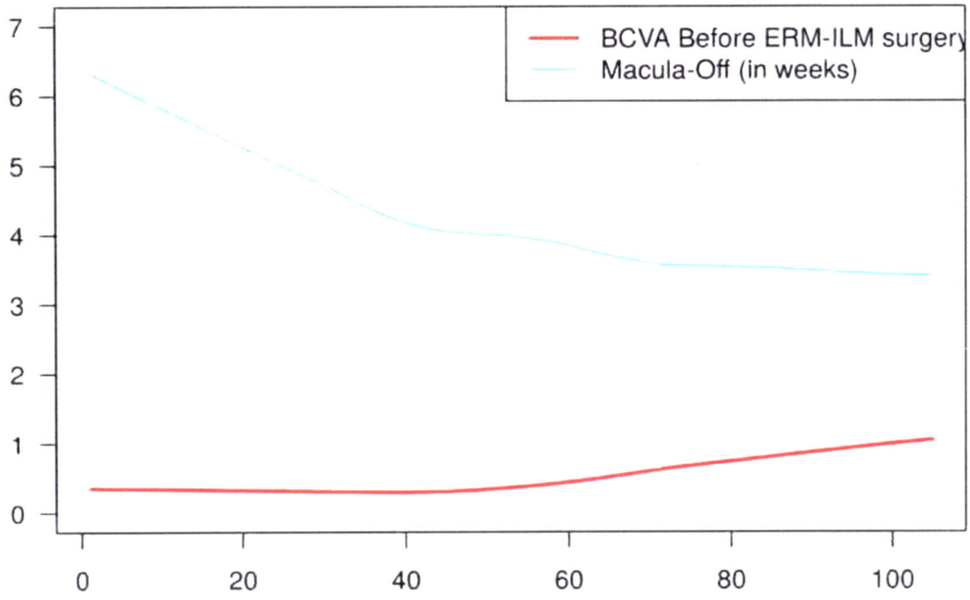

Additional Fig. S3. Postoperative BCVA was significantly negatively associated when only vitrectomy (nonpeeling group) was performed in the first surgery variable (coefficient = -0.23, p<0.01) and significantly negatively associated with the variable preoperative period of macula-off in weeks (coefficient= -0.02, p<0.05).

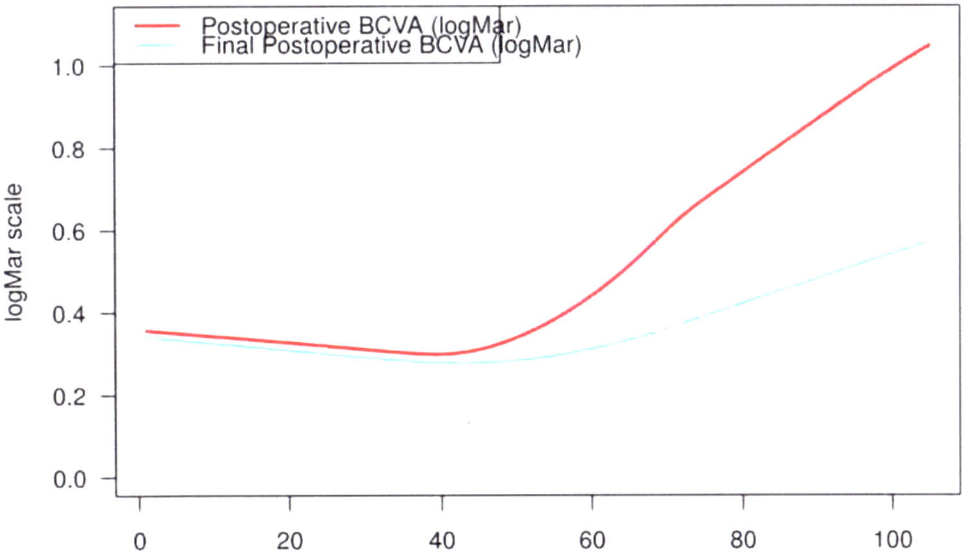

Additional Fig. S4. The GLM for the final BCVA in log MAR units after ERM proliferation removal showed that it was significantly positively associated (p>0.01) with the postoperative.

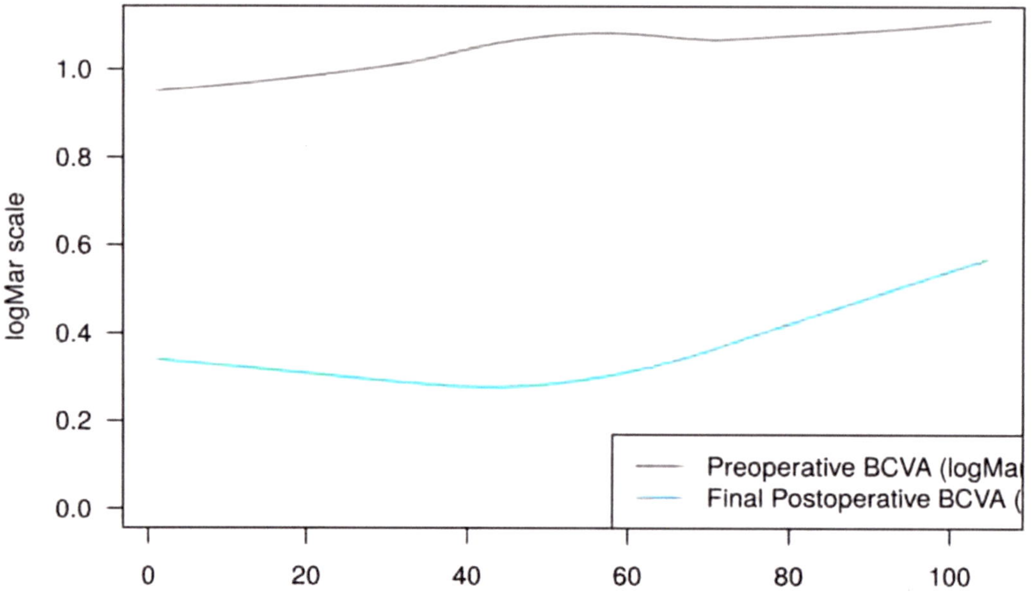

Additional Fig. S5. Shows when only vitrectomy was the first surgery variable, and with the preoperative BCVA.

SUBJECT INDEX

D

I

L

M

N

O

P

R

S

T

V

Y

Made in the USA
Las Vegas, NV
03 November 2026

57423613R00186